CANCER MORTALITY

Environmental and Ethnic Factors

Academic Press Rapid Manuscript Reproduction

CANCER MORTALITY

ENVIRONMENTAL AND ETHNIC FACTORS

by

Dorothy Gaites Wellington
Eleanor J. Macdonald
Patricia F. Wolf
Department of Epidemiology
The University of Texas System
Cancer Center
Texas Medical Center
Houston, Texas

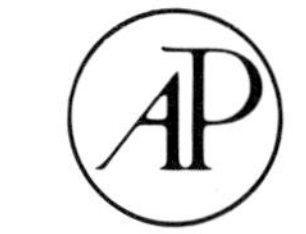

ACADEMIC PRESS
NEW YORK SAN FRANCISCO LONDON 1979
A Subsidiary of Harcourt Brace Jovanovich, Publishers

ACADEMIC PRESS, INC.
111 Fifth Avenue, New York, New York 10003

United Kingdom Edition published by
ACADEMIC PRESS, INC. (LONDON) LTD.
24/28 Oval Road, London NW1 7DX

Library of Congress in Cataloging in Publication Data

Wellington, Dorothy Gaites.
Cancer mortality.

1. Cancer—Mortality. 2. Carcinogenesis.
3. Epidemiology. I. Macdonald, Eleanor J., joint
author. II. Wolf, Patricia F., joint author.
III. Title. [DNLM: 1. Neoplasms—Mortality—United
States. 2. Environmental health—United States.
3. Ethnic groups—United States. QZ200.3 W452c]
RC261.W44 616.9'94'071 79-10560
ISBN 0-12-745850-6

PRINTED IN THE UNITED STATES OF AMERICA

79 80 81 82 9 8 7 6 5 4 3 2 1

CONTENTS

FOREWORD

In Dante Alighieri's search for St. Peter's Gate, geologists' search for oil, and epidemiologists' search for cancer etiology, geographic exploration is a necessary starting point. Stratigraphic exploration of hell under Virgil's expert guidance led Dante to an understanding of the route to salvation. Topographic, stratigraphic, and geomorphic maps of the earth's crust are essentially crude models of the association of local geographic features with the presence of petroleum. These models have on the whole proved to be useful guides in the search for petroleum deposits, even though they not infrequently lead to dry holes and to (pleasant) surprises, such as the recent Chinese and Mexican discoveries.

Systematic search for the many causes of the many cancers is reasonably analogous: crude descriptions of the macroepidemiology of the cancer family suggest strategies for investigations of next level, microepidemiology of individual cases, which in turn lead to laboratory studies of organs, cells, nuclei, and molecules in the search for explanatory mechanisms (''causes'').

In the recent generation of epidemiologic science quantum leaps in the technological capability at all levels have set off a new wave of highly refined research that has engendered a new optimism about our ability ultimately to understand cancer processes.

Macdonald, who has spent a lifetime of infinite care developing and refining cancer registries as the foundation of modern microepidemiology, has turned now, with the statistical collaboration of Wellington, to drawing the zipper around the contemporary bag of best available and highest current analytical technology applicable to the macroepidemiology of cancer(s). While several recent studies have updated the classical macroepidemiology of cancer with detailed geographic mapping of mortality rates, by type and site of cancer, various levels of aggregation (in time and space), and have reconnoitered demographic and environmental correlates, Wellington, Macdonald, and Wolf have achieved a synthesis of the available data in a unified, comprehensive model, which step by step addresses the shortcomings of previous analyses.

The multitude of options as to data and analytic method were carefully sifted and tested before selection of an optimum model:

Particular U.S. mortality, demographic, and environmental variates are selected as, overall, of the highest quality available.

States (vis-a-vis counties and SMSAs) are selected as the optimum aggregation level for segregation of 25 cancer types and sites and for meaningful impact of demographic and environmental correlates thereon.

The 20 years (1950 to 1969) are selected as the optimum time window—a period long enough to generate numbers sufficient for detailed subcategory analysis, late enough to assure uniformly high-quality data, and early enough (though barely) to escape the massive homogenization of U.S. culture that is rapidly obliterating regional variation in possible correlates of cancer. (The "cost" of this 20-year average choice, of course, is the foregone exploration of time trends. Such exploration, however desirable, is severely limited by the small frequencies occurring in short-time intervals.)

By exhaustive analysis of the components of variation in 23 demographic variables, 6 income, 11 climate, 37 air contamination, 3 radiation, 20 consumption (cigarettes, alcohol, water, milk), and 74 ethnic variables, a "best" explanatory set of four major "factor pools" associated with variation in cancer mortality is teased out (three environmental variables, one income, four consumption, and four ethnic variables). These 12 variables appropriately combined account for 30% (in female trachea, bronchus, and lung specified as primary) to 90% (in male rectum) of the observed variation in cancer mortality. With only slight loss of explanatory power the model can be reduced to six variables, which in turn reduce to two global constellations of urban factors and population density and its concomitants.

Finally, best-fitting multiple regression models with standardized coefficients, developed for uniform application to the 25 site/types, by sex, permit examination of the *net* effects of individual causal variables with others "held constant" and exploration of possible causal pathways. These models are appropriately corrected for the well-known latency, nonnormality, collinearity, and aliasing that have so persistently dogged previous studies.

If, as it may seem to most readers, the substantive findings merely confirm what we already knew or suspected or simply raise more of the same kind of vexing questions for which we have no immediate answer—or even access—it can nevertheless now be said that all that is to be learned from cross-section geographic analysis of available data on cancer mortality and its many possible correlates has been extracted. Further advances will require descent to minute investigation on lower levels of aggregation, for the exploration of which this study may serve epidemiology as Virgil served Dante. "Now let us onward, for the way is long . . . . Long is the journey and the road is rough . . . ."

Carl E. Hopkins
Professor of Public Health
School of Public Health
University of California
Los Angeles, California

PREFACE

The study of death records has been a long-time concern of one of the authors (EJM), who published the first definitive paper evaluating the accuracy of cancer mortality records 40 years ago. The regional patterns of cancer mortality rates have been of special interest to the authors since their studies at M. D. Anderson Hospital in the early 1960s revealed the geographic relationship betweeen degree of urbanization and mortality level for some of the major types of cancer. In that project the age-adjusted death rates were calculated for each category of cancer mortality available in the national vital statistics reports by state and by subpopulation group for each year from 1940 through 1959. Time trends were calculated for three periods: 1940–1948, 1949–1959, and 1940–1959. Some of the results were presented at the IX International Cancer Congress in Japan in 1966, and were summarized in an article in *Cancer,* 1967. Not until 1975 were the authors able to direct their attention again to this study. At that time Mason and McKay made available age-adjusted death rates averaged over the period 1950–1969, and it was decided to base further analysis on this later data set, using the results from the earlier period for comparability.

In spite of the problems involved in deriving models based on vital statistics and the available data on economic and sociological variables, preliminary results proved to be reasonable and consistent, and at the same time posed questions that stimulated more detailed and more comprehensive investigation. The goal of this book has been to present in an organized and comprehensive manner the sets of factors whose joint by-state variation best explain the state patterns of cancer mortality and to explore the nonconformation of individual states to the national models. The authors hope that not only will the factor effects that emerge in the models be of interest but that attention may be called to potential etiologies that are implicated through their association with the model effects, such as a nutrition habit that underlies an ethnic effect.

Without the assistance of Alan Romano in managing the data bank and providing computer services, it would not have been possible to accomplish the very large amount of computer analysis with such ease, speed, and flexibility. Paul Callen, Hugh Bray, Jacqueline Wheat, and Lynn Hayward were also helpful in the early stages of the computer programming. Of great importance was the continual availability of sufficient computer time, which enabled unrestricted analysis of the data and immediate investigation into new leads as they arose in the analysis.

The authors are appreciative of those who aided in the preparation of this work: Evelyn B. Heinze, Margaret C. Murphy, Margaret Jansen, John Hanna, Eleanor Hassett, Kay Hermes, Kaye Reed, and Miriam Toloudis.

This project was supported in part by The University of Texas System Cancer Center, USPHS Grant FR-00254, NCI Grant CS-9299, Texas State Department of Health, American Cancer Society, Texas Division, Regional Medical Program Grants RMA-00007 and RMD-00007, Special Project of the Council for Tobacco Research, U.S.A., Inc., T. D. Wellington, Princeton, New Jersey, and The Clayton Fund, Houston, Texas.

Dorothy Gaites Wellington
Eleanor J. Macdonald
Patricia F. Wolf

TABLES

Chapter 1
Description and Purpose of the Study

I Background and Purpose of the Study

In the United States there are large differences among the states in death rates from different types of cancer and also from other causes of death. In an early study by Macdonald *et al.* (1) the by-state distributions of the age-adjusted death rates for selected primary cancer sites indicated that these differences are largely regional, while states within the same geographic region have similar rates, and even adjacent regions experience closer mortality levels than those farther apart. Large differences among counties within a state do occur, however, as shown in Mason and McKay's publication of cancer death rates by state and by county (2), but frequently the high-risk counties are found in contiguous clusters (3). The very small population base of many counties will produce more volatile estimated rates, especially for the less common cancer primary sites, and when population subsets are involved, such as white males, the chance variation increases. Even an entire state, if it is as sparsely populated as Nevada, will exhibit extremes of high and low death rates not exhibited by the more populous states. The volatility of these estimated rates is modified and their large variance decreased when they are combined into 10- or 20-year averages, as they are in the Macdonald and the Mason and McKay projects cited above.

In recent years it has been recognized that a person's risk of developing cancer is influenced by environmental, consumption, and genetic factors, and by his response to those factors. His risk of dying from cancer also is influenced by the medical facilities available to him. Because of the complex of potentially interactive factors, an individual person is the natural unit for investigating the etiology of each type of cancer mortality, and many studies have been made on comparatively small numbers of individuals with the purpose of associating one or more factors with the incidence of, or mortality from, particular cancer primaries. The knowledge gained from these studies can be supplemented or reinforced by more generalized population studies. Just as microeconomics, the study of the individual firm or the individual consumer, and macroeconomics, the study of mass flows of prices, income, and spending in large populations, combine to explain economic processes, so a "microepidemiology" that deals with the experience of samples of individuals chosen to represent larger populations can be combined with a "macroepidemiology" that analyzes the experience of the target populations themselves, to delineate etiological factors of disease. The data in the microstudies must be gathered with a high degree of accuracy and under explicit rules of sampling so that inferences to the parent population can be made, and they entail great expense. Statistical estimates derived from the larger data masses used in macrostudies are less vulnerable to the errors in individual records unless those errors result from a strong bias in collection or recording. In the vital statistics of large and complete populations there are massive flows that, like the ocean currents, may be rippled by disturbances, but are usually not diverted from their overall patterns. Since data of this kind are continuously provided by governmental bodies, it behooves researchers to put them to maximum use, as urged in a 1977 editorial in the American Journal of Public Health (4).

The purpose of this study has been to carry out a systematic analysis of state patterns of cancer mortality in all categories of malignant neoplasms for which the data were available and to determine the syndrome of state characteristics associated with a high level of each type of cancer mortality in its population (white). Previously McDonald and Schwing (5) had combined multiple linear regression and ridge regression techniques for considering a large number of factor variables in a model for state variation in death rates, but only one category of mortality was analyzed—deaths from all causes in the total population. Later Breslow and Enstrom (6) used multiple linear regression models to explain the state variation in selected cancer death rates, but with a limited set of factor variables from which to draw the mortality models. Carnow and Meier (7) considered multiple regression inadequate for identifying the factors responsible for differing lung cancer death rates because the intercorrelation among the factor variables and their close relationship with an overall urban or population density factor would lead to "aliasing," i.e., the disguising of one factor's effect under the label of another. Instead they chose a measure of one of the common air pollutants, benzo[*a*]pyrene, as a single index of pollution "to represent the effects of all of the correlated pollution variables combined" (7) and combined it with a per capita measure of cigarette sales in a two-factor multiple regression model of lung cancer mortality. Since the publication of the cancer mortality rates by county as well as by state (2) several studies have employed the epidemiologic technique of geographic correlation between death rate and potential etiologic factors using either selected counties (8-10) or all 3056 of them (11). In another study, Lave and Seskin (12) derived multiple regression models using data from 117 Standard Metropolitan Statistical Areas (SMSAs).

In the all-counties study a multiple regression model relates lung cancer mortality to county demographic and occupational indices that include a percentage urban factor in addition to a redundant percentage rural factor. The SMSA study includes variables measuring both population size and density. The insertion of a variable representing either urbanization or population density into epidemiological mortality models has become almost as standard a procedure as including an income variable in econometric models, but the usage is quite different. The income effect has been thoroughly investigated in economic theory and adjustment for its influence is well understood. On the other hand the urban effect in mortality models has been observed but not well analyzed, and its influence attributed to a number of associated characteristics ranging from measurable and specific to unmeasurable and vague, such as "tension, stress, and unhealthy personal habits" (12). The inclusion of an urban variable in order to adjust for all its associated factors, both known and unknown, essentially begs the question. What is needed is to determine which components of the urban factor, and in what combinations and relative strengths, best explain the state mortality patterns for different types of cancer. When such a factor is adjusted for the overall urban effect of which it is a part, it is thereby partially corrected for itself, weakening or obliterating its potential effect in the model. It is akin to adjusting the factors of beer or wine consumption for the variable comprising total consumption of alcohol.

Further confusion of model effects has arisen when the urban variable has been replaced by a measure of population density with which it is only weakly correlated. The rationale attending the use of a population density variable is even less clearly defined, and the subfactors cited to be associated with it are fewer. The intention of the study presented here is to explain the strong effects that both these generalized variables display in multiple regression models of mortality patterns by *replacing* them with their associated component factors. In this study a very wide range of factor variables were tested in preliminary modeling, and from them were chosen four sets of variables to make up the four variable pools. Each variable pool was used to derive the multiple regression models for every type of cancer mortality *in order to provide a comparability of model effects across all categories of cancer deaths.* In additional analysis these four variable pools, which were constructed specifically for the derivation of cancer mortality models, were also used to derive models of state mortality patterns for all the major categories of death. These served as a type of control, providing the contrast that profiled those factor combinations specifically characteristic of the cancer mortality patterns.

II Statistical Methodology and Computer Programs

For each mortality pattern multiple regression models were derived by linear least squares methodology and the stability of the coefficient estimates was tested by ridge regression techniques. Subset models were chosen from each of the four variable pools by two computer program packages, which employed different criteria for choosing the "best" set of factor variables to explain each mortality pattern. One was the stepwise multiple regression program 2R from the Biomedical Computer Programs of UCLA (15), referred to henceforth as BMD, and the other the LINCUR regression program (16) developed and described by Daniel and Wood (17), referred to as LIN. In the former, the F value to enter the model was set at 1.5 and the F to remove at 1.0, with the tolerance level set at .01, thereby excluding variables 99% of whose variation could be expressed in linear terms of the variables already entered. The LINCUR choice of the best set of variables was guided by the plot proposed by Mallows (18) of the C_p-statistic versus p, the number of coefficient estimates. The C_p-statistic is an estimate of the standardized "total squared error," the sum of the squared random errors of the dependent variable plus the squared bias at each point due to estimating that point by the derived model rather than by the "true" equation. Only the models with the lowest C_p values were examined, and the patterns of factors entering these models were taken into consideration in the choice. When the chosen LIN model was not the one with the smallest C_p value but rather with the second or third lowest, it is indicated in the text as "second or third LIN." If the model's C_p value was greater than p, indicating some bias, it was usually not chosen, and the few cases included are so notated.

When the best subset models were decided upon either by the stepwise procedure of the BMD program or the minimum C_p-statistic of the LINCUR program or both, each was run as a full model in the LINCUR program to obtain an analysis of the distribution of its residuals. Included in the LINCUR printout are plots of the cumulative distribution of residuals, of the residuals against estimated mortality rate, and of component effect plus residual against factor value for each independent variable in the model. The component effect of the ith factor on the response variable after correction for all the other factor effects, measured at the jth observation, is $b_i(x_{ij} - \bar{x}_i)$, where b_i is the estimated coefficient of factor i in the model, x_{ij} is the value of the ith factor at the jth observation, and $\bar{x}_i$ is the mean value of the ith factor. As suggested by Wood (19) these plots were used to estimate the influence of individual observations working through each factor variable in the model, and to detect outlier observations with respect to each model effect. These are similar to the partial residual plots that Larsen and McCleary (20) compare with the usual residual plot against factor variable in that the latter show deviations from linearity while the former show "both the extent of the deviation from linearity and the extent and the direction of the linearity" (20). Individual states that represented residuals of extreme value were examined for their ranking in factor values and mortality rate to learn why they did not conform to the general model. Besides the outliers in the residual distributions, potential outliers in the influence space were also identified by the LINCUR output of weighted squared standardized differences. The specific influence on the chosen model of any state that constituted an extreme value in the space of model effects was determined by the changes in model effects when that state was excluded from the derivation.

The intercorrelation that is unavoidable among factor variables of the kind used in this study can lead to unstable coefficient estimates and inflated standard errors when least squares procedures are used. Ridge regression analysis, first proposed by Hoerl and Kennard (21, 22) controls the variance resulting from high collinearity by augmenting the diagonal of the normal equations' matrix by small increasing values, producing slightly biased but more stable coefficient estimates. Although variables are not eliminated by this procedure, those whose coefficient estimates decrease almost to zero as the augmentation increases are considered not to maintain their effect in the model in competition against related factors with more stable traces of their coefficient estimates. This technique was applied only to the largest variable pool, examining the plotted trace of the estimated coefficients for each of the variables to determine the relative strength and stability of the model effects chosen for each mortality pattern.

The computer program used for the ridge regression analysis was provided by S. Radhakrishnan of Shell Oil Company.

There are 49 data points in each regression model: the 48 continental states and the District of Columbia. Since these 49 cases constitute the whole population of interest, the statistics in multiple regression, which were developed to enable inference from a sample to the whole population, were used primarily as guidelines to relative judgment about the size or importance of the coefficient of a model factor. Even though, in one sense, the model coefficients are themselves the population coefficients, and thus techniques such as F tests, C_p-statistics, and ridge traces of their stability as estimates appear unnecessary, these statistical procedures served as tools in choosing the best subsets of factors for each mortality pattern, in indicating the relative importance of each factor and in focusing on those factors whose effects were the most stable in the face of strong collinearity.

The aim of the statistical methodology was not predictive per se, since the particular conjuncture of circumstances covering those years under study will never reoccur, but rather it was to find which combinations of factors best explained each cancer mortality pattern and which individual factors showed strength or consistency in both the male and the female mortality patterns for a particular cancer primary, or in the mortality patterns that are related by type of cancer primaries, such as those of the digestive organs.

III The Data

The dependent or response variables are the death rates of white males and of white females for each of the continental 48 states and the District of Columbia. The rates used in deriving the cancer mortality models were Mason and McKay's (2) age-adjusted death rates for each state averaged over the 20-year period 1950-1969. The one exception was the division of the deaths from cancer of the trachea, bronchus, and lung into those specified to be the primary site and those neither specified as primary nor secondary. The rates for these two subcategories are given by Burbank (13) and are averages of the 18-year period 1950-1967. The mortality models for the major categories of death were derived from age-adjusted rates averaged over the 11-year period 1949-1959, which were part of an earlier study at The University of Texas System Cancer Center M. D. Anderson Hospital (1). Also included in the preliminary analysis but not in the final models of this study were age-adjusted cancer death rates averaged over the 9-year period 1940-1948, the 11-year period 1949-1959, and the 20-year period 1940-1959, all of which were done in a previous M. D. Anderson study (1).

Data for the independent or factor variables were gathered from all the available sources, stored in a working data matrix in a CDC 6400 computer, and were continuously on call, enabling the maximum amount of test modeling and immediate feedback in the preliminary stages of determining the most effective pools of variables from which to choose the cancer mortality models. A listing of the basic data and sources from which the factor variables were drawn is given in Table I. A list of the dependent variables, the state age-adjusted death rates, and sources is given in Table II.

Natural logarithms were taken of the values of all the independent variables in order to normalize their generally skewed distributions due to the concentration of a few very high values in a very few states and the completely urban District of Columbia. The natural logarithm values were standardized by subtracting their mean (centering) and dividing by their standard deviation (scaling). Marquardt and Snee (14) point out that centering removes the nonessential ill-conditioning and some of the inflated variance of the coefficient estimates that accompanies collinearity. Strong intercorrelation among the factor variables in this study required this adjustment for mean values. The scaling forced all variances to the value of 1, standardizing the coefficient estimates, and thereby enabling the relative size of each coefficient to reflect the relative importance of each factor within each model. When a principal components analysis was used to combine several factor variables into a single composite factor variable, the calculations were made on the transformed values of the composing variables. The resultant first principal component scores were themselves standardized in order to maintain homogeneity of variances in the independent variables.

TABLE I
Factor Variables[a]

Population Distribution Variables	
	Urban white population as percentage of state white population
URBW30	1930 (18)
URBW40	1940 (18)
URBW50	1950–old urban definition (18)
URBW5N	1950–new urban definition (18)
URBW60	1960 (19)
URBW70	1970 (20)
	Urban white male population as percentage of state white male population
URWM30	1930 (18)
URWM40	1940 (18)
URWM50	1950–old urban definition (18)
URWM5N	1950–new urban definition (18)
URWM60	1960 (19)
URWM70	1970 (20)
	Urban white female population as percentage of state white female population
URWF30	1930 (18)
URWF40	1940 (18)
URWF50	1950–old urban definition (18)
URWF5N	1950–new urban definition (18)
URWF60	1960 (19)
URWF70	1970 (20)
	Population density
DENS40	1940 total population per square mile land area (7)
DENS50	1950 total population per square mile land area (8)
DENS60	1960 total population per square mile land area (4)
DENS70	1970 total population per square mile land area (4)
WDEN50	Weighted average of area densities with area populations as weights = (density of central city x percentage of population in central city) + (density of urban fringe x percentage of population in urban fringe) + (density of outside city x percentage of population in outside city) + (density of rural area x percentage of population in rural area)
Climate Variables	
TMPJAN	Mean January temperature for period of record through 1947 (7)
TMWMAX	Mean January maximum temperature 1921-1950 (8)
TMWMIN	Mean January minimum temperature 1921-1950 (8)
TMPJUL	Mean July temperature for period of record through 1947 (7)
TMSMAX	Mean July maximum temperature 1921-1950 (8)
TMSMIN	Mean July minimum temperature 1921-1950 (8)
TMPDIF	Difference between mean July temperature and mean January temperature (7)
TEMP[b]	Temperature: first principal component score combining TMPJAN and TMPJUL
PRECIP	Annual precipitation 1921-1950 (8)
ELEVAT	Mean elevation (14)
PRELEV[b]	Precipitation/elevation: first principal component score combining PRECIP and ELEVAT (high score connotes high precipitation and low elevation; low score connotes low precipitation and high elevation.

[a] For footnote *a*, table references, see p. 12.
[b] Included in final variable pools.

TABLE I (continued)

Air Contamination Variables	
BNZAPY	Benzo[a]pyrene emissions per cubic meter air weighted by urban and rural populations, quarterly average for 1969 (3)
	Particulate matter emissions 1970 (22)
PARKIL	Per square kilometer land area
PARTIC	Per square kilometer land area weighted by population
PARCAP	Per capita
PARTC2	Per capita weighted by land area
	Sulfur dioxide emissions 1970 (22)
SULKIL	Per square kilometer land area
SULFDI	Per square kilometer land area weighted by population
SULCAP	Per capita
SULFC2	Per capita weighted by land area
	Carbon monoxide emissions 1970 (22)
CARKIL	Per square kilometer land area
CARBMO	Per square kilometer land area weighted by population
CARCAP	Per capita
CARBC2	Per capita weighted by land area
	Hydrocarbon emissions 1970 (22)
HYDKIL	Per square kilometer land area
HYDRCA	Per square kilometer land area weighted by population
HYDCAP	Per capita
HYDRC2	Per capita weighted by land area
	Nitric oxide emissions 1970 (22)
NITKIL	Per square kilometer land area
NITROX	Per square kilometer land area weighted by population
NITCAP	Per capita
NITRC2	Per capita weighted by land area
	Combinations of emission data (22)
PSUKIL	PARKIL + SULKIL: Particulate matter plus sulfur dioxide per square kilometer land area
CHNKIL	CARKIL + HYDKIL + NITKIL: Carbon monoxide plus hydrocarbon plus nitric oxide per square kilometer land area
HDOVNX	HYDKIL/NITKIL: Hydrocarbon divided by nitric oxide per square kilometer land area
POLLUT[b]	Air pollution: first principal component score combining BNZAPY, PARTIC, SULFDI, CARBMO, HYDRCA, and NITROX
	Vehicle miles
TVMS40	1940 per square mile land area (1)
WVRU40	1940 per square mile land area weighted by rural and urban white population (1)
UVUW40	1940 urban miles per capita urban white population (1)
TVMS62	1962 per square mile land area (2)
WVRU62	1962 per square mile land area weighted by 1960 rural and urban white population (2)
UVUW62	1962 urban miles per capita 1960 urban white population (2)
HHCOAL	Percentage of house heating utilizing coke/coal 1970 (15)

[b] Included in final variable pools.

TABLE I (continued)

Variable	Description
	Employment
MAGR40	1940 males employed in agriculture as percentage of all employed males (16)
MMIN40	1940 males employed in mining as percentage of all employed males (16)
	Males employed in manufacturing as percentage of all employed males
MMFR40	1940 (16)
MMFR50	1950 (17)
FMFR50	1950 females employed in manufacturing as percentage of all employed females (17)
Radiation Variables	
RADIAT	Average dose equivalent (mrem/year) from natural background sources, both cosmic and terrestrial, weighted by resident populations 1958-1963 (9)
RADCOS	Average dose equivalent (mrem/year) from natural background sources, cosmic radiation, weighted by resident populations 1958-1963 (9)
RADTER	Average dose equivalent (mrem/year) from natural background sources, terrestrial radiation, weighted by resident populations 1958-1963 (9)
Income Variables	
	Per capita personal income
INCM40	1940 (13)
INCM50[b]	1950 (14)
INCM60	1960 (14)
INCM65	1965 (14)
	1949 median income (17)
MDIW49	White population
NFMDIW	White urban and rural nonfarm population
Consumption Variables	
	Cigarette consumption per capita (10)
CIGS55[b]	1955
CIGS60	1960
CIGS65	1965
CIGS70	1970
CIGS71	1971
	Malt beverage consumption
MALT40	Per capita 1940 (11)
MALT4A	Per capita adult 1940 (11)
MALT50	Per capita 1950 (11)
MALT5A[b]	Per capita adult 1950 (11)
MALT55	Per capita 1955 (11)
MALT66	Per capita 1966 (12)
MALT6A	Per capita adult 1966 (12)
WINE6A[b]	Wine consumption per capita adult 1966 (12)
DISP6A[b]	Distilled spirits consumption per capita adult 1966 (12)
ALCO[b]	Alcohol consumption: first principal component score combining MALT5A, WINE6A, and DISP6A

[b] Included in final variable pools.

TABLE I (continued)

	Drinking water (14)
DWFLUR	Percentage of population using fluoridated drinking water 1969
DWPUBL	Percentage of population using public drinking water 1969
	Surface water (14)
INWATR	Inland water as percentage of total area in state
TOTWAT	All water as ratio to total area in state
MIPR74	Milk production 1974 (21)
Ethnic Variables	
	State percentage of total foreign white stock in the U.S.
SPFS40	1940 (13)
SPFS50	1950 (13)
SPFS60	1960 (14)
	Total foreign-born white as percentage of state white population
FNBW40	1940 (13)
FNBW50	1950 (13)
FNBW60	1960 (14)
	Urban foreign-born white as percentage of state white population: those born in England and Wales, Scotland, Ireland, Netherlands, Belgium, France, Germany, Poland, Czechoslovakia, Austria, Hungary, Yugoslavia, Russia, Lithuania, Greece, Italy, and the Latin American countries other than Mexico
UFBW40	1940 (7, 16)
UFBW50	1950 (17)
UFBW60	1960 (19)
	Native white of foreign or mixed parentage as percentage of state white population
FMPW40	1940 (13)
FMPW50	1950 (13)
FMPW60	1960 (14)
	Foreign-born white as percentage of state white population by country(ies) of birth:
	England and Wales
ENWA40	1940 (7)
ENWA50	1950 (17)
	Scotland
SCOT40	1940 (16)
SCOT50	1950 (17)
	Northern Ireland
NIRE40	1940 (16)
NIRE50	1950 (17)
	Ireland
EIRE40	1940 (7)
EIRE50	1950 (17)
	France
FRAN40	1940 (7)
FRAN50[b]	1950 (17)

[b] Included in final variable pools.

TABLE I (continued)

	Germany
GERM40	1940 (7)
GERM50	1950 (17)
	Netherlands and Belgium
NEBE40	1940 (16)
NEBE50	1950 (17)
	Italy
ITAL40	1940 (7)
ITAL50	1950 (17)
	Austria
AUST40	1940 (7)
AUST50	1950 (17)
	Czechoslovakia
CZEC40	1940 (7)
CZEC50	1950 (17)
	Poland
POLA40	1940 (7)
POLA50	1950 (17)
	Hungary
HUNG40	1940 (7)
HUNG50	1950 (17)
	Yugoslavia
YUGO40	1940 (16)
YUGO50	1950 (17)
	Greece
GREC40	1940 (7)
GREC50	1950 (17)
	Russia
RUSS40	1940 (7)
RUSS50	1950 (17)
	Lithuania
LITH40	1940 (16)
LITH50	1950 (17)
	Norway
NORW40	1940 (7)
NORW50	1950 (17)
	Sweden
SWED40	1940 (7)
SWED50	1950 (17)
	Denmark
DENM40	1940 (7)
DENM50	1950 (17)
	Finland
FINL40	1940 (7)
FINL50	1950 (17)
	Mexico
MEXI40	1940 (16)
MEXI50	1950 (17)

TABLE I (continued)

	Latin America other than Mexico
OLAM40	1940 (16)
OLAM50	1950 (17)
	Canada, French
CAFR40	1940 (16)
CAFR50	1950 (17)
	Canada, other than French
OCAN40	1940 (16)
OCAN50	1950 (17)
	Canada, total
CAND40	1940 (16)
CAND50	1950 (17)
	British Isles: England and Wales, Scotland, Ireland and Northern Ireland
BRIT40	1940 (7, 16)
BRIT50 [b]	1950 (17)
	Scandinavia: Norway, Sweden, and Denmark
SCAN40	1940 (7)
SCAN50 [b]	1950 (17)
OTHEUR [b]	Other Europe: first principal component score combining ITAL50, GERM50, RUSS50, POLA50, AUST50, CZEC50, HUNG50, NEBE50, LITH50, and JWTP51.
	Germanic: Germany, Austria, Netherlands, Belgium
GERM	1950 (17)
	Slavic: Poland, Russia, Czechoslovakia
SLAV	1950 (17)
	Jewish population
JWTP17	1917 as percentage of 1930 state white population (7)
JWTP27	1927 as percentage of 1930 state white population (7)
JWTP37	1937 as percentage of 1940 state white population (7)
JWTP51	1951 as percentage of 1950 state white population (5)
JWTP58	1958 as percentage of 1960 state white population (6)

[b] Included in final variable pools.

[a] Key to table references:

1. Automobile Manufacturers Association. "Automobile Facts and Figures." Detroit, Michigan, 1941.
2. Automobile Manufacturers Association. "Automobile Facts and Figures." Detroit, Michigan, 1965.
3. Carnow, B. W., and Meier, P. Air pollution and pulmonary cancer. *Arch. Environ. Health 27*:207-218, 1973. (Larsen and Clements, unpublished data.)
4. Delury, G. E., ed. "The World Almanac 1974 and Book of Facts." Newspaper Enterprise Association, New York, 1974.
5. Fine, M., ed. "American Jewish Yearbook," Vol. 52. American Jewish Committee and the Jewish Publication Society of America, New York, 1951.

TABLE I (continued)

6. Fine, M., ed. "American Jewish Yearbook," Vol. 59. American Jewish Committee and the Jewish Publication Society of America, New York, 1959.
7. Hansen, H., ed. "The World Almanac 1950 and Book of Facts." New York World-Telegram and The Sun, New York, 1950.
8. Hansen, H., ed. "The World Almanac 1960 and Book of Facts." New York World-Telegram and The Sun, New York, 1960.
9. Oakley, D. T. "Natural Radiation Exposure in the United States." U. S. Environmental Protection Agency Publication No. ORP/SID 72-1, Washington, D. C., 1972; reprinted October 1974.
10. Tobacco Tax Council, Inc. "The Tax Burden on Tobacco," Volume 9: Historical Compilation. Richmond, Virginia, 1974.
11. U. S. Brewers Association. "Brewer's Almanac 1956." New York, 1956.
12. U. S. Brewers Association. "Brewer's Almanac 1974." New York, 1974.
13. U. S. Bureau of the Census. "Statistical Abstract of the United States: 1960," 81st ed. USGPO, Washington, D. C., 1960.
14. U. S. Bureau of the Census. "Statistical Abstract of the United States: 1970," 91st ed. USGPO, Washington, D. C., 1970.
15. U. S. Bureau of the Census. "U. S. Census of Housing; 1970. Detailed Characteristics," HC(1)B1. USGPO, Washington, D. C., 1971.
16. U. S. Bureau of the Census. "U. S. Census of Population: 1940," Vol. II, Characteristics of the Population, Part 1, United States Summary. USGPO, Washington, D. C., 1943.
17. U. S. Bureau of the Census. "U. S. Census of Population: 1950," Vol. II, Characteristics of the Population, Part 1, United States Summary. USGPO, Washington, D. C., 1953.
18. U. S. Bureau of the Census. "U. S. Census of Population: 1950," Vol. II, Characteristics of the Population, Parts 2-50. USGPO, Washington, D. C., 1952.
19. U. S. Bureau of the Census. "U. S. Census of Population: 1960," General Population Characteristics, United States Summary, Final Report PC(1)-1B. USGPO, Washington, D. C., 1961.
20. U. S. Bureau of the Census. "U. S. Census of Population: 1970," Vol. I, Characteristics of the Population, Part 1, United States Summary, Section 1. USGPO, Washington, D. C., 1971.
21. U. S. Department of Agriculture. "Dairy Situation." Economic Research Service Publ. No. DS-354, Washington, D. C., 1975.
22. U. S. Environmental Protection Agency. "The National Air Monitoring Program: Air Quality and Emissions Trends, Annual Report," Volume II. Publ. No. EPA-450/1-73-001b, USGPO, Washington, D. C., 1973.

TABLE II
Response Variables: State Age-Adjusted Death Rates

Code Number[a]	Site	
1950-1969[b]		ICD 1948
M/ F100	All malignant neoplasms	140-205
M/ F140	Buccal cavity and pharynx	140-148
M/ F150	Esophagus	150
M/ F151	Stomach	151
M/ F153	Large intestine excluding rectum	153
M/ F154	Rectum	154
M/ F155	Biliary passages and liver specified as primary and unspecified	155, Unspec. Part of 156
M/ F157	Pancreas	157
M/ F161	Larynx	161
M/ F166	Trachea, bronchus, and lung	162-163
M/ F170	Breast	170
F171	Cervix uteri	171
F172	Corpus and other parts of uterus, and uterus unspecified	172-174
F175	Ovary	175
M177	Prostate	177
M/ F180	Kidney	180
M/ F181	Bladder and other urinary organs	181
M/ F190	Malignant melanoma of skin	190
M/ F191	Other malignant neoplasms of skin	191
M/ F193	Brain and other parts of the nervous system	193
M/ F194	Thyroid	194
M/ F200	Lymphosarcoma and reticulosarcoma	200, 202, 205
M/ F201	Hodgkin's disease	201
M/ F203	Multiple myeloma	203
M/ F204	Leukemia and aleukemia	204
1950-1967[c]		
M/ F162	Trachea, and bronchus and lung specified as primary	162
M/ F163	Bronchus and lung unspecified as to primary or secondary	163
1949-1959[d]		
M/ F100B	All malignant neoplasms	140-205
M/ F140B	Buccal cavity and pharynx	140-148
M/ F150B	Esophagus	150
M/ F151B	Stomach	151
M/ F153B	Intestines excluding rectum	152-153
M/ F154B	Rectum	154

[a] M, white male. F, white female.

[b] Mason, T. J., and McKay, F. W. "U. S. Cancer Mortality by County: 1950-1969." DHEW Publ. No. (NIH) 74-615, USGPO, Washington, D. C., 1973.

[c] Burbank, F. Patterns in cancer mortality in the United States: 1950-1967. *Nat. Cancer Inst. Monogr. 33:* 199-216, 1971.

[d] U. S. Public Health Service. "Vital Statistics of the United States," Vols. II and III, Mortality Data, 1949-1959. USGPO, Washington, D. C., 1951-1962.

TABLE II (Continued)

Code Number[a]	Site	
M/ F158B	Biliary passages and liver	155-156
M/ F155B	Biliary passages and liver specified as primary	155
M/ F156B	Biliary passages and liver secondary and unspecified	156
M/ F157B	Pancreas	157
M/ F161B	Larynx	161
M/ F166B	Trachea, bronchus, and lung	162-163
M/ F162B	Trachea, and bronchus, and lung specified as primary	162
M/ F163B	Bronchus and lung unspecified as to primary or secondary	163
M/ F170B	Breast	170
F171B	Cervix uteri	171
F172B	Corpus and other parts of uterus, and uterus unspecified	172-174
F175B	Ovary	175
M177B	Prostate	177
M/ F180B	Kidney	180
M/ F181B	Bladder and other urinary organs	181
M/ F189B	Skin including melanoma	190-191
M/ F193B	Brain and other parts of the nervous system	193
M/ F194B	Thyroid	194
M/ F200B	Lymphosarcoma and reticulosarcoma and other forms of lymphoma	200-203, 205
M/ F201B	Hodgkin's disease	201
M/ F204B	Leukemia and aleukemia	204
1960[e]		ICD 1955
M/ F256	Gallbladder	155.1
Major Disease Categories		
1949-1959[f]		ICD 1948
M/ F010B	Tuberculosis	001-019
M/ F050B	Infectious and parasitic except influenza and tuberculosis	020-138
M/ F400B	Circulatory system	400-468
M/ F470B	Respiratory system except influenza and asthma	470-475, 490-527
M/ F480B	Influenza	480-483
M/ F500B	Genito-urinary system	590-637
M/ F530B	Digestive system	530-587
M/ F800B	Accidental and violent causes	E800-E999
M/ F900B	All deaths	001-E999

[e] U. S. Public Health Service. "Vital Statistics of the United States," Vol. II, Mortality Data, 1960. USGPO, Washington, D. C., 1963.

[f] U. S. Public Health Service. "Vital Statistics of the United States," Vols. II and III, Mortality Data, 1949-1959. USGPO, Washington, D. C., 1951-1962.

Chapter 2
The Factor Variable Pools

I Correlations Between Response Variables

The simple correlation coefficient between any two cancer mortality patterns indicates the degree to which those states with high death rates from one type of cancer also have high death rates from the other. High correlation between the male and female state patterns for the same cancer mortality indicates a parallelism between the sexes in the high-, medium-, and low-mortality risk states in that type of cancer. Since significance levels are used only as guidelines throughout the study and since in this case almost all the correlation coefficients qualified as significantly different from zero at the 5% level, an arbitrary criterion was chosen to demark the stronger associations of mortality, that is, a coefficient of determination equal to .50 or more, indicating that the two state patterns of death rates have at least 50% of their variation in common. Thus any two mortality patterns with a correlation coefficient of at least .7071 were considered to be strongly related and are listed in Table III.

It can be seen that a cancer mortality pattern is frequently most correlated with the same cancer mortality in the opposite sex. Those cancer primaries in which the mortality pattern for either sex has its highest correlation with that of the other sex are trachea, and bronchus and lung, specified primary; bronchus and lung, unspecified primary; stomach; large intestine; rectum; pancreas; brain; lymphosarcoma; leukemia; melanoma (of the skin); and other malignant skin cancer. For the combined category of specified primary and unspecified trachea, bronchus, and lung, the male mortality pattern is most highly correlated with that of male laryngeal cancer, and next most with its counterpart in female mortality, while the latter has its highest association with its male counterpart. Although it is not shown in the table because their common variation is a little less than 50%, the mortality pattern of female cancer of the larynx is most highly correlated with that of female cancer of the esophagus, and next most with

TABLE III

Coefficients of Determination[a] for Each Male Site

Male site	Correlated site	Coefficient
Buccal cavity and pharynx		
	M-Larynx	91.3
	M-Esophagus	74.1
	M-T, B & Lung	59.6
	F-Bladder	56.5
	M-Lg. Intestine	50.0
Larynx		
	M-Buc Cav & Ph.	91.3
	M-Esophagus	74.5
	M-T, B & Lung	71.0
	F-Bladder	64.8
	M-B & L Unspec.	55.4
	M-Bladder	53.7
	M-Lg. Intestine	52.0
Trachea, bronchus and lung		
	M-Larynx	71.0
	F-T, B & Lung	68.6
	M-B & L Unspec.	66.1
	M-Buc Cav & Ph.	59.6
	F-Bladder	52.6
Trachea and bronchus and lung specified primary		
	F-T, B & L Spec.	76.4
Bronchus and lung unspec. as primary or secondary		
	F-B & L Unspec.	81.0
	M-T, B & Lung	66.1
	M-Larynx	55.4
Esophagus		
	M-Lg. Intestine	77.1
	M-Larynx	74.5
	M-Buc Cav & Ph.	74.1
	F-Breast	71.2
	M-Bladder	69.9
	M-Rectum	69.1
	F-Lg. Intestine	62.8
	F-Bladder	61.4
	F-Rectum	60.2
	F-Ovary	51.4
Stomach		
	F-Stomach	92.3
	M-Kidney	52.1
Large intestine exc. rectum		
	F-Lg. Intestine	92.6
	M-Rectum	91.0
	F-Breast	86.5
	F-Rectum	80.9
	M-Bladder	77.6
	M-Esophagus	77.1
	F-Ovary	69.4
	M-Kidney	60.3
	M-Larynx	52.0
	F-Bladder	50.7
	M-Buc Cav & Ph.	50.0
Rectum		
	F-Rectum	92.6
	F-Breast	91.0
	M-Lg. Intestine	91.0
	F-Lg. Intestine	88.9
	M-Bladder	82.5
	F-Ovary	71.0
	M-Kidney	70.6
	M-Esophagus	69.1
	M-Lymphosarcoma	51.8
	F-Hodgkin's Dis.	51.0
Pancreas		
	F-Pancreas	51.0
Kidney		
	F-Breast	78.0
	F-Ovary	74.9
	M-Rectum	70.6
	F-Rectum	63.2
	M-Lg. Intestine	60.3
	F-Lymphosarcoma	58.3
	F-Hodgkin's Dis.	58.1
	M-Bladder	57.9
	F-Lg. Intestine	56.2
	F-Other Skin	52.7[b]
	M-Stomach	52.1
	M-Other Skin	51.5[b]
	M-Lymphosarcoma	51.2
Bladder and other urinary organs		
	M-Rectum	82.5
	F-Breast	80.9
	M-Lg. Intestine	77.6
	F-Rectum	76.5
	M-Esophagus	69.9
	F-Lg. Intestine	69.3
	F-Bladder	58.3
	M-Kidney	57.9
	F-Ovary	56.0
	M-Larynx	53.7
Brain and other parts nervous system		
	F-Brain	63.7
Lymphosarcoma		
	F-Lymphosarcoma	71.9
	F-Breast	58.7
	F-Ovary	54.3
	M-Rectum	51.8
	M-Kidney	51.2
Leukemia		
	F-Leukemia	60.8
Melanoma of skin		
	F-Melanoma	62.2
	M-Other Skin	55.1
	F-Buc Cav & Ph.	54.9
Other skin		
	F-Other Skin	70.2
	F-Melanoma	60.4
	M-Melanoma	55.1
	M-Kidney	51.5[b]
Sites with all coefficients of determination less than 50%		
	Hodgkin's Disease	
	Prostate	
	Liver *et al.*	

[a] Coefficient of determination equals coefficient of correlation squared times 100.
[b] Negative correlation.

Cancer Sites with More than 50% Common Variation in State Mortality Rates

Coefficients of Determination[a] for Each Female Site

Site	Coefficient
Buccal cavity and pharynx	
M-Melanoma	54.9
F-Other Skin	52.9
Trachea, bronchus and lung	
M-T, B & Lung	68.6
F-B & L Unspec.	58.4
Trachea and bronchus and lung specified primary	
M-T, B & L Spec.	76.4
Bronchus and lung unspec. as primary or secondary	
M-B & L Unspec.	81.0
F-T, B & Lung	58.4
Stomach	
M-Stomach	92.3
Large intestine exc. rectum	
M-Lg. Intestine	92.6
M-Rectum	88.9
F-Rectum	85.1
F-Breast	77.8
M-Bladder	69.3
F-Ovary	64.8
M-Esophagus	62.8
M-Kidney	56.2
F-Bladder	51.4
Rectum	
M-Rectum	92.6
F-Lg. Intestine	85.1
M-Lg. Intestine	80.9
F-Breast	79.8
M-Bladder	76.5
M-Kidney	63.2
M-Esophagus	60.2
F-Ovary	59.0
F-Bladder	54.8
F-Hodgkin's Dis.	54.7
Pancreas	
M-Pancreas	51.0
Bladder and other urinary organs	
M-Larynx	64.8
M-Esophagus	61.4
M-Bladder	58.3
M-Buc Cav & Ph.	56.5
F-Rectum	54.8
M-T, B & Lung	52.6
F-Lg. Intestine	51.4
M-Lg. Intestine	50.7
Brain and other parts nervous system	
M-Brain	63.7
Lymphosarcoma	
M-Lymphosarcoma	71.9
F-Ovary	60.0
M-Kidney	58.3
F-Breast	55.5
Hodgkin's disease	
M-Kidney	58.1
F-Rectum	54.7
M-Rectum	51.0
Leukemia	
M-Leukemia	60.8
Breast	
M-Rectum	91.0
M-Lg. Intestine	86.5
F-Ovary	82.5
M-Bladder	80.9
F-Rectum	79.8
M-Kidney	78.0
F-Lg. Intestine	77.8
M-Esophagus	71.2
M-Lymphosarcoma	58.7
F-Lymphosarcoma	55.5
Ovary, fallopian tubes, and broad ligament	
F-Breast	82.5
M-Kidney	74.9
M-Rectum	71.0
M-Lg. Intestine	69.4
F-Lg. Intestine	64.8
F-Lymphosarcoma	60.0
F-Rectum	59.0
M-Bladder	56.0
M-Lymphosarcoma	54.3
M-Esophagus	51.4
Melanoma of skin	
M-Melanoma	62.2
M-Other Skin	60.4
F-Other Skin	54.8
Other skin	
M-Other Skin	70.2
F-Melanoma	54.8
F-Buc Cav & Ph.	52.9
M-Kidney	52.7[b]
Sites with all coefficients of determination less than 50%	
Larynx	
Esophagus	
Liver *et al.*	
Kidney	
Cervix Uteri	
Corpus Uteri	

that of male laryngeal cancer. However, the patterns of male mortality from cancer of the larynx, of the buccal cavity and pharynx, of the esophagus, and of the combined specified primary and unspecified category of trachea, bronchus, and lung are all most closely related to each other. In addition to the female mortality patterns of the three categories of lung cancer (specified primary, unspecified, and combined), the pattern of female mortality from cancer of the bladder is most related to this set of male cancer mortalities. The digestive cancer mortality patterns, except for those of the liver and pancreas, are closely related to each other and to male bladder cancer mortality, while mortality from cancer of the liver, pancreas, brain, and prostate, and from lymphosarcoma, leukemia, and Hodgkin's disease occurs in more individualized patterns. The death rates from cancer of the breast and the ovary are highly correlated and they are also closely related to the digestive cancer mortality patterns. Melanoma and other malignant skin cancer deaths are most closely related to each other and to female mortality from cancer of the buccal cavity and pharynx.

The basic structure underlying the mortality models is the set of correlations between the mortality patterns and the factor variables, but in their simple form these correlations can be misleading. Associations may be exhibited that are artificial, the occurrence due solely to statistical association with a third variable. Because a strong collinearity among the sociological, economic, ethnic, and even climatic factors involved in this study is unavoidable, it is imperative that only the adjusted effect of each factor be considered. For this reason the mortality models are derived by multiple regression techniques that determine the *net* effect of each factor on a mortality pattern after correction for its relationship, and that of the death rate, with all the other factors brought into the model.

II Choosing the Factor Variable Pools[a]

A Urbanization and Population Density Factors

The choice of the four basic sets of variables that constitute the four variable pools used in the derivation of all the mortality models was arrived at by determining the correlation patterns between the death rates and the factor variables, analyzing the structure of the interrelationships among the factor variables, and testing a succession of variable pools and the mortality models resulting from them.

Most of the initial models chosen by the computer programs contained one or the other of two independent variables that represented the degree of urbanization and the population density. The two variables URBW5N, the percentage of white population living in an urban area in 1950, and DENS50, the 1950 total

[a]Definitions of the variables referred to and their sources are found in Table I.

population per square mile in 1950, are two facets of an urban density concept that has been of recent interest as a factor in cancer and other mortality patterns. Three approaches to measuring this concept are (1) the percentage of the white population of each state that lives in urban areas as defined by the Bureau of the Census, (2) total population per square mile of area in a state, (3) a weighted average of the population density in different types of area, the weights being the relative proportions of the population living in each area. The first variable, URBW5N, urban percentage white, reflects the degree to which the white population of any state lives in urban as opposed to rural areas, and its negative aspect indicates the rural character of the white population. This variable shows high correlations with income level and with consumption and ethnic variables such as the per capita consumption of alcoholic beverages and the percentage of foreign born in the white population. It was an influential factor in the first mortality models derived for major cancers such as the digestive cancers and cancer of the breast. The second variable, DENS50, is a crude measurement of the overall degree of crowding of a state's total population, white and nonwhite, and does not differentiate between a large state whose population lives primarily in cities surrounded by large areas of open territory and a small state whose population is evenly spread across its land in moderate sized towns. To refine this variable in order to reflect a state population's relative exposure to crowding, a third variable was calculated, WDEN50. This is a weighted average of the population densities of four areas–central city, urban fringe, outside city, and rural–weighted by the proportion of total state population living in each area. For this study a preferable average would have involved the density of the total population in each area weighted by the proportion of the state's *white* population living in that area, but the latter data were not available. Neither of these two measures of population density, surprisingly, is closely correlated with the measure of urbanization or its related sociological factors, but instead they show a closer association with the climatic factors and the pollution measures, a higher degree of density found with higher pollution levels and in wetter climates at lower elevation levels. The population density measures entered significantly the initial mortality models for the respiratory cancers and for cancer of the upper, partially exposed sites such as the buccal cavity and pharynx and the larynx.

It was recognized that this dichotomy in the urban/density pattern between an urban-ethnic-consumption variation and a density-climate-pollution variation among the states should be represented in both its aspects in the final choice of variable pools. The need was to discover which elements in an urban and in a densely populated environment were responsible for the importance of urbanization and population density in the mortality models. Higher pollution levels, higher levels of consumption of cigarettes and alcohol, greater proportions of European foreign born, as well as differing climatic conditions are clearly associated with higher values of the urban/density variables. All of these components evolved as important factors in themselves.

B Factors of Climate and Geography

The physical environment is reflected in the final factor structure by two measures, one for average temperature and one for a combination of average precipitation and average elevation. The mean temperatures in January and in July were combined with equal weights into a single measure of state climate, TEMP. It would have been preferable if a state average of sectors of contrasting climate, each weighted by its resident population, could have been calculated for those states that extend from warm to cold climates such as California and Texas, or states where the population is concentrated in the northern (Illinois) or the southern (New York) sector. The variables representing precipitation and elevation were too strongly correlated (negatively) to function as separate factors. Therefore a single variable, PRELEV, combining both factors by means of their first principal component scores was used to reflect in its positive aspect an environment of high rainfall and low elevation, and in its negative aspect one of low rainfall and high elevation.

C Air Contamination Variables

1 Pollutant Emission Measures

Individual pollution variables representing the air content of suspended particulate matter, sulfur dioxide, carbon monoxide, hydrocarbon, and nitric oxide were derived from EPA measurements for each station monitoring any segment of a state. The form of the variable chosen as most appropriate was constructed to represent the exposure of a state's population to each pollutant. Each pollution variable is calculated as the weighted average over all segments within a state of the amount per kilometer measured for each segment and weighted by the resident population. Since the EPA considered each segment and its population to be under the province of a single station, it was possible to assign to each state its fractional share when one station covered segments from more than one state. This was all that the EPA would make available on request, and its use necessitates keeping the following shortcomings in mind.

(1) The state of technology employed in taking these measurements was still not very good and, moreover, differed greatly from state to state.

(2) The year of measurement was 1970 (some stations reported for 1966, 1968, and 1969) while the mortality data covered the period 1950-1969. Since pollution effects may be the result of long-term as well as current exposure, the fallacy in the direct inference of measurable increments in mortality resulting

from incremental changes in pollution level is evident. Instead, the assumption was made that the *relative position or rank* of each state in industrial and economic development and hence in pollution levels did not change radically over the period of interest. This was borne out by the very close correlations between time periods in other variables reflecting this type of development. For example, the 1940 state percentage of males in manufacturing was very highly correlated with the 1950 figures ($r = .983$).

(3) The populations at risk given by the EPA were combined white and nonwhite, whereas the mortality rates in this book are only for the white portion. The assumption is made that the distribution of whites among segments this large parallels the distribution of the total population, and, since the whites are in the majority, it is a workable premise.

(4) The average level of each type of pollutant over a year's period may not be the crucial measure of exposure, but rather the peak levels and their duration. The assumption had to be that where the average over time was high, the maximum levels were the highest.

Each of these pollution variables was primarily an index of a state's relative position with respect to its population's exposure to that pollutant. The five variables representing the five basic types of air pollutant were found to be so closely correlated that their individual use in models was misleading and their individual effects were inseparable. Therefore a principal components analysis was made combining these five variables with a sixth variable, a measure of benzo[*a*] pyrene, similarly weighted by resident populations. The first principal component, which accounted for 80% of the joint variation of the six measures of air pollutants, was chosen as the variable POLLUT to represent the degree of a state population's exposure to overall air pollution. The state pattern of benzo[*a*] pyrene was not closely related to the other five pollutant variables, nor was it as individually effective in the preliminary modeling. It was included in a general pollution score rather than as a separate variable, although in one study (7) it was considered sufficient to "represent the effects of all the correlated pollution variables combined." Its weight in the first principal component scoring was somewhat less than those of the other five pollutant measures, among which the weighting was almost equal.

2 *Vehicle Miles Traveled*

Another variable in this category considered in the initial models was TVMS62, vehicle miles traveled in 1962 per square mile of land area. It entered many models very significantly and appeared to be an even more important factor than the pollution variables, all of which outweighed the urbanization and the population density variables in most of the models. Although this variable was chosen to reflect a state population's relative exposure to the pollutants emitted by vehicles, it is strongly confounded with population density, since the vehicle miles driven per square mile of area are directly related to the population of that area. A per capita version of this variable was tried but it could not be justified logically as a measure either of individual or of group exposure to auto pollutants.

3 Household Use of Coal or Coke

The number of households using coal or coke was also considered, but its distribution was extremely skewed, concentrating in only a very few states, and no effect on the mortality patterns was indicated. The burning of coal releases benzo[*a*]pyrene into the air (23), a contaminant that is represented in the combination variable, POLLUT.

4 Employment in Manufacturing

Two other variables that showed important effects in the preliminary modeling were the percentage of males, and the percentage of females, employed in manufacturing in each state. These differed in their regional patterns, the percentages of males employed in manufacturing being highest in the midwestern states while those of females were highest in New England. These variables entered some of the initial cancer mortality models (male buccal cavity and pharynx, larynx, and rectum; female bladder, large intestine, and corpus uteri) as strongly as the variables measuring vehicle miles traveled, and were similarly omitted from the final variable pools. The variable representing male employment in manufacturing was closely correlated with vehicle miles traveled and with the population density and the pollution variables. It was considered to be similar to vehicle miles traveled as a secondary measure of air contaminants. The degree to which it reflected individual workers' exposure within their factories was too general to warrant its use instead of or in addition to a pollution measure.

D Radiation

In a study published by the EPA Oakley (24) presents an estimate of the average dose equivalent of each state population's exposure to the radiation from natural background sources, both cosmic and terrestrial. This index is an average of the total external radiation exposure rates of a state's area segments, urbanized and nonurbanized, weighted by the resident populations. Although the level of cosmic radiation is positively related to both latitude and altitude, the influence of the former within the United States is negligible while that of the latter is almost completely determinant. Therefore the dose exposures of the ionizing and of the neutron components of cosmic radiation were calculated from the average elevation of each area segment in accordance with the known relationships between altitude and each cosmic radiation component.

Estimates of population exposure to terrestrial radiation were derived from applying population maps to information from aerial surveys conducted by the U. S. Atomic Energy Commission, and three major regions of radiation level were found: the Atlantic and Gulf coastal plains with low dose equivalent levels (22.8 mrem/year), the Colorado Front Range, including Denver, with the highest level (89.7 mrem/year), and the rest of the U. S. falling between these levels (45.6 mrem/year). To illustrate the importance of exposure to naturally occurring radiation within the U. S., Oakley estimates that the dose equivalent to the gonads and bone marrow from cosmic sources is 44 mrem/year, from terrestrial sources (after correcting for housing and screening factors) 26 mrem/year, and from internal (body) sources 18 mrem/year, totaling 88 mrem/year compared with an estimated average X-ray exposure of 55 mrem/year. Moreover, the range of dose exposure due to cosmic radiation is from 41.0 mrem/year in Florida to 80.5 mrem/year in Wyoming, and the range due to terrestrial radiation is from 22.3 mrem/year in Florida to 65.8 mrem/year in Colorado. Therefore, although this data set was received after the major part of the statistical analysis was completed, the quality of its method of derivation, the potential of its importance in cancer mortality, and its close association ($r = -.807$) with the strongest effect in the cancer mortality models—the precipitation/elevation factor PRELEV—warranted additional analysis focused on its possible role. The variable representing this radiation index, RADIAT, was tested in a different manner from the others and its analysis is discussed separately.

E Income

Two measures of a state's relative position with respect to personal income level were considered, the average income of the total state population and the median income of its white population. Although the mortality models are derived only for the white population, a measure characterizing the entire state was chosen for the final variable pool. The per capita personal income of the whole population, INCM, was considered to reflect both the personal wealth of the majority and the state's relative position with respect to availability of medical facilities and services.

F Consumption Factors

Since product consumption is not given by race or by sex, the alcohol consumption variables were calculated as per capita adult (21 and over) in each state, thereby adjusting for different state age distributions. It had to be assumed that the relative state level of female consumption of alcohol mirrored that of the males, and that the pattern of state consumption was due to the racial majority. The state consumption patterns of the two types of alcoholic beverage consumed, wine and distilled spirits, are more closely related (r = .763) than each is with the third type, malt (.537, .553). In order to represent a general alcohol consumption factor all three components were combined into a single first principal component score and this variable, ALCO, was used in two of the final variable pools. However, marked differences in the models arose among these three alcohol component variables and sufficient additional variance was explained by their division to maintain all three as separate factors in the other two final pools.

The cigarette consumption figures available were per capita for the entire state population and did not include other types of tobacco use.

In the measures of consumption factors the year used was the earliest for which complete and comparable state data were available, but it was usually too recent for determining etiological effects, which are generally assumed to be long-term. In order to include these essential factors it had to be assumed that each state's relative position in each type of consumption changed little over the period in question. The high correlations of state consumption rates between different time periods permitted this assumption.

A recent study (25) found significantly higher male mortality rates from cancer of the stomach, bladder, and all neoplasms in Ohio counties where the source of drinking water was surface rather than ground. Although adjustment was made for five social and demographic variables, important factors such as alcohol consumption were not among these. Without detailed state data on drinking water sources and population usage, a variable measuring inland water as a percentage of total state area was used to reflect the prevalence and potential importance of surface water sources. Neither this variable nor one measuring the percentage of total water area, coastal as well as inland, to total area indicated strength in the preliminary modeling, but their rough representation of the consumption patterns of interest could have been the cause of their nonproductivity.

The variable measuring the percentage of population using public drinking water showed some strength but was too connected with urban development to be able to stand alone. A fluoridated drinking water variable was carefully tested because of popular interest in this additive but it did not enter any of the models. Since this measure does not include the duration of exposure to fluoridation of each consuming population group, and since communities have entered the fluoridation ranks in different years, it is not likely to reflect well the dose-exposure of each state population. Unlike the ongoing consumption of wine or beer, the large-scale consumption of fluoridated water is recent, with times of inception and duration varying from town to town, so that any study of its effects must focus on individual communities rather than entire states.

G Ethnic Variation

The importance of ethnic variables such as the percentage of the white population who were foreign born, or the native white of foreign or mixed parentage, or the combination of the two into foreign white stock, became evident in the initial models. When the foreign born were broken down by country of origin, 25 countries were chosen as the largest sources of white immigration into the U. S. The regional distributions of most of these ethnic categories were highly related to the urbanization variable, either positively or negatively, and similarly related to each other. When a principal components analysis was made on these ethnic proportions, the first principal component evolved as a linear combination with weightings equivalent to the degree of urbanization of each ethnic category, resulting in just another measure of the urban factor.

Needed was a picture of basic ethnic differences condensed into a minimum number of variables. The British influence being the strongest in the United States, the foreign born from the five countries England, Wales, Scotland, Northern Ireland, and Ireland were combined into one population subgroup, and its percentage of the white population of each state calculated for 1940 and 1950. This measurement for the year 1950 was chosen as one of the four ethnic variables in the final variable pool and is referred to as BRIT. Although the state percentages born in France were very small compared with other ethnic proportions, this variable presented such strong individual effects in many of the models and maintained a sufficiently different regional pattern from the British-born, that it was added to the variable pool as the only single-nation ethnic variable. It is referred to as FRAN and does not include the French Canadians, an immigrant group so large that its numbers would overwhelm the basic French figures. The Canadians, both French and "other," were the largest white immigrant populations in the U. S., although, if the Mexicans were correctly enumerated, they might have been. The distribution of the other Canadians is completely in the states along the northern border and therefore yields a variable totally confounded with the climate variable TEMP. The French Canadians are located in New England almost exclusively, and that ethnic variable is therefore similarly confounded with the characteristics of a particular region. The heavy distribution of the Mexican population in the southwestern border states confounds this ethnic factor with the climate and sociological factors of that area. Although the Mexican ethnic variable was not included in the basic variable pools, it was tested as an additional factor in selected mortality patterns, as described in Chapter 8.

The third ethnic variable added to the pool combined the three foreign-born populations from Norway, Sweden and Denmark into a single percentage of a state's white population. This variable, SCAN, has some correlation with TEMP

($r = -.692$), but the relationship was not strong enough to produce an unmanageable confounding. This ethnic variable, like FRAN, demonstrated such individualized and strong effects in the preliminary models that it was kept as a basic variable.

The fourth ethnic variable had to carry the heavy burden of representing a major portion of the European immigration into the U. S. Excluded from this European subpopulation were, besides the countries represented in the other three ethnic variables, the Balkans, the Iberian peninsula, the upper Baltic, and Finland. The ten European countries included represent *mittel Europa* and Russia, a combination of Germanic, Slavic, and Italian ethnic categories. Principal components analysis was used to combine these ethnics into one variable representing an "other European" ethnicity, OTHEUR. The percentages of foreign born from each of the ten countries plus the Jewish proportion of the white population in each state were combined into a first principal component score in order to represent as much of the variation as possible in the distribution of the ethnic categories from these European countries. The Jewish component was included since these countries represented the major source of Jewish immigration into the U. S.

This combination ethnic variable proved to be so important in the cancer mortality models that it was divided into three variables GERM, ITAL, and SLAV representing its three major components. Replacing OTHEUR with these three more specific ethnic variables, the cancer mortality models were rederived solely to dissect the other European effects that had entered. These three variables were not incorporated into the basic variable pools, however, because of the need to restrict the number of factor variables and the multicollinearity among them.

It is necessary to point out that it is not the foreign born alone that are of interest in this study, but the relative proportion of each ethnic *stock* in a state's white population. Since in the past new immigrants tended to settle where there were concentrations of earlier immigrants from the same European country or even the same European village, it could be expected that a state's relative position with respect to each ethnic stock could be represented by its relative position with respect to the foreign born of that ethnic. In confirmation of this relationship it was found that the variables representing foreign born and foreign stock were so highly correlated as to be almost identical.

It is interesting to note that, of the 25 individual ethnic percentages of foreign born, those most correlated with the malt consumption variable were the Austrians, Germans, and Irish; with the wine consumption variable were the French, Latin Americans other than Mexicans, and Italians; with the distilled spirits consumption variable were the French, Greeks, and Irish; and with the cigarette consumption variable were the French, Irish, Scotch, and English. The ethnics most correlated with urbanization were the Jewish, Italians, French, and British.

III Final Variable Pools

Four final variable pools were chosen for the derivation of all the mortality models to ensure comparability of model effects across mortality patterns. The smallest, the 6-variable pool, is made up of the basic variables TEMP, PRELEV, POLLUT, INCM, CIGS, and ALCO, the total alcohol consumption variable. The 8-variable pool divides ALCO into its three components, MALT, WINE, and DISP. The 10-variable pool adds to the 6-variable pool the four ethnic variables FRAN, BRIT, SCAN, and OTHEUR, and the 12-variable pool adds these ethnic variables to the 8-variable pool (Table IV).

TABLE IV The Variable Pools

6-VAR	8-VAR	10-VAR	12-VAR
TEMP	TEMP	TEMP	TEMP
PRELEV	PRELEV	PRELEV	PRELEV
POLLUT	POLLUT	POLLUT	POLLUT
INCM	INCM	INCM	INCM
CIGS	CIGS	CIGS	CIGS
	MALT		MALT
ALCO	WINE	ALCO	WINE
	DISP		DISP
		FRAN	FRAN
		BRIT	BRIT
		SCAN	SCAN
		OTHEUR	OTHEUR

Observation of the changes in effects entering the mortality models as variables were added to each pool afforded insight into the interrelationships and primacy of the chosen factors. This procedure provided information to determine whether alcohol consumption as a whole, ALCO, was a factor, or whether one type of alcohol was responsible for this general effect. It also allowed non-ethnic factors to show their effects on the mortality patterns before the complications of ethnicity were introduced, since the association between the consumption and the ethnic variables is strong. This sequence of pools assumed that the path of causation is most commonly from ethnicity to consumption habits to mortality effect. The alternative path of consumption to ethnicity is impossible. The possibility of ethnicity directly affecting mortality, while producing incidentally a spurious association between consumption and mortality, is, however, a statistical possibility. The progression of models arising from each pool of variables permitted a careful consideration of these paths of causation for each type of mortality.

IV Collinearity in the Variable Pools

The correlation matrix of the 12 variables chosen to comprise the largest variable pool is shown in Table V. The highest correlations exist among the

TABLE V

Correlation Matrix of the Factor Variables

	Environmental factors				Consumption factors					Ethnic factors			
	Climatic					Alcoholic							
	TEMP	PRELEV	POLLUT	INCM	CIGS	ALCO	MALT	WINE	DISP	FRAN	BRIT	SCAN	OTHEUR
TEMP	1.000	.354	.171	–.406	–.321	–.318	–.515	–.064	–.274	–.246	–.475	–.692	–.429
PRELEV	.354	1.000	.538	–.158	.005	–.053	–.177	–.034	.057	–.086	–.092	–.443	–.004
POLLUT	.171	.538	1.000	.407	.228	.395	.326	.368	.330	.302	.289	–.126	.487
INCM	–.406	–.158	.407	1.000	.698	.806	.831	.622	.656	.806	.809	.660	.842
CIGS	–.321	.005	.228	.698	1.000	.756	.631	.583	.746	.742	.686	.342	.566
ALCO	–.318	–.053	.395	.806	.756	1.000	.790	.896	.903	.842	.759	.500	.723
MALT	–.515	–.177	.326	.831	.631	.790	1.000	.537	.553	.712	.765	.659	.834
WINE	–.064	–.034	.368	.622	.583	.896	.537	1.000	.763	.776	.615	.301	.548
DISP	–.274	.057	.330	.656	.746	.903	.553	.763	1.000	.697	.604	.367	.523
FRAN	–.246	–.086	.302	.806	.742	.842	.712	.776	.697	1.000	.855	.515	.717
BRIT	–.475	–.092	.289	.809	.686	.759	.765	.615	.604	.855	1.000	.675	.821
SCAN	–.692	–.443	–.126	.660	.342	.500	.659	.301	.367	.515	.675	1.000	.661
OTHEUR	–.429	–.004	.487	.842	.566	.723	.834	.548	.523	.717	.821	.661	1.000

ethnic variables, between the ethnic variables and income level, and between the ethnic and the consumption variables. In a principal components analysis of the 12 variables, the first principal component, which explained 56% of the joint variation, could be considered to represent a general urban factor with high weights on income level, the French, British and Other European ethnic percentages, and on malt and cigarette consumption levels. The second principal component, explaining an additional 18% of the variation, appears to represent the population density factor with high weights on pollution level and climate factors. When the state scores for all 12 principal components were used as pseudofactor variables in a multiple regression on the cancer death rates, the first principal component, or general urban factor, was the most influential in state mortality patterns of both sexes for cancer of the stomach, the large intestine and the rectum, lymphosarcoma and Hodgkin's disease, as well as for cancer of the kidney, bladder, and esophagus in males and cancer of the pancreas, breast, and ovary in females. The second principal component or pollution/climate factor was the most influential in the mortality patterns of both sexes for cancer of the buccal cavity and pharynx, larynx, and trachea, bronchus, and lung, as well as for cancer of the liver and pancreas in males and cancer of the bladder and cervix in females. This general division in cancer sites with respect to the factor sets that are most influential in their state mortality patterns is borne out in the more direct regression analysis involving the primary factor variables.

V Relating Ethnic Effects to European Mortality Patterns

Segi (26), in the fifth volume of his study "Cancer Mortality for Selected Sites in 24 Countries," ranks the 1964-1965 age-adjusted cancer death rates for males and for females in 24 countries. After dropping U. S. nonwhite, Japan, Australia, New Zealand, and South Africa as not representing sources of U. S. white ethnicity, the remaining 20 national rates were reranked for each type of cancer mortality. These ranks are used throughout this study as indices of the relative risk level in each country for specified cancer mortalities, and they are compared with the associated ethnic effects in the U. S. cancer mortality models. Considered are the ranks of individual countries in each group, as well as an average group rank, weighted by the relative proportions of each member's foreign born in the U. S. The British group are the same as the components of the ethnic variable BRIT: Scotland, Northern Ireland, Ireland, England and Wales. The Scandinavian group are those of the ethnic variable SCAN: Norway, Sweden, and Denmark. Of the countries comprising the Other European group in the ethnic variable OTHEUR, Austria, Belgium, Germany (the Federal Republic), Italy, and the Netherlands are also in Segi's ranking. For a few major cancer sites Segi includes Bulgaria, Czechoslovakia, Hungary, and Poland in a ranking of 40 countries, but he indicates that their rates are not strictly comparable with the basic set of 24 national ranks. However, the relative ranking of these eastern European countries was considered wherever possible in judging the combined rank of the Other European group.

In the concluding chapter a summary comparison between ethnic factors in the models and foreign mortality levels includes cancer mortality data taken from an official Soviet journal and adjusted to Segi's rates. Because of the limited number of cancer sites covered and questionable comparability, the Russian rates were not incorporated into the main body of analysis.

Some types of cancer mortality are not treated by Segi and reference is then made to the world cancer *incidence* rates compiled by the International Union against Cancer (27). Unfortunately the comparison of 60 incidence rates in this reference cannot be used more frequently for comparison with the ethnic effects in the U. S. mortality models for the following reasons: (1) many individual nations have multiple rates covering a wide range of values; (2) as in Segi's larger listing of countries, many rates are of nonwhite populations; (3) the incidence rates of important nations such as France and Italy are not included; and (4) a nation's rank in incidence rate may not reflect its rank in mortality rate.

It can be deduced that if the ethnic factor does carry over into the foreign experience, that is, if the model effect is paralleled by the associated national ranking, then it is due either to genetic factors or to habits of consumption or other cultural characteristics. On the other hand, the failure of an ethnic effect to be matched by foreign ranking can be due to one of three possibilities: the actual etiological factor is environmental and that population subgroup markedly changed the conditions of its environment after migration; the etiology is a pattern of consumption or other cultural custom that the population subgroup altered after migration; or the etiological factor is one of the consumption factors included in the model, which, because of its strong association with that population subgroup, replaced or "aliased" its ethnic effect in the model.

For corroboration of the U. S. ethnic effects, reference is frequently made to Haenszel's (28) study of relative risk of cancer death in foreign-born whites from 12 countries (England and Wales, Ireland, Norway, Sweden, Germany, Austria, Czechoslovakia, Poland, USSR, Italy, Canada, Mexico) compared to native-born U. S. whites.

Chapter 3
The Cancer Mortality Models

I Introduction

The cancer mortality models presented in this chapter are the best subset models chosen from the four variable pools by the stepwise regression and smallest C_p-statistic methods described in Chapter 1. The factor effects that emerge in these models are compared with their relative strength and stability in the ridge trace of the coefficient estimates for the full model from the largest variable pool. Tables VI-XIII serve as reference guides to the discussion of the models in this chapter and Chapter 6.

Table VI summarizes the factor variables comprising the variable pools and their interpretation as model effects.

A schematic summary of the best subset models derived for each cancer mortality pattern is presented in Tables VII-X. Under the heading for each variable are listed the standardized coefficients of the effects chosen to be in each model, with their *p*-values indicated. As has been stated, in this study significance level is used as a concomitant indicator with the standardized coefficient size to reflect the relative importance of each model effect. These tables are presented for the factor patterns they reveal, for the similarities and contrasts among the different cancer mortalities in the model effects chosen to represent them. The tables are designed to display the progression of model effects that emerge for each mortality pattern as the variable pools are increased in size, first by the division of alcohol consumption into its three components and then by the addition of the ethnic variables.

The coefficient patterns for the major categories of death are given in Table XI for comparison with those of the cancer mortalities, but they are discussed in Chapter 6.

The results of the ridge regression analysis are presented in Table XII with an evaluation of the strength of each variable as the set of coefficient estimates stabilizes in the full 12-variable model of each cancer mortality pattern. Judgment of the relative strength of an effect, whether positive or negative, depended on the following: the distance of a coefficient trace from the zero line, i.e., the magnitude of the effect when all or most of the coefficients were stabilized; the

TABLE VI

	Independent variable
TEMP	First principal component score combining mean January temperature for period of record through 1947, mean July temperature for period of record through 1947.
PRELEV	First principal component score combining average annual precipitation 1921-1950, mean elevation.
POLLUT	First principal component score combining suspended particulate matter per square kilometer land area weighted by population 1970, sulfur dioxide per square kilometer land area weighted by population 1970, carbon monoxide per square kilometer land area weighted by population 1970, hydrocarbon per square kilometer land area weighted by population 1970, nitric oxide per square kilometer land area weighted by population 1970, benzo[*a*]pyrene per cubic meter air weighted by population 1969.
INCM	Personal income per capita 1950.
CIGS	Cigarette consumption per capita 1955.
MALT	Malt beverage consumption per capita adult 1950.
WINE	Wine consumption per capita adult 1966.
DISP	Distilled spirits consumption per capita adult 1966.
ALCO	First principal component score combining malt beverage consumption per capita adult 1950, wine consumption per capita adult 1966, distilled spirits consumption per capita adult 1966.
FRAN	Percentage of white population in 1950 born in France.
BRIT	Percentage of white population in 1950 born in England and Wales, Scotland, Ireland, and Northern Ireland.
SCAN	Percentage of white population in 1950 born in Norway, Sweden, and Denmark.
OTHEUR	First principal component score combining percentage of white population in 1950 born in Italy, Germany, Russia, Poland, Austria, Czechoslovakia, Hungary, Netherlands and Belgium, Lithuania, Jewish population in 1951 as percentage of 1950 white population.

Interpretation of Factor Effects in the Mortality Models

Positive effect	Negative effect
High January temperature and high July temperature	Low January temperature and low July temperature
High precipitation and low elevation	Low precipitation and high elevation
High pollution level	Low pollution level
High income level	Low income level
High cigarette consumption	Low cigarette consumption
High malt beverage consumption	Low malt beverage consumption
High wine consumption	Low wine consumption
High distilled spirits consumption	Low distilled spirits consumption
High alcohol consumption	Low alcohol consumption
High French ethnicity	Low French ethnicity
High British ethnicity	Low British ethnicity
High Scandinavian ethnicity	Low Scandinavian ethnicity
High Other European ethnicity	Low Other European ethnicity

TABLE VII

Variable pool	Program	Percent R^2 Full eq'n	Model	TEMP	PRELEV	POLLUT	INCM
M140–Buccal Cavity and Pharynx							
6 VAR	BMD = LIN	81.21	80.02		.89***	.33*	
8 VAR	BMD = 2nd LIN	81.48	81.01		.80***	.41**	
	LIN	81.48	80.21		.80***	.41**	
10 VAR	BMD = LIN	84.14	83.42		.86***	.43**	
12 VAR	BMD = LIN	84.67	83.99[a]		.78***	.36**	
M161–Larynx							
6 VAR	BMD = 2nd LIN	83.08	82.77	.12*	.39***	.14*	
8 VAR	BMD = LIN	83.24	81.88		.40***	.19**	
10 VAR	BMD = LIN	87.55	86.98		.38***	.12	
12 VAR	BMD = 2nd LIN	87.81	86.72[a]		.36***	.13*	
	LIN	87.81	86.18		.34***	.17**	
M166–Trachea, Bronchus, and Lung							
6 VAR	BMD = LIN	78.14	78.02	3.05***	3.51***		
8 VAR	LIN	81.47	80.35	2.19***	3.85***		
10 VAR	LIN	85.82	85.22	1.77**	3.69***	−1.51	
12 VAR	BMD = LIN	86.38	84.35[a]	1.68*	3.47***		
M162–Trachea, and Bronchus and Lung Specified as Primary							
6, 12 VAR 8, 10 VAR	BMD = LIN } BMD }	44.26	36.15	2.02***	.82		1.70**
8 VAR	LIN	40.42	37.75[a]	1.87**	.82		1.23
10 VAR	LIN	39.30	37.65[a]	2.39***		1.13*	
M163–Bronchus and Lung Unspecified as to Primary or Secondary							
6 VAR	BMD = LIN	56.66	56.23	.92	2.36***		−1.71
8 VAR	LIN	58.10	55.31		2.77***		−2.21
10 VAR	BMD = LIN	69.93	68.73		2.74***	−2.31**	
12 VAR	BMD = 2nd LIN	71.89	71.43[a]		2.40***	−1.78*	−2.01
	LIN	71.89	66.81		2.96***	−1.62*	
M150–Esophagus							
6 VAR	BMD = LIN	80.14	79.82	−.25*	.51***	.39**	
8 VAR	BMD = 3rd LIN	80.33	79.95	−.25	.53***	.37**	
	LIN } tie	80.33	79.05	−.30*	.57***	.36**	
	LIN } tie	80.33	80.02	−.28*	.53***	.39**	
10 VAR	BMD = LIN	84.31	82.47		.53***	.17	
12 VAR	BMD = LIN	84.85	82.68[a]		.46***	.21	
M151–Stomach							
6 VAR	LIN	65.68	64.35	−1.97***			
8 VAR	BMD = LIN	75.50	74.64	−2.09***	.41		
10 VAR	LIN	77.23	74.89	−1.69***			−.99*
12 VAR	BMD = 2nd LIN	80.52	80.08[a]	−1.84***			−1.19**
	LIN	80.52	79.25	−1.95***			−.98*

[a] Best models. *, $.01 < p < .05$; **, $.001 < p < .01$; ***, $p < .001$.

Coefficient Patterns in the Cancer Mortality Models–Males

CIGS	(ALCO)			FRAN	BRIT	SCAN	OTHEUR
	MALT	WINE	DISP				
	–	(.68***)	–	–	–	–	–
.20		.30	.24	–	–	–	–
		.30	.39*	–	–	–	–
	–	(.40*)	–	.52**			–.27
			.33*	.54***		–.20	
.10	–	(.39***)	–	–	–	–	–
.18**		.29***		–	–	–	–
	–	(.29**)	–	.29***		–.20**	
	.10		.18**	.35***		–.22**	
			.18**	.38***		–.18**	
2.21**	–	(2.76***)	–	–	–	–	–
3.17***		3.23***	–1.39	–	–	–	–
	–	(1.81*)	–	3.63***		–3.10**	1.81
1.21		1.06		3.47***		–1.61**	
		.66		–	–	–	–
.88	–	( )	–			.99	
1.67	–	(3.02**)	–	–	–	–	–
1.93*	1.43	2.01**		–	–	–	–
	–	(1.90)	–	2.44*		–3.68***	1.98
	1.64		1.38	3.22***		–3.50***	2.02
	1.94*			3.59***		–3.11***	
	–	(.68***)	–	–	–	–	–
	.29*	.30	.21	–	–	–	–
	.31*	.45***		–	–	–	–
.18	.22	.38**		–	–	–	–
	–	(.50***)	–				.47***
			.41***				.60***
–.59	–	(1.11**)	–	–	–	–	–
	.89**	1.21**	–1.27**	–	–	–	–
	–	( )	–				1.98***
	.55	.95**	.80*				1.52***
		1.00**	–.81*				1.74***

TABLE VII

Variable pool	Program	Percent R^2 Full eq'n	Model	TEMP	PRELEV	POLLUT	INCM
M153–Large Intestine excluding Rectum							
6 VAR	BMD = LIN	77.50	77.48	−1.24***	1.46***	1.07*	1.16*
8 VAR	BMD = LIN	82.67	81.79	−.89**	1.52***	.93*	
10 VAR	BMD = 3rd LIN	88.04	87.60	−.69*	1.25***	.77*	−.67
	LIN	88.04	87.04	−.70*	1.43***	.62	
12 VAR	BMD = LIN	89.68	89.63[a]	−.41	1.24***	.84*	−.82
M154–Rectum							
6 VAR	BMD = LIN	77.00	76.83	−1.21***	.68**	.69**	
8 VAR	LIN	81.81	80.45	−.93***	.83***	.49*	
10 VAR	BMD = LIN	89.91	89.79	−.76***	.54**	.48*	−.99**
12 VAR	BMD = LIN	90.59	90.58[a]	−.69***	.59**	.46*	−1.11***
M155–Biliary Passages and Liver							
6 VAR	BMD = LIN	34.93	33.92		.15	.30**	
8 VAR	BMD = LIN	44.44	42.69		.20	.26*	−.25
10 VAR	LIN	64.26	61.44	−.20*	.12		
12 VAR	LIN	70.41	69.57[a]	−.19	.16*		
M157–Pancreas							
6 VAR 10 VAR	BMD = LIN LIN }	41.79	34.16		.28**		−.26
8 VAR	BMD = 2nd LIN	40.22	38.51		.38***	−.14	
8, 12 VAR	LIN, 2nd LIN	46.29	36.33		.31***		
12 VAR	LIN	46.29	43.01[a]		.37***		−.29*
M180–Kidney							
6 VAR	BMD = LIN	74.13	73.98	−.26***	.12**		.17*
8 VAR	BMD = LIN	76.42	75.45	−.20***	.11*		
10 VAR	BMD = LIN	83.70	82.63	−.11*	.12*		
12 VAR	LIN } tie	84.31	82.61[a]	−.11*	.10*		
	LIN	84.31	82.60	−.15**	.11*		
M181–Bladder and Other Urinary Organs							
6 VAR	BMD = LIN	79.94	79.35	−.34**	.62***		.39*
8 VAR	BMD = LIN	82.27	81.57	−.31*	.63***		
10 VAR	BMD	89.43	87.78		.61***	−.24	
	LIN	89.43	88.86	−.24*	.53***		−.27
12 VAR	BMD = LIN	89.93	89.45[a]	−.17	.52***		−.36

[a]Best models. *, $.01 < p < .05$; **, $.001 < p < .01$; ***, $p < .001$.

(Continued)

CIGS	(ALCO)			FRAN	BRIT	SCAN	OTHEUR
	MALT	WINE	DISP				
.75	–	( )	–	–	–	–	–
.67*	1.65***			–	–	–	–
.62	–	( )	–		1.11*		1.60**
.42	–	( )	–		.99*		1.31**
.65*	.84*	–.56			1.33**		1.21*
.53	–	(.62)	–	–	–	–	–
.52*	.97**			–	–	–	–
.58**	–	( )	–		.91***		1.20***
.51**	.47				.92***		.98**
	–	( )	–	–	–	–	–
	.36*			–	–	–	–
	–	( )	–	.30*	–.45*	–.57***	.67***
–.21*	.37**			.34*	–.39*	–.63***	.44**
	–	(.47**)	–				
		.38***		–	–	–	–
		.32***					
		.43***				.24	
	–	(.18*)	–	–	–	–	–
	.25***		.15**	–	–	–	–
.12	–	(.21**)	–	–.19*		.19*	.19**
	.12		.19***	–.12		.14*	.19*
.09			.13*		–.16*	.18*	.26***
	–	(.81***)	–	–	–	–	–
.28	.65***	.45**		–	–	–	–
	–	(.56***)	–		.58***		.45**
	–	(.42*))	–	.44*	.36		.42*
	.33		.26*	.49*	.37		.38

TABLE VIII

Variable pool	Program	Percent R^2 Full eq'n	Model	TEMP	PRELEV	POLLUT	INCM
F140–Buccal Cavity and Pharynx							
6 VAR	LIN	46.37	46.03	.14**		.08	–.18**
8 VAR	BMD = LIN	60.26	58.96	.08		.09*	
10 VAR	BMD	58.28	52.95		.08		
	LIN	58.28	52.26			.09	
12 VAR	BMD	66.31	61.37			.06	
	LIN	66.31	64.76[a]			.13***	–.11
F161–Larynx							
6 VAR	BMD = LIN	49.61	48.05		.02	.02	–.05**
8 VAR	LIN } tie	54.92	54.01		.02	.02	–.03
	LIN } tie	54.92	51.74		.02	.02	–.04**
10 VAR	BMD	60.73	58.26		.02	.02	–.04*
	LIN	60.73	58.90		.02*	.03*	–.04*
12 VAR	BMD = LIN	63.88	61.21[a]		.01	.02	–.05*
F166–Trachea, Bronchus and Lung							
6 VAR	BMD = LIN	61.28	60.29	.45***	.19		
8 VAR	BMD = LIN	65.57	62.84	.34**	.22*		
10 VAR	BMD = LIN	70.76	68.16				
12 VAR	BMD = 3rd LIN	72.49	69.99[a]				
	LIN	72.49	68.67				
F162–Trachea, and Bronchus and Lung Specified as Primary							
6 VAR 10 VAR	BMD = LIN } LIN }	27.06	20.86	.26**			.23**
8 VAR	BMD = LIN	27.17	23.91	.21*			.37**
10 VAR	BMD = 2nd LIN	27.06	24.27	.27**			.38**
12 VAR	BMD = LIN	36.33	28.53[a]	.24**			.37**
F163–Bronchus and Lung Unspecified as to Primary or Secondary							
6 VAR	BMD = LIN	44.04	43.79	.15	.16		–.37*
8 VAR	BMD = LIN	46.40	45.84	.17	.19		–.49*
10 VAR	BMD = 2nd LIN	59.36	53.82				–.23
12 VAR	BMD = LIN	62.33	59.51[a]				–.42*
F150–Esophagus							
6 VAR 10 VAR	BMD = LIN } LIN – tie }	60.77	58.22		.05	.10**	–.14***
8, 12 VAR	BMD = LIN	71.61	71.32[a]	–.06*	.06*	.11**	–.11*
10 VAR	BMD	60.77	50.00		.10***		
	LIN – tie	60.77	56.14			.14***	–.18***
F151–Stomach							
6 VAR	BMD = LIN	54.60	50.72	–1.07***		.29	
8 VAR	BMD = LIN	64.97	63.96	–1.08***	.28		
10 VAR	BMD = LIN	65.52	62.71	–.86***			–.74**
12 VAR	BMD = 2nd LIN	69.12	68.07[a]	–.92***			–.80**
	LIN	69.12	67.02	–.99***			–.68*

[a]Best models. *, $.01 < p < .05$; **, $.001 < p < .01$; ***, $p < .001$.

Coefficient Patterns in the Cancer Mortality Models–Females

CIGS	(ALCO)			FRAN	BRIT	SCAN	OTHEUR
	MALT	WINE	DISP				
.14**	–	( )	–	–	–	–	–
.12*	–.26***	.06		–	–	–	–
	–	( )	–	.16**		–.15**	–.15*
	–	( )	–	.16**		–.14*	–.20*
	–.23***			.19***		–.14**	
.10*	–.24***			.25***	–.15*		
.02	–	(.04*)	–	–	–	–	–
.02*	–.02	.03**		–	–	–	–
.02		.03**		–	–	–	–
	–	(.02)	–	.04**		–.02	
	–	(.02)	–	.05**			–.03*
			.02*	.04**		–.02	
.28	–	(.47**)	–	–	–	–	–
.35**		.43***		–	–	–	–
	–	(.33*)	–	.62**	–.34	–.67***	.36*
.17		.30*		.50*	–.37	–.60***	.41**
		.30*		.59**	–.31	–.63***	.41**
	–	( )	–	–	–	–	–
	–.19			–	–	–	–
	–	( )	–	–.18			
		.19		–.33*			
.28	–	(.55**)	–	–	–	–	–
.36*	.40*	.29*		–	–	–	–
	–	(.47*)	–	.43*		–.47***	
	.48**		.25*	.50**		–.55***	
.17***	–	( )	–				
.18***	–.11**	.13***	–.08				
.11***	–	( )	–			–.06*	
.18***	–	( )	–				
	–	( )	–	–	–	–	–
–.33	.52*	.59*	–.58*	–	–	–	–
	–	( )	–				1.09***
	.33	.47*	–.47*				.83**
		.50*	–.47*				.96***

TABLE VIII

Variable pool	Program	Percent R^2 Full eq'n	Percent R^2 Model	TEMP	PRELEV	POLLUT	INCM
F153–Large Intestine excluding Rectum							
6 VAR	BMD = LIN	73.35	72.90	–1.44***	1.01**	1.10***	
8 VAR	BMD = LIN	81.08	80.73	–1.08***	1.34***	.73*	
10 VAR	BMD = LIN	82.27	81.24	–1.02**	1.08***		
12 VAR	BMD = 2nd LIN	85.93	84.31	–.91**	1.18***		
	3rd LIN	85.93	85.04[a]	–.65*	.95**	.81*	–1.17*
F154–Rectum							
6 VAR	BMD = LIN	71.84	71.06	–.59***	.30*	.31*	
8 VAR	BMD = LIN	76.88	76.02	–.56***	.29*	.34*	–.43*
10 VAR	BMD = 2nd LIN	84.44	83.37	–.42***	.13	.36**	–.75***
12 VAR	BMD = 2nd LIN	85.10	84.34[a]	–.39***	.16	.35**	–.82***
	LIN	85.10	82.78	–.41***		.45***	–.85***
F155–Biliary Passages and Liver							
6 VAR	BMD = LIN	38.56	38.51	–.47***	–.27	.54***	
8 VAR	BMD = 2nd LIN	60.88	59.56	–.34**	–.17	.43**	–.38*
10 VAR	BMD = LIN	61.36	58.96	–.46***	–.31**		
12 VAR	BMD = LIN	75.11	74.31[a]	–.44***	–.19*		
F157–Pancreas							
6 VAR	BMD = LIN	43.13	42.99	–.12*		.15*	–.19*
8 VAR	BMD = LIN	44.43	43.39	–.18**		.16**	–.12
10 VAR	BMD = 2nd LIN	48.82	43.86			.18**	–.28*
12 VAR	BMD	51.49	43.32				–.25*
	LIN	51.49	46.71[a]	–.14*		.12	–.22*
F180–Kidney							
6 VAR	BMD = 2nd LIN	50.88	47.41	–.23***	.05		
8 VAR	LIN	60.34	58.46	–.15***			
10 VAR	BMD = LIN	71.24	67.98	–.19***	.07		
12 VAR	BMD = LIN	74.14	71.54[a]	–.15***	.07*		
F181–Bladder and Other Urinary Organs							
6 VAR	BMD = LIN	77.73	77.73	–.09*	.13**	.16**	–.24***
8 VAR	BMD = LIN	77.73	77.73	–.09	.13**	.16**	–.24**
10 VAR	BMD = LIN	81.99	79.88	–.16***	.17***		
12 VAR	BMD	82.24	80.08	–.15**	.17***		
	LIN	82.24	80.76[a]	–.11*	.12**	.07	–.12

[a] Best models. *, $.01 < p < .05$; **, $.001 < p < .01$; ***, $p < .001$.

(Continued)

CIGS	(ALCO)			FRAN	BRIT	SCAN	OTHEUR
	MALT	WINE	DISP				
1.07***	–	( )	–	–	–	–	–
1.10**	1.18**		–.77*	–	–	–	–
.63	–	( )	–	–.77	1.22*	–.97*	1.57***
.39	.93*	–.69*			.99*	–1.08**	1.07*
.93**	1.01*	–.72*			.92*		.77
.29	–	(.28)	–	–	–	–	–
.36*	.50**	.22		–	–	–	–
.42**	–	( )	–		.52**		.51**
.38**	.26				.53**		.39*
.46***					.53**		.53**
	–	(–.29*)	–	–	–	–	–
	.63***		–.41**	–	–	–	–
	–	( )	–	–.46***		–.70***	.96***
–.16	.64***		–.22	–.33*		–.72***	.56***
	–	(.31***)	–	–	–	–	–
		.24***		–	–	–	–
	–	(.31***)	–			.18*	
		.12	.14				.29**
		.23**					.17
	–	( )	–	–	–	–	–
–.11*	.15**	–.14*	.12	–	–	–	–
	–	( )	–		–.24***	.13*	.17**
	.10			–.10	–.17*	.13*	.11
.16**	–	(.25***)	–	–	–	–	–
.17**	.09	.10	.10	–	–	–	–
	–	(.28***)	–		.11	–.28***	
	.11*	.08	.14*		.11	–.28***	
	.14*		.21***		.16**	–.24***	

TABLE IX

Variable pool	Program	Percent R^2 Full eq'n	Percent R^2 Model	TEMP	PRELEV	POLLUT	INCM
M193–Brain and Other Parts of the Nervous System							
6 VAR; 8 VAR	BMD = LIN; BMD = 2nd LIN	35.02	28.01		.09	.14	
10 VAR	BMD	49.44	43.49		.18*	.25**	
	LIN	49.44	47.48	.16*	.16*	.27**	
12 VAR	BMD	60.14	48.25[a]		.13	.24**	
F193–Brain and Other Parts of the Nervous System							
6, 8 VAR	BMD = LIN	31.89	26.23	–.09*		.14**	
10 VAR	LIN	42.79	39.50			.24***	
12 VAR	BMD = LIN	50.63	45.69[a]			.22***	
M200–Lymphosarcoma and Reticulosarcoma							
6 VAR	BMD = LIN	47.54	44.27	–.20**		.24**	.09
8 VAR	BMD	51.88	46.25	–.16*		.22**	
	LIN	51.88	47.67	–.17*	.08	.17*	
10, 12 VAR	BMD	64.41	61.65[a]		.10	.16	
	LIN	64.41	59.23			.25**	–.22*
F200–Lymphosarcoma and Reticulosarcoma							
6, 8 VAR	LIN	54.30	51.83	–.15**		.09	.15**
10, 12 VAR	BMD = LIN	70.48	67.95[a]			.12*	
M201–Hodgkin's Disease							
6 VAR; 8 VAR	BMD = LIN; LIN	42.48	32.94	–.11**			
	BMD = 2nd LIN	42.48	35.37	–.11**			
10 VAR	LIN (tie)	50.20	48.37	–.06		.08	–.22**
	LIN (tie)	50.20	45.79			.08	–.23**
12 VAR	BMD	55.16	44.24	–.09*			–.10
	LIN (tie)	55.16	52.33[a]	–.08		.11**	–.23**
	LIN (tie)	55.16	49.76			.09*	–.23**
	LIN (tie)	55.16	47.28			.11**	–.21**
F201–Hodgkin's Disease							
6 VAR	BMD = LIN	47.37	45.21	–.15***	.06	.06*	
8 VAR	BMD = LIN	49.50	45.96	–.12***	.10**		
10, 12 VAR	BMD = LIN	63.33	61.13[a]	–.07*	.05	.13**	–.18**
M204–Leukemia and Aleukemia							
6, 8 VAR	LIN	21.82	12.19				.27*
10, 12 VAR	BMD = LIN	49.56	47.29[a]		.21*		.22
F204–Leukemia and Aleukemia							
6, 8 VAR	BMD = LIN	24.90	20.27				.24**
10, 12 VAR	BMD = LIN	39.41	31.49[a]			.19**	

[a] Best models. *, $.01 < p < .05$; **, $.001 < p < .01$; ***, $p < .001$.

Coefficient Patterns in the Cancer Mortality Models–Males and Females

CIGS	(ALCO)			FRAN	BRIT	SCAN	OTHEUR
	MALT	WINE	DISP				
–.17**				–	–	–	–
–.18**	–	( )	–			.34**	–.24
	–	( )	–	–.22**		.47***	–.21
–.13	–.28**					.32***	
–.14**				–	–	–	–
	–	( )	–	–.16**		.25***	–.13
	–.17**			–.13*		.26***	
	–	( )	–	–	–	–	–
	.14			–	–	–	–
	.17*			–	–	–	–
				–.20*	.16	.22*	.15
						.28**	.23
				–	–	–	–
				–.11*		.23***	.16*
.07*				–	–	–	–
.12*			–.06	–	–	–	–
.12*	–	( )	–		.09	.13*	
.13**	–	( )	–		.09	.18**	
.10			–.06		.14*		
.17**			–.10*	.08		.17**	
.18**			–.08		.08	.19**	
.22***			–.09			.23***	
	–	( )	–	–	–	–	–
	.07*			–	–	–	–
.09*						.19***	
–.27*				–	–	–	–
					–.59***	.57***	
–.21**				–	–	–	–
					–.26**	.31***	

TABLE IX

Variable pool	Program	Percent R^2 Full eq'n	Model	TEMP	PRELEV	POLLUT	INCM
F170–Breast							
6 VAR	BMD = LIN	83.23	83.21	–1.65***	1.02**	.85*	1.21**
8 VAR	BMD = LIN	84.31	84.21	–1.57***	1.13***	.76*	.97*
10 VAR	BMD	89.45	88.91	–1.24***	.85**	.67*	
12 VAR	BMD	89.46	88.85	–1.19***	.77**	.70*	
	LIN	89.46	89.05[a]	–1.10***	.83**	.81*	
F175–Ovary							
6, 8 VAR	BMD = LIN	79.29	78.11	–.56***	.24*	.24	.60***
10 VAR	BMD = 2nd LIN	88.76	88.60[a]	–.26**	.19*	.22	.18
10, 12 VAR	LIN	89.15	88.31	–.25*	.16	.27*	
F171–Cervix Uteri							
6, 8 VAR	BMD = LIN	49.79	46.30			.67***	–1.56***
10, 12 VAR	BMD = LIN	71.52	68.88[a]	–.51**			
F172–Corpus and Other Parts of Uterus							
6 VAR	BMD = 2nd LIN	40.46	40.20	–.38**	.31*	.30*	
8 VAR	LIN	46.06	43.75	–.38**	.39**	.24	
10 VAR	BMD = 2nd LIN	64.77	62.58	–.45***	.19		
12 VAR	BMD = LIN	68.02	63.81[a]	–.41***	.18		
M177–Prostate							
6 VAR	BMD = 2nd LIN	48.49	43.78	–.98***			–.26
8 VAR	BMD = LIN	54.88	51.00	–.87***			–.34
10 VAR	BMD = LIN	58.13	51.21	–.85***	.41*		
12 VAR	BMD = LIN	62.06	54.67[a]	–.63**			–.57*

[a]Best models. *, $.01 < p < .05$; **, $.001 < p < .01$; ***, $p < .001$.

(Continued)

CIGS	(ALCO)			FRAN	BRIT	SCAN	OTHEUR
	MALT	WINE	DISP				
	–	(.87*)	–	–	–	–	–
	.85	.52		–	–	–	–
	–	(.52)	–		.82*		1.24**
			.39		.88*		1.37**
			.38		.83*	.35	1.17*
				–	–	–	–
.28*	–	( )	–	–.42**		.32*	.57***
.33**				–.39**		.38**	.61***
.91***				–	–	–	–
.38**						–1.68***	
.26	–	(–.36)	–	–	–	–	–
.30			–.41*	–	–	–	–
	–	(–.27)	–	–.29	.60**	–.77***	.50**
		–.39***			.45**	–.79***	.47**
	–	( )	–	–	–	–	–
		–.45	.62*	–	–	–	–
	–	( )	–			.60*	–.60**
		–.49*	.70**			.45	

TABLE X

Variable pool	Program	Percent R^2 Full eq'n	Percent R^2 Model	TEMP	PRELEV	POLLUT	INCM
M190–Malignant Melanoma of Skin							
6 VAR	BMD	61.73	59.27	.25***			–.06
	LIN	61.73	61.69	.25***	.08*	–.06	
8 VAR	BMD = 2nd LIN	72.24	70.86	.18***	.04		
	LIN	72.24	69.56	.19***			
10 VAR	BMD = 2nd LIN	70.35	68.54	.19***	.07*		
	LIN	70.35	67.53	.18***	.08*		
12 VAR	BMD	76.27	73.15[a]	.15***	.05		
	LIN	76.27	72.85	.16***	.08*		.12
F190–Malignant Melanoma of Skin							
6 VAR	BMD = LIN	67.17	64.30	.13***			–.09***
10 VAR	BMD = 3rd LIN	70.08	68.96	.10***	.04		
	LIN	70.08	69.21	.11***	.05*		
8, 12 VAR	LIN } tie	77.05	71.81	.11***			
	LIN } tie	77.05	73.06[a]	.10***	.03		
M191–Other Malignant Neoplasm of Skin							
6 VAR	BMD = LIN	73.32	72.76	.27***	.16**	–.13*	
8 VAR	BMD = LIN	75.17	73.08	.27***	.19***	–.16**	
10 VAR	BMD = LIN	81.91	81.26	.13*	.14**	–.11*	
12 VAR	LIN	84.57	82.90[a]	.12*	.17***	–.13**	
F191–Other Malignant Neoplasm of Skin							
6 VAR	BMD = 2nd LIN	69.87	69.40	.07**	.05*		–.12**
8 VAR	BMD = LIN	72.07	71.35	.05	.06*		–.09*
10 VAR	BMD = LIN	77.21	77.11		.05		–.07
12 VAR	BMD	78.10	74.11		.04		
	LIN	78.10	76.62[a]		.05*		
4 VAR Pool							
M190	BMD = LIN	59.06	56.56	.23***	.05		
F190	BMD = LIN	65.41	64.30	.13***			–.09***
M191	BMD = LIN	70.53	70.53	.27***	.15*	–.12*	–.13*
F191	BMD = LIN	66.30	66.25	.07*	.05*		–.16***

[a] Best models. *, $.01 < p < .05$; **, $.001 < p < .01$; ***, $p < .001$.

Coefficient Patterns in Skin Cancer Mortality Models–Males and Females

CIGS	(ALCO)			FRAN	BRIT	SCAN	OTHEUR
	MALT	WINE	DISP				
.10*	–	( )	–	–	–	–	–
.07*	–	( )	–	–	–	–	–
.10*	–.17***	.07		–	–	–	–
.11**	–.18***	.07		–	–	–	–
.05	–	( )	–	.11			–.16***
	–	( )	–	.15**			–.16***
.08	–.17***			.18**	–.11		
	–.15*			.13**			–.14*
	–	( )	–	–	–	–	–
	–	( )	–		–.06		–.05
–.05	–	( )	–				–.08**
	–.12***						
	–.12***						
	–	(–.15**)	–	–	–	–	–
			–.14**	–	–	–	–
	–	(–.17*)	–	.24**	–.22*	–.13*	
			–.15**	.23**	–.24**	–.14*	
.05	–	(–.09*)	–	–	–	–	–
.06	–.08		–.07	–	–	–	–
	–	(–.11**)	–	.13**	–.09	–.09**	
	–.08**		–.05*			–.11***	
	–.09*		–.07*	.09*	–.08	–.09*	
–	–	–	–	–	–	–	–
–	–	–	–	–	–	–	–
–	–	–	–	–	–	–	–
–	–	–	–	–	–	–	–

TABLE XI

Sex	Var. pool	Program[a]	Percent R^2 Full eq'n	Percent R^2 Model	Intercept	TEMP	PRELEV	POLLUT	INCM
All malignant neoplasms–ICD 140-205 (1950-1969)									
M	8	B = L	83.90	82.79	164.81		12.05***		
	12	B = L	88.45	87.43			10.98***		–5.83*
F	8	B = L	84.54	83.47	124.37	–5.06***	3.99***	4.82***	–2.40
	12	B = L	88.27	87.11		–5.90***	3.98***	1.55	
All malignant neoplasms–ICD 140-205 (1949-1959)									
M	8	B = L	81.86	81.00	145.01	–4.14*	12.41***		
	12	L	87.08	85.33		–3.16*	11.37***		
F	8	B	83.86	82.15	121.87	–5.79***	4.05**	5.17***	–2.41
	12	B = L	87.50	86.23		–6.63***	3.99***	1.77	
Circulatory system–ICD 400-468 (1949-1959)									
M	8	B = L	66.92	66.42	430.05	–8.98	15.25**	17.12**	
	12	B = L	73.10	72.02		–9.78	14.50*	10.93	
F	8	B = L	71.13	70.03	254.41	–15.50***	16.03***	13.49**	
	12	L	80.90	80.20		–18.22***	13.55**	8.21	
Respiratory system excluding influenza and asthma–ICD 470-475, 490-527 (1949-1959)									
M	8	L	56.52	55.11	43.69	1.99	–7.09***	3.89*	–3.40
	12	B = L	61.11	56.58			–6.72***	1.89	
F	8	B = L	40.13	38.60	25.43		–3.51***	2.63**	–3.93***
	12	B	48.38	44.71			–3.36***	1.03	
Digestive system–ICD 530-587 (1949-1959)									
M	8	B = L	72.21	70.73	41.34		–1.92*	2.82**	
	12	B	79.01	78.54			–2.45**	2.00*	
F	8	B = L[b]	56.21	50.41	26.43		–1.67**		
	12	B = L	67.19	65.89			–2.73***		
Genito-urinary system–ICD 590-637 (1949-1959)									
M	8	B	48.55	48.16	43.49	2.21		3.29**	
	12	L	66.17	63.61					5.76***
F	8	L	35.80	31.24	28.70			3.04***	
	12	L	56.52	50.67					4.86***
Infectious and parasitic excluding tuberculosis and influenza–ICD 020-138 (1949-1959)									
M	8	B = L	38.20	34.61	9.31	1.04***	–.99***		
	12	B	67.27	65.16		.29	–.90***		.50
F	8	B = L	49.61	46.96	5.86	.69**	–.90***		–1.03**
	12	B = L	69.22	66.05			–.87***	–.40	
Accidental and violent causes–ICD E800-E999 (1949-1959)									
M	8	B = L	63.58	62.17	109.08	11.35***	–16.02***	–6.79*	
	12	B = L	79.58	76.19			–15.08***		
F	8	B = L	56.48	52.16	40.93	2.07**	–4.57***		
	12	L	75.76	74.36		1.31	–3.94***		
All Causes–ICD 001-E999 (1949-1959)									
M	6	B = L	54.25	53.55	1055.15		–16.73	33.53**	–35.80*
	8	B = L	55.28	54.12			–19.97	36.12**	–29.27*
	10	B = L	71.22	70.12		–21.75*	–13.39	20.81*	
	12	B = L	73.36	70.95		–18.58*	–18.24*	15.58*	
F	6	B = L	57.98	57.81	700.36	–28.16***		34.74***	–14.48
	8	B = L	64.07	62.53		–22.51**		32.68***	–29.07**
	10	B = 2dL	74.37	73.82		–38.62***		14.17*	
		L	74.37	72.61		–38.76***		20.42***	
	12	B = 2dL	79.31	78.90		–35.50***		15.02**	
		L	79.31	78.05		–35.30***		14.16**	

[a] B = BMD, L = LIN.

[b] $C_p > p$, model with bias. *, $.01 < p < .05$; **, $.001 < p < .01$; ***, $p < .001$.

Coefficient Patterns in the Mortality Models for the Major Categories of Death

CIGS	(ALCO)			FRAN	BRIT	SCAN	OTHEUR
	MALT	WINE	DISP				
3.26	8.56***	5.23**		–	–	–	–
2.85	5.09*	2.66		6.01*			6.58*
2.90*	4.78**			–	–	–	–
	2.83*				2.55	–5.35***	4.79*
	10.12***	5.96***		–	–	–	–
	3.92			6.72***			5.92*
2.82*	4.54**			–	–	–	–
	2.33				2.67	–5.55***	5.11*
12.69			11.46	–	–	–	–
			13.34*		24.72***	–14.91	
	14.79**			–	–	–	–
–7.41	12.18*				25.26***	–18.47**	
2.91*		3.22*		–	–	–	–
		3.29**			2.65	–4.98**	
		1.59*		–	–	–	–
		2.02*		–1.91		–2.65**	
1.79*		3.63***		–	–	–	–
	1.39	1.59	1.39	3.19**		–3.05**	
	.89	2.06***		–	–	–	–
	1.97**	1.55**			1.34	–3.05***	
2.04	–2.96*	–3.73*	2.20	–	–	–	–
	–2.15	–3.52**	2.37*			–6.96***	
2.42*	–2.64*	–2.23*		–	–	–	–
		–2.39**				–5.81***	
.40				–	–	–	–
	1.07**			.99*	–1.23*	–.93*	–.84
	.71*			–	–	–	–
	.91***				–.55*	–1.30***	
		–6.18	8.86*	–	–	–	–
4.04				15.06***	–14.86**		–11.63***
1.50*				–	–	–	–
	2.11*	–2.84**	1.58	5.70***	–3.41**		–2.75*
35.66**	–	(28.08*)	–	–	–	–	–
33.55**			24.40*	–	–	–	–
	–	(28.51*)	–	39.97**		–46.02***	–20.25
			25.18**	37.94***		–53.95***	
18.10*	–	( )	–	–	–	–	–
16.00*	23.08*			–	–	–	–
	–	( )	–		26.25**	–47.35***	14.49
	–	( )	–		31.94***	–40.92***	
	23.84**		–6.50		25.91***	–48.60***	
	22.55**				23.01**	–48.14***	

TABLE XII

	Very strong	Strong
MALES		
Buc Cav & Ph	PRELEV, POLLUT	DISP, –SCAN, FRAN
Larynx	PRELEV, POLLUT	FRAN, DISP, WINE, –SCAN
T, B, & Lung	PRELEV, TEMP, FRAN	–SCAN, CIGS, WINE
T, B, & L Spec.	TEMP	POLLUT, WINE, PRELEV
B & L Unspec.	PRELEV	FRAN, –SCAN
Esophagus	PRELEV, POLLUT	OTHEUR, DISP, BRIT, WINE
Stomach	–TEMP	OTHEUR, MALT, SCAN
Lg. Intestine	PRELEV, OTHEUR, POLLUT, BRIT	MALT, CIGS, –TEMP
Rectum	OTHEUR, BRIT, PRELEV	–TEMP, MALT, POLLUT, CIGS
Liver *et al.*	–SCAN	MALT, POLLUT, PRELEV, OTHEUR
Pancreas	PRELEV	WINE
Kidney	OTHEUR, –TEMP, SCAN, DISP, MALT	PRELEV, CIGS, INCM
Bladder	PRELEV, BRIT	OTHEUR, FRAN, MALT
Brain	POLLUT, SCAN, PRELEV	–CIGS
Lymphosarcoma	OTHEUR, POLLUT, SCAN	PRELEV, BRIT
Hodgkin's Dis.	–TEMP	BRIT, CIGS, SCAN
Leukemia	SCAN	–BRIT
Prostate	–TEMP	SCAN, DISP
Melanoma	TEMP	–MALT, PRELEV, –OTHEUR
Other Skin	TEMP, –SCAN	PRELEV, –DISP, –BRIT, –OTHEUR

[a] Solid underline, very stable, little change from linear least squares solution; broken underline, stable, moderate change from linear least squares solution.

Stabilized Effects in the Ridge Trace for Each Type of Cancer Mortality[a]

Moderate	Weak	Minimal or null
BRIT, WINE, CIGS, TEMP	OTHEUR	MALT, INCM
CIGS, OTHEUR, TEMP	MALT	INCM, BRIT
POLLUT	DISP, OTHEUR, MALT	–INCM, BRIT
INCM, CIGS, FRAN	–DISP, –MALT	–SCAN, OTHEUR, BRIT
CIGS, DISP, WINE	TEMP, MALT, –INCM, OTHEUR	POLLUT, BRIT
CIGS, MALT	INCM, –TEMP	–SCAN, FRAN
	WINE, –DISP, FRAN	–CIGS, –INCM, POLLUT, –PRELEV, BRIT
INCM	SCAN, DISP	–WINE, FRAN
	SCAN, DISP	WINE, INCM, FRAN
FRAN, –BRIT	WINE	DISP, TEMP, CIGS, INCM
–INCM, FRAN, DISP	POLLUT, OTHEUR, –MALT, SCAN	CIGS, BRIT, TEMP
BRIT		–FRAN, WINE, POLLUT
DISP, CIGS, –TEMP, WINE	POLLUT, INCM	SCAN
–MALT, –FRAN	–DISP	WINE, TEMP, OTHEUR, –BRIT, INCM
MALT, –TEMP	–DISP, –FRAN, INCM	WINE, CIGS
–INCM, MALT, PRELEV	–DISP, FRAN	OTHEUR, –POLLUT, WINE
–CIGS, INCM, OTHEUR	–FRAN, PRELEV	DISP, –TEMP, –POLLUT, –WINE, MALT
–WINE, –FRAN, BRIT, –INCM, –OTHEUR		MALT, PRELEV, CIGS, POLLUT
WINE, –BRIT, FRAN, CIGS	DISP, POLLUT	–INCM, SCAN
–MALT	–INCM, –POLLUT	FRAN, CIGS, WINE

TABLE XII

	Very strong	Strong
FEMALES		
Buc Cav & Ph	–MALT	–SCAN, TEMP
Larynx	PRELEV, –SCAN	POLLUT, WINE, DISP, FRAN
T, B, & Lung	WINE	–SCAN, TEMP, FRAN, CIGS
T, B, & L Spec.	TEMP	INCM, WINE, POLLUT
B & L Unspec.	–SCAN	FRAN
Esophagus	PRELEV, CIGS	POLLUT, WINE, –SCAN
Stomach	–TEMP	OTHEUR, MALT, SCAN
Lg. Intestine	PRELEV	OTHEUR, –TEMP, MALT, POLLUT, BRIT, CIGS
Rectum	–TEMP, BRIT	OTHEUR, PRELEV
Liver *et al.*	MALT	–TEMP, OTHEUR
Pancreas	WINE	POLLUT, DISP, OTHEUR
Kidney	–TEMP	SCAN, MALT, OTHEUR, –FRAN
Bladder	PRELEV, DISP, POLLUT, –SCAN, CIGS	WINE
Brain	POLLUT, SCAN	–CIGS
Lymphosarcoma	SCAN, OTHEUR	POLLUT, –TEMP, INCM, MALT
Hodgkin's Dis.	–TEMP	SCAN, PRELEV
Leukemia	SCAN	INCM
Breast	OTHEUR, –TEMP, POLLUT, BRIT, PRELEV	MALT, SCAN
Ovary	OTHEUR, –TEMP	SCAN, POLLUT, INCM

(Continued)

Moderate	Weak	Minimal or null
–OTHEUR, PRELEV, FRAN, WINE, CIGS, POLLUT	–INCM, –BRIT	DISP
–MALT, –INCM, –OTHEUR, BRIT, CIGS		TEMP
PRELEV, POLLUT, DISP, MALT, OTHEUR		BRIT, INCM
–MALT	SCAN, –BRIT, –FRAN, CIGS	–PRELEV, –DISP, OTHEUR
CIGS, MALT, WINE, DISP, PRELEV	–INCM, TEMP	POLLUT, –BRIT, OTHEUR
–MALT, –INCM, BRIT, DISP		–TEMP, OTHEUR, FRAN
–CIGS, –DISP	WINE, –INCM	POLLUT, PRELEV, FRAN, BRIT
–WINE	FRAN, INCM	–SCAN, DISP
CIGS, MALT, POLLUT	WINE, DISP, –INCM	SCAN, FRAN
POLLUT, –DISP	–FRAN, –WINE, –SCAN, –PRELEV	–CIGS, INCM, BRIT
–TEMP	–INCM, SCAN, MALT, CIGS, FRAN	BRIT, PRELEV
–WINE	DISP, –BRIT, PRELEV	–CIGS, –POLLUT, INCM
–TEMP, BRIT, MALT, OTHEUR	–INCM	FRAN
–FRAN	PRELEV, –MALT, OTHEUR, –TEMP	–DISP, –BRIT, WINE, INCM
–FRAN	BRIT	WINE, DISP, –CIGS, PRELEV
POLLUT	OTHEUR, MALT, BRIT, CIGS, –INCM	DISP, WINE, FRAN
–CIGS, POLLUT, –FRAN, OTHEUR, –BRIT	PRELEV	–TEMP, –WINE, –DISP, MALT
INCM, DISP, CIGS	WINE	FRAN
PRELEV, CIGS, DISP, BRIT		–WINE, –FRAN, MALT

TABLE XII

	Very strong	Strong
Cervix Uteri	–SCAN	CIGS
Corpus Uteri	PRELEV	–TEMP
Melanoma	TEMP	–MALT
Other Skin	–SCAN	–MALT, –INCM

(Continued)

Moderate	Weak	Minimal or null
–OTHEUR, –INCM, POLLUT, PRELEV	DISP, –BRIT, –WINE	MALT, –TEMP, FRAN
–SCAN, BRIT, OTHEUR, –WINE, POLLUT	CIGS, –DISP	–FRAN, INCM, MALT
–BRIT, PRELEV, –OTHEUR	–CIGS, WINE, –INCM	–DISP, –FRAN, POLLUT, SCAN
PRELEV, –BRIT, TEMP, –DISP	–WINE	–CIGS, –FRAN, POLLUT, OTHEUR

TABLE XIII

	Very strong	Strong
All Malignant Neoplasms 1950-1969		
Male	PRELEV	POLLUT, OTHEUR, BRIT, FRAN, CIGS, WINE, MALT
Female	PRELEV, POLLUT, –TEMP, OTHEUR	MALT, BRIT
All Malignant Neoplasms 1949-1959		
Male	PRELEV	OTHEUR, POLLUT, BRIT, MALT, FRAN
Female	PRELEV, –TEMP, POLLUT, OTHEUR	MALT, BRIT, CIGS
Diseases of Circulatory System 1949-1959		
Male	PRELEV, POLLUT	BRIT, DISP, FRAN, CIGS
Female	PRELEV, POLLUT, BRIT	–TEMP, OTHEUR, MALT
Diseases of Respiratory System 1949-1959		
Male	–PRELEV	WINE
Female	–PRELEV	–SCAN, WINE
Diseases of Digestive System 1949-1959		
Male	WINE, FRAN	POLLUT, DISP, –SCAN
Female	–PRELEV	WINE
Diseases of Genito-Urinary System 1949-1959		
Male	–SCAN	
Female	–SCAN	
Infectious and Parasitic Diseases 1949-1959		
Male	–PRELEV	–SCAN
Female	–PRELEV	–SCAN
Accidental and Violent Causes 1949-1959		
Male	–PRELEV	–OTHEUR, –POLLUT
Female	–PRELEV	–OTHEUR
All Deaths 1949-1959		
Male	–SCAN, DISP, CIGS, FRAN	POLLUT
Female	–TEMP, POLLUT	MALT, –SCAN

[a] Solid underline, very stable, little change from linear least squares solution; broken underline, stable, moderate change from linear least squares solution.

Stabilized Effects in the Ridge Trace for Each Major Category of Mortality[a]

Moderate	Weak	Minimal or null
DISP	–SCAN	–TEMP, INCM
CIGS		DISP, INCM, –SCAN, WINE, FRAN
DISP, CIGS, WINE, –TEMP	SCAN	INCM
		–SCAN, FRAN, DISP, WINE, INCM
–SCAN, –TEMP	OTHEUR, WINE, MALT	INCM
–SCAN, CIGS	DISP, INCM	WINE, FRAN
–SCAN, TEMP, DISP, FRAN	MALT, CIGS, POLLUT, BRIT	INCM, OTHEUR
–BRIT, –INCM	–FRAN, POLLUT	MALT, –CIGS, TEMP, DISP, OTHEUR
–PRELEV, CIGS, MALT	INCM, BRIT	OTHEUR, TEMP
MALT, FRAN, –SCAN	CIGS, BRIT, INCM	TEMP, –POLLUT, OTHEUR, DISP
POLLUT	TEMP, PRELEV, –OTHEUR, –WINE	INCM, CIGS, –MALT, –FRAN, DISP, BRIT
PRELEV, POLLUT	–WINE, INCM, CIGS, –OTHEUR	–MALT, –FRAN, –BRIT, DISP, TEMP
TEMP, –BRIT	–OTHEUR, MALT, FRAN, CIGS, INCM, –POLLUT	–DISP, WINE
–BRIT, –OTHEUR, MALT, –POLLUT, TEMP, –DISP	WINE, –INCM, CIGS	FRAN
–BRIT	TEMP, FRAN, CIGS, DISP	–MALT, INCM, WINE, SCAN
FRAN	–BRIT, CIGS, INCM, TEMP, MALT, DISP	–WINE, –SCAN, POLLUT
WINE	MALT, –OTHEUR, INCM	–PRELEV, –TEMP, BRIT
BRIT	CIGS, OTHEUR, PRELEV	INCM, WINE, DISP, FRAN

stability of that coefficient trace before the point of general stabilization; and, to a lesser degree, the magnitude of the effect as k approached 1. The stability of those factors whose coefficient estimates changed very little from their least squares values is indicated by a solid underscore. Those whose least squares coefficient estimates showed moderate changes but stabilized very quickly are underscored with a broken line. For comparability Table XIII gives the same presentation of coefficient strengths and stability in the mortality patterns of the major categories of death.

II The Models of Male Cancer Mortality

1 Buccal Cavity and Pharynx, Males–M140 (ICD 140-148)

6 VAR, BMD and LIN

$$Y(M140) = 5.204 + \overset{***}{.886}\ PRELEV + \overset{*}{.332}\ POLLUT + \overset{***}{.679}\ ALCO$$

8 VAR, BMD and Second LIN

$$Y(M140) = 5.204 + \overset{***}{.804}\ PRELEV + \overset{**}{.408}\ POLLUT + .202\ CIGS + .299\ WINE + .242\ DISP$$

8 VAR, LIN

$$Y(M140) = 5.204 + \overset{***}{.798}\ PRELEV + \overset{**}{.407}\ POLLUT + .305\ WINE + \overset{*}{.389}\ DISP$$

10 VAR, BMD and LIN

$$Y(M140) = 5.204 + \overset{***}{.861}\ PRELEV + \overset{**}{.431}\ POLLUT + \overset{*}{.400}\ ALCO + \overset{**}{.515}\ FRAN - .270\ OTHEUR$$

12 VAR, BMD and LIN

$$Y(M140) = 5.204 + \overset{***}{.775}\ PRELEV + \overset{**}{.361}\ POLLUT + \overset{*}{.332}\ DISP + \overset{***}{.541}\ FRAN - .195\ SCAN$$

Both the BMD and the LINCUR programs choose the same best model for male mortality from cancer of the buccal cavity and pharynx from the 6-variable pool. With just three of the variables, PRELEV, POLLUT, and ALCO, the model accounts for 80.02% of the states' variation in this type of mortality (Table VII) compared with 81.21% explained by the complete model with all six variables. The chosen model indicates that higher mortality rates occurred in those states with positive scores in all three factors, i.e., those with more precipitation and at lower altitude, with higher levels of alcohol consumption, and with higher pollution levels.

When the alcohol consumption variable ALCO is divided into its three components MALT, WINE, and DISP, it is replaced by WINE and DISP in the models, but these individual components have weaker coefficient weights. Cigarette consumption also enters the BMD model, also with a weak coefficient.

When the four ethnic variables FRAN, BRIT, SCAN, and OTHEUR are added to the 6-variable pool, the chosen model indicates that French ethnicity is a strongly positive factor, while the Other European ethnic effect enters the model negatively and nonsignificantly. When ALCO is again divided into its components, the model chosen from the resulting 12-variable pool by both programs accounts for 83.99% of the mortality variation with only five factors compared with just 84.67% explained by the complete 12-variable model. This final model indicates that, after adjusting for all model effects, those states that are wet and low, that have a larger proportion of French ethnicity in their white population, high levels of pollution, high consumption of distilled spirits, and a smaller proportion of Scandinavians, also have the highest male mortality rates from cancer of the buccal cavity and pharynx. Among all the individual ethnic variables, the one showing the highest correlation with WINE, with DISP, and with CIGS was FRAN. Since FRAN displaced WINE and CIGS in the final model, ethnicity is indicated as being the stronger variable, but its effect can be due to its associated patterns of wine consumption and smoking. The continuation of DISP in the model maintains the importance of this type of alcohol consumption, even after adjustment for ethnic effects.

When the ethnic effects in the above models are compared with the corresponding national ranking in this type of male cancer mortality using Segi's data as described in Chapter 2, a striking parallelism is evident. In mortality from cancer of the buccal cavity and pharynx males in France ranked the highest among those from the 20 countries considered, matching the highly significant positive effect of FRAN in the models. On the other hand males in Sweden and in Denmark ranked low, sixteenth and seventeenth respectively, paralleling the negative effect of SCAN in the model. Since males in Norway held a middle rank of eleventh, the combined Scandinavian ranking was modified, and the nonsignificance of the negative coefficient for SCAN would be a reflection of this diminished effect. Similarly, of the countries listed in Segi that belong to the Other European group, all but one, Italy, ranked below the median, matching the negative coefficient of OTHEUR in the model from the 10-variable pool. The very high rank (third) of Italy, which represents a major sector of this ethnic grouping, partially offsets the very low ranking of Germany (nineteenth) and the Netherlands (eighteenth), modifying the low combined rank for this group of countries. This is paralleled by the nonsignificance of the negative coefficient of OTHEUR, and its omission from the final model. In Table XIV, which displays the results of dividing OTHEUR into its major components, it can be seen that it is the negative GERM effect that leads to the negative OTHEUR effect, matching the low ranking of the Germanic countries in Segi.

In Haenszel's study of ethnic mortality in the United States Swedish and Russian men were found to be at low risk of mortality from cancer of the buccal cavity and pharynx, which is in line with the negative effects of SCAN and OTHEUR in the models.

Males in England and Wales, Scotland, and Northern Ireland ranked in the middle third (tenth, ninth, eighth) in this type of cancer mortality, but males in Ireland had somewhat higher death rates, ranking sixth. Haenszel found an excess risk of death from this type of cancer in Irish men in the U. S., particularly from cancer of the tongue, but no excess risk for those from England and Wales. The combined rank of the countries in the British Isles is a middle one, and its counterpart is the null British effect implied by the omission of BRIT from these models.

The ridge trace of the coefficient estimates for all 12 variables in the largest pool reveals that the most important effect, PRELEV, is also the most unstable, but in spite of continuous decreases, its coefficient weight remains the largest in magnitude. The FRAN and DISP effects decrease before stabilizing, while the POLLUT effect is constant, surpassing them in importance. The BRIT and negative SCAN effects both decrease in magnitude before stabilizing, while the CIGS and WINE effects increase.

In comparison with the chosen subset models, ridge regression confirms the importance of PRELEV but shows its effect to be unstable, while it gives greater importance to POLLUT and shows its effect to be stable. DISP is confirmed to be the important component of alcohol consumption, and WINE of moderate importance. The ridge regression gives much more importance to the negative SCAN effect and shows it to be stable, while it decreases the weight of the very strong FRAN effect. CIGS is maintained as a factor of moderate importance, and BRIT and a very stable TEMP effect are added as factors that should be included. The addition of a positive TEMP effect brings male mortality from cancer of the buccal cavity and pharynx into line with the female mortality pattern for this cancer, as well as with the mortality patterns of closely related cancer sites such as larynx, and trachea, bronchus, and lung.

It should also be noted that the weak negative OTHEUR effect in one of the subset models becomes weakly positive in the stabilized pattern of the ridge trace.

TABLE XIV
Results of Dividing the Other European Variable into Its Component Ethnic Effects:[a] Germanic,[b] Italian, and Slavic[c]

	Male Cancer Mortality Models		Female Cancer Mortality Models	
	OTHEUR effect before division	Component effects	OTHEUR effect before division	Component effects
Buc Cav & Ph.		(–)GERM		(–)GERM**
Larynx		SLAV*		(–)GERM*
T, B & Lung			**	SLAV**
T, B, & L Spec.				
B & L Unspec.	n.s.	SLAV		SLAV
Esophagus	***	ITAL*, SLAV***		
Stomach	***	ITAL, SLAV**	**	SLAV**
Lg. Intestine	*	SLAV**	n.s.	ITAL**, SLAV*
Rectum	**	GERM, ITAL, SLAV	*	ITAL*, SLAV*
Liver *et al.*	**	SLAV***	***	GERM*, SLAV
Pancreas			n.s.	(–)GERM**, SLAV***
Kidney	*	SLAV**, (–)ITAL	n.s.	(–)GERM*, (–)ITAL***, SLAV***
Bladder	n.s.	GERM*, ITAL		ITAL**
Brain		(–)ITAL		
Lymphosarcoma	n.s.	(–)GERM, SLAV**	*	SLAV**
Hodgkin's Dis.		ITAL		(–)GERM, SLAV
Leukemia				ITAL
Melanoma		(–)GERM*		
Other Skin		(–)GERM**, ITAL		
Prostate			–	–
Breast	–	–	*	GERM, SLAV
Ovary	–	–	***	GERM*, SLAV*
Cervix Uteri	–	–		(–)GERM, ITAL*
Corpus Uteri	–	–	**	SLAV

[a] All effects are positive except where indicated to be negative by (–), and their coefficient significance is annotated by n.s., nonsignificant; *, $.01 < p < .05$; **, $.001 < p < .01$; ***, $p < .001$.

[b] Born in Germany, Austria, Belgium, Netherlands.

[c] Born in Poland, Russia, Czechoslovakia.

2 *Larynx, Males–M161 (ICD 161)*

6 VAR, BMD and Second LIN

$$Y(M161) = 2.297 + \overset{*}{.117}\ TEMP + \overset{***}{.391}\ PRELEV + \overset{*}{.142}\ POLLUT + .102\ CIGS + \overset{***}{.391}\ ALCO$$

8 VAR, BMD and LIN

$$Y(M161) = 2.297 + \overset{***}{.396}\ PRELEV + \overset{**}{.188}\ POLLUT + \overset{**}{.178}\ CIGS + \overset{***}{.294}\ WINE$$

10 VAR, BMD and LIN

$$Y(M161) = 2.297 + \overset{***}{.377}\ PRELEV + .117\ POLLUT + \overset{**}{.294}\ ALCO + \overset{***}{.293}\ FRAN - \overset{**}{.201}\ SCAN$$

12 VAR, BMD and Second LIN

$$Y(M161) = 2.297 + \overset{***}{.357}\ PRELEV + \overset{*}{.133}\ POLLUT + .104\ MALT + \overset{**}{.179}\ DISP + \overset{***}{.346}\ FRAN - \overset{**}{.223}\ SCAN$$

12 VAR, LIN

$$Y(M161) = 2.297 + \overset{***}{.343}\ PRELEV + \overset{**}{.168}\ POLLUT + \overset{**}{.185}\ DISP + \overset{***}{.380}\ FRAN - \overset{**}{.175}\ SCAN$$

The models for male mortality from cancer of the larynx and from cancer of the buccal cavity and pharynx are very similar, as is to be expected since these male mortality patterns are highly correlated, their correlation coefficient of .956 indicating that they have 91% of their state variation in common. According to the models the mortality rates for both types of cancer are higher in those states that have more precipitation and lower elevation, higher levels of pollution, more cigarette and alcohol consumption, a relatively large proportion of French and a relatively small proportion of Scandinavian ethnicity.

For male mortality from laryngeal cancer the best model chosen from the 6-variable pool by BMD is equivalent to the LIN model with the second lowest C_p. The LIN model with the lowest C_p drops the variable CIGS, but its C_p value is greater than its p value, indicating some bias. Alcohol consumption and the precipitation/elevation factor are of equally high significance and weight in this model. The model from the 8-variable pool concentrates the ALCO effect on WINE and shows a significant contribution by CIGS. However, when the ethnic variables enter the variable pools, FRAN and negative SCAN take on a high level of significance in the models, while CIGS is dropped and alcohol consumption is concentrated on DISP. The BMD model and the second-best LIN model from the 12-variable pool are equivalent, both including a nonsignificant MALT effect, whereas the best LIN model explains almost the same amount of variation in mortality without the MALT.

Again the ranking in Segi parallels the ethnic effects in the mortality models, with males in France ranking highest in mortality from cancer of the larynx, and those in all three Scandinavian countries ranking the lowest. The males in the British countries rank in the middle, matching their null effect in the models. Males in the Other European countries have mixed ranks, from high to low, with Italy ranked very high (second) as it was in cancer of the buccal cavity and pharynx. And just as in the mortality models for cancer of the buccal cavity and pharynx the importance of WINE as a factor is partially absorbed into the ethnic variable FRAN. The strength of FRAN in the male mortality models for both cancer categories, buccal cavity and pharynx and larynx, may be due to its close association with the three consumption factors DISP, WINE, and CIGS, which are important positive effects in these models.

As the chosen subset models are very similar for male mortality from cancer of the buccal cavity and pharynx and cancer of the larynx, the ridge traces are equally similar. For laryngeal cancer the important alcoholic component effects DISP and WINE are more stable, and the latter is confirmed to be more important than in cancer of the buccal cavity and pharynx. Both the FRAN and negative SCAN effects are unstable, decreasing in magnitude, but remain strong factors. CIGS is shown to be a factor of moderate strength, as are the stable effects OTHEUR and TEMP. Compared with the final subset models the ridge regression analysis increases the importance of POLLUT, decreases that of FRAN, brings TEMP, WINE, and CIGS back in as viable factors and adds the positive ethnic effect, OTHEUR.

3 Trachea, Bronchus, and Lung, Males–M166 (ICD 162, 163)

6 VAR, BMD and LIN

$$\begin{aligned} Y(M166) = {} & 35.513 + \overset{***}{3.052}\ \text{TEMP} + \overset{***}{3.506}\ \text{PRELEV} + \overset{**}{2.213}\ \text{CIGS} \\ & + \overset{***}{2.761}\ \text{ALCO} \end{aligned}$$

8 VAR, LIN

$$\begin{aligned} Y(M166) = {} & 35.513 + \overset{***}{2.187}\ \text{TEMP} + \overset{***}{3.850}\ \text{PRELEV} + \overset{***}{3.172}\ \text{CIGS} \\ & + \overset{***}{3.229}\ \text{WINE} - 1.388\ \text{DISP} \end{aligned}$$

10 VAR, LIN

$$\begin{aligned} Y(M166) = {} & 35.513 + \overset{**}{1.766}\ \text{TEMP} + \overset{***}{3.685}\ \text{PRELEV} - 1.514\ \text{POLLUT} \\ & + \overset{*}{1.813}\ \text{ALCO} + \overset{***}{3.634}\ \text{FRAN} - \overset{**}{3.097}\ \text{SCAN} + 1.811\ \text{OTHEUR} \end{aligned}$$

12 VAR, BMD and LIN

$$\begin{aligned} Y(M166) = {} & 35.513 + \overset{*}{1.675}\ \text{TEMP} + \overset{***}{3.475}\ \text{PRELEV} + 1.215\ \text{CIGS} \\ & + 1.060\ \text{WINE} + \overset{***}{3.468}\ \text{FRAN} - \overset{**}{1.608}\ \text{SCAN} \end{aligned}$$

4 Trachea, and Bronchus and Lung Specified as Primary, Males–M162 (ICD 162)

6 and 12 VAR, BMD and LIN; 8 and 10 VAR, BMD

$$Y(M162) = 14.941 + \overset{***}{2.018}\ \text{TEMP} + .822\ \text{PRELEV} + \overset{**}{1.703}\ \text{INCM}$$

8 VAR, LIN

$$Y(M162) = 14.941 + \overset{**}{1.869}\ \text{TEMP} + .824\ \text{PRELEV} + 1.233\ \text{INCM} + .658\ \text{WINE}$$

10 VAR, LIN

$$Y(M162) = 14.941 + \overset{***}{2.390}\ \text{TEMP} + \overset{*}{1.131}\ \text{POLLUT} + .882\ \text{CIGS} + .988\ \text{SCAN}$$

5 Bronchus and Lung Unspecified as to Primary or Secondary, Males–M163 (ICD 163)

6 VAR, BMD and LIN

$$Y(M163) = 18.252 + .925\ TEMP + \overset{***}{2.364}\ PRELEV - 1.715\ INCM + 1.674\ CIGS + \overset{**}{3.019}\ ALCO$$

8 VAR, LIN

$$Y(M163) = 18.252 + \overset{***}{2.774}\ PRELEV - 2.211\ INCM + \overset{*}{1.930}\ CIGS + 1.430\ MALT + \overset{**}{2.010}\ WINE$$

10 VAR, BMD and LIN

$$Y(M163) = 18.252 + \overset{***}{2.742}\ PRELEV - \overset{**}{2.308}\ POLLUT + 1.899\ ALCO + \overset{*}{2.438}\ FRAN - \overset{***}{3.676}\ SCAN + 1.975\ OTHEUR$$

12 VAR, BMD and Second LIN

$$Y(M163) = 18.252 + \overset{***}{2.396}\ PRELEV - \overset{*}{1.779}\ POLLUT - 2.009\ INCM + 1.638\ MALT + 1.380\ DISP + \overset{***}{3.216}\ FRAN - \overset{***}{3.504}\ SCAN + 2.022\ OTHEUR$$

12 VAR, LIN

$$Y(M163) = 18.252 + \overset{***}{2.958}\ PRELEV - \overset{*}{1.622}\ POLLUT + \overset{*}{1.943}\ MALT + \overset{***}{3.588}\ FRAN - \overset{***}{3.111}\ SCAN$$

Three sets of models were derived for the respiratory cancers (other than laryngeal cancer), one set for the deaths recorded to be from cancer of the trachea and of the bronchus and lung specified to be primary, one set for those deaths recorded to be from cancer of the bronchus and lung unspecified as primary or secondary, and one set for the combination of these deaths. The last category of mortality, deaths from cancer of the trachea, and bronchus and lung both specified and unspecified, is in most common use [Mason and McKay (2), Segi (26), Haenszel (28)] but is seen to combine two very different patterns of mortality. Burbank's (13) breakdown of these deaths into the specified primary and the unspecified categories, though covering a slightly different period of time from those of Mason and McKay's rates, is used to illustrate these two types of recorded deaths from lung cancer. The correlation between male death rates for the specified and for the unspecified categories is only .022, showing that they have almost no state variation in common. It should be noted here that a small negative correlation (–.322) exists between the female death rates for these two categories, implying a slight complementarity. On the other hand there is close correlation between the male and female death rates within each category, .874 for the specified primary lung cancer mortality and .900 for the unspecified.

A strong contrast in the models for both categories is the positive INCM effect in the specified primary mortality models and the negative INCM effect in those for the unspecified category. This same contrast is found in the female mortality models, and with greater significance in the coefficients. An explanation of this income effect could be in the relationship of a state's relative income level to its relative level of sophistication of medical services or of medical records, so that in the wealthier states the specific diagnosis of "lung cancer stated to be primary" would be more frequently made or recorded on the death certificate, while in the poorer states the less precise diagnosis of unspecified lung cancer would more frequently occur. However, this does not mean that the two categories are strictly complementary and their sum the total mortality from cancer of the trachea, bronchus, and lung, because the unspecified category of lung cancer deaths includes those which are metastatic from other primary sites.

The male mortality models for cancer of the trachea, bronchus, and lung specified primary indicate only one highly significant factor besides INCM, and that is the strongly positive effect TEMP, a characteristic shared only by the corresponding female mortality models and by the skin cancer mortality models for both sexes. A positive TEMP effect is shown to be a factor in male and female mortality from cancer of the buccal cavity and pharynx and in male mortality from cancer of the larynx, but not with coefficients as consistently significant. POLLUT also enters as a significant factor, but only when INCM is not in the model, indicating a possible interchange between these two effects. This appears to be even more the case in the models for the unspecified category where an uninterpretable negative POLLUT effect alternates with a negative INCM effect. The correlation between these two variables is not large (.407) but the variation that they have in common could represent specifically those state differences that produce the varying quality in medical diagnosis and records.

PRELEV, a strong positive effect in most of the cancer mortality models, is notably weak in the models for primary lung cancer in males, and does not even enter the female mortality models for this cancer category. A few of the consumption and ethnic factors enter these models positively but weakly: CIGS, WINE, and SCAN. It is clear that the variable pools do not contain all the factors needed to explain sufficiently the variation in this category since only 44.26% is accounted for by the full 12-variable equation. However, the chosen models explain a large proportion of this percentage.

The model for male mortality in the unspecified category of lung cancer chosen from the smallest variable pool includes, in addition to the income factor, two very significant positive effects, PRELEV and ALCO, and two less important, TEMP and CIGS. The division of ALCO brings two of its components into the model, WINE with a very significant coefficient, and MALT with a nonsignificant one. Addition of the ethnic variables to the pools brings into the models those ethnic effects that are also in the models for buccal cavity and pharynx and for larynx–positive FRAN and negative SCAN–both with very significant coefficients. And just as in the models for those cancer sites, the addition of these ethnic factors decreases the importance of alcohol consumption, shifting the effect from WINE to DISP and MALT, and wipes out the smoking effect. This similarity in consumption and ethnic effects as well as in the TEMP and PRELEV effects indicates that the unspecified category of lung cancer deaths may contain deaths from primary cancers of the buccal cavity and pharynx or larynx that metastasized to the lung. The importance of MALT and the inclusion of OTHEUR in the models for the unspecified category of lung cancer point to the digestive cancers as other primary sites that metastasized to the lung and may be included in the unspecified lung cancer category, esophageal cancer in particular.

The models for the combination of the specified primary and the unspecified categories of lung cancer mortality chiefly reflect the model effects of the unspecified component, not surprisingly since it is the larger in size. The high level of significance of the positive TEMP effect in the models for the combined category derives from the model effects for the specified primary category, but the remaining model effects are derived from those of the unspecified category. The income effect is null in the combined category since it serves only to differentiate between the component categories. The divergence between the models for specified primary lung cancer and those for the commonly used combined category points up the invalidity of the latter as a measure of the former.

Since international mortality rates are given only for the combined category of lung cancer, it is not possible to determine international comparability with respect to death rates from primary cancer of the lung.

In male mortality for the combined category of lung cancer the men in France are ranked low in Segi, one of the few examples of complete divergence between foreign ranking and ethnic effect in the mortality models. Men in Norway and Sweden rank very low and men in Denmark rank in the middle, the low combined Scandinavian rank paralleling the negative SCAN effect in the models. Haenszel ranked men from Sweden and Norway lowest in mortality for this combined category of lung cancer, confirming the SCAN effect. Men in the Other European countries listed in Segi rank high except those in Italy, matching the positive OTHEUR effect. Haenszel found men from Poland, Russia, Austria, and Czechoslovakia to be at higher risk from this category of cancer mortality than their U. S. native-white counterparts, corroborating the ethnic effect in the models. Men in Scotland and in England and Wales are ranked the highest, but men in the Irelands rank in the middle, producing a combined British ranking that is moderately high. However, Haenszel ranks the men from Ireland very low in this mortality, which probably offsets high death rates in the English and Scotch ethnic groups, thereby neutralizing the BRIT effect in the U. S. models. Thus only the French ethnic effect in the male mortality models for the combined category of lung cancer is contrary to its counterpart experience abroad.

The ridge regression analysis shows the TEMP effect, the most important in the specified primary category, to be unstable, decreasing continually but still maintaining its top position of importance. The POLLUT and PRELEV effects are relatively stable, decreasing only very gradually and maintaining their relative importance. The WINE, INCM, and CIGS effects are unstable, decreasing sharply before stabilizing, but are given greater importance than in the subset models. It is interesting that the model that emerges in the ridge regression is a combination of the two strongly different model subsets chosen by the other programs.

The SCAN effect, which is strongly positive at the least squares solution, becomes negative as it stabilizes, while the reverse is true for the OTHEUR effect, which goes from strongly negative to positive in the stable pattern. FRAN, which is not chosen in the subset models, is given more importance by the ridge regression analysis.

For the unspecified category the ridge trace is similar to those for cancer of the buccal cavity and pharynx and cancer of the larynx just as their subset models are similar. The PRELEV effect is more stable in this mortality but decreases continually although holding its major role. The FRAN and negative SCAN effects are very unstable but also maintain their importance. The DISP effect loses some of its strength while the WINE and CIGS effects gain before stabilizing. While the subset models pick and choose among CIGS, DISP, and WINE, the ridge trace shows all three to be contributing net effects. Although the negative INCM effect loses its strength in competition with the other factors, it does remain negative, while the negative POLLUT effect, puzzling in the subset models, becomes positive after stabilizing in the ridge trace.

Similarly, in the combined lung cancer category POLLUT becomes a positive effect when it stabilizes. The other effects shown to be important in the ridge trace of the combined category are the strongest factors in each of the component categories–TEMP in specified primary and PRELEV in unspecified–as well as those the two subcategories have in common–CIGS, WINE, and FRAN. The TEMP, CIGS, and WINE effects are especially stable.

6 Esophagus, Males–M150 (ICD 150)

6 VAR, BMD and LIN

$$Y(M150) = 3.529 - \overset{*}{.254}\ TEMP + \overset{***}{.508}\ PRELEV + \overset{**}{.387}\ POLLUT + \overset{***}{.679}\ ALCO$$

8 VAR, BMD and Third LIN

$$Y(M150) = 3.529 - .248\ TEMP + \overset{***}{.531}\ PRELEV + \overset{**}{.366}\ POLLUT + \overset{*}{.290}\ MALT + .303\ WINE + .210\ DISP$$

8 VAR, LIN

$$Y(M150) = 3.529 - \overset{*}{.301}\ TEMP + \overset{***}{.572}\ PRELEV + \overset{**}{.362}\ POLLUT + \overset{*}{.307}\ MALT + \overset{***}{.454}\ WINE$$

$$Y(M150) = 3.529 - \overset{*}{.280}\ TEMP + \overset{***}{.530}\ PRELEV + \overset{**}{.393}\ POLLUT + .225\ MALT + \overset{**}{.380}\ WINE + .181\ CIGS$$

10 VAR, BMD and LIN

$$Y(M150) = 3.529 + \overset{***}{.526}\ PRELEV + .173\ POLLUT + \overset{***}{.503}\ ALCO + \overset{***}{.473}\ OTHEUR$$

12 VAR, BMD and LIN

$$Y(M150) = 3.529 + \overset{***}{.457}\ PRELEV + .209\ POLLUT + \overset{***}{.410}\ DISP + \overset{***}{.605}\ OTHEUR$$

The models for cancer of the esophagus combine the important model effects for cancer of the buccal cavity and pharynx and of the larynx, specifically WINE and DISP, with those for the digestive system cancers, specifically MALT, OTHEUR, and negative TEMP. The positive effects PRELEV and POLLUT are common to the mortality models for both groups of cancers.

The model from the 6-variable pool indicates that a high level of alcohol consumption is the most important factor in high mortality levels, with wet climate at low altitude, high pollution level, and colder temperature following in that order. The division of ALCO brings all three of its components into the BMD model, only MALT and WINE into one of the best LIN models, and MALT, WINE, and CIGS into the other best LIN model. In the models from the nonethnic variable pools the only difference between those for cancer of the esophagus and those for cancer of the buccal cavity and pharynx and cancer of the larynx is the cold temperature factor and the increased importance of MALT in the former. The pattern of ethnic effects, however, is completely different, shifting cancer of the esophagus into the digestive cancer group, with a very significant positive coefficient for OTHEUR, and without the positive FRAN and negative SCAN effects. Since the correlation between MALT and OTHEUR is very high, .834, it is not surprising that the consumption factor MALT is displaced by the ethnic factor OTHEUR, just as in the buccal cavity and pharynx and the larynx models WINE was partially or wholly displaced by FRAN. This does not decrease the importance of MALT as a factor in esophageal cancer since it may be the consumption habit that underlies the ethnic importance of the Other European factor.

Reference to Segi shows that the same world pattern of male mortality from cancer of the buccal cavity and pharynx and cancer of the larynx holds for cancer of the esophagus, namely, that the men in France rank first, the men in Scandinavia rank lowest, and the men in the British and the Other European countries have mixed or middle ranks. Thus the male mortality models for esophageal cancer, in which the only ethnic effect is positive OTHEUR, are not matched by the international ranking of male death rates from cancer of the esophagus.

Haenszel found that all the foreign-born males in his study suffered much higher mortality rates from esophageal cancer than the native born, the men from Poland, Czechoslovakia, and Ireland the highest. The high risk for the first two ethnic groups confirms the positive OTHEUR effect in the models, while Table XIV affirms that it is the SLAV effect that underlies it. The high Irish immigrant risk concurs with the high rank of Ireland in Segi.

The ridge trace again shows, as it does in the models for cancer of the buccal cavity and pharynx and the larynx, the instability of the most important effect, PRELEV, which continually decreases though remaining the largest in magnitude, and the stability of the POLLUT effect, which becomes second largest in the stabilized pattern. The OTHEUR effect, which is the largest in the least squares solution, shows the greatest instability, decreasing very sharply but third in magnitude in the stable pattern. The BRIT, WINE, and CIGS coefficient estimates are very stable while the MALT estimate increases slightly before stabilizing early. On the other hand, the negative TEMP effect, which appears significantly in the nonethnic subset models, is very unstable, decreasing considerably in magnitude.

It will be seen that the ethnic pattern in the male mortality models for stomach cancer, which is similar to that for esophageal cancer, does reflect the international ranking of stomach cancer death rates in males. And while the esophageal cancer mortality models are closer to those for stomach cancer in ethnic patterns, the international mortality pattern of esophageal cancer concurs with that of cancer of the buccal cavity and pharynx and the larynx. In their nonethnic effects the mortality models for cancer of the esophagus are divided, sharing PRELEV, POLLUT, positive CIGS, and positive DISP with the buccal cavity and pharynx and the larynx models, negative TEMP and positive MALT with the stomach cancer models. Table XV illustrates this division in the factor sets for male mortality from cancer of the esophagus.

7 *Stomach, Males–M151 (ICD 151)*

6 VAR, LIN

$$Y(\text{M151}) = 14.361 - \overset{***}{1.973}\ \text{TEMP} - .587\ \text{CIGS} + \overset{**}{1.108}\ \text{ALCO}$$

8 VAR, BMD and LIN

$$Y(\text{M151}) = 14.361 - \overset{***}{2.093}\ \text{TEMP} + .411\ \text{PRELEV} + \overset{**}{.891}\ \text{MALT} + \overset{**}{1.213}\ \text{WINE} - \overset{**}{1.266}\ \text{DISP}$$

10 VAR, LIN

$$Y(\text{M151}) = 14.361 - \overset{***}{1.690}\ \text{TEMP} - \overset{*}{.993}\ \text{INCM} + \overset{***}{1.982}\ \text{OTHEUR}$$

12 VAR, BMD and Second LIN

$$Y(\text{M151}) = 14.361 - \overset{***}{1.842}\ \text{TEMP} - \overset{**}{1.191}\ \text{INCM} + .550\ \text{MALT} + \overset{**}{.946}\ \text{WINE} - \overset{*}{.797}\ \text{DISP} + \overset{***}{1.523}\ \text{OTHEUR}$$

12 VAR, LIN

$$Y(\text{M151}) = 14.361 - \overset{***}{1.948}\ \text{TEMP} - \overset{*}{.982}\ \text{INCM} + \overset{**}{.995}\ \text{WINE} - \overset{*}{.809}\ \text{DISP} + \overset{***}{1.740}\ \text{OTHEUR}$$

From the 6-variable pool the LIN model for male mortality from cancer of the stomach gives the greatest importance to cold temperature and a high level of alcohol consumption as factors in high death rates. A negative CIGS is also included but not significantly, and is not in any of the other models. The BMD model is not listed since it is the equivalent of only the third-best LIN model. Both programs choose the same model from the 8-variable pool, dropping CIGS and adding a positive but nonsignificant PRELEV effect. The division of ALCO into its components leads to very significant positive coefficients for MALT and WINE, but also a very significant negative coefficient for DISP.

When the ethnic variables are added to the pools the sole ethnic effect is OTHEUR, with a highly significant positive coefficient in each model. Negative INCM also enters the models significantly, and negative TEMP continues as the most important effect in male mortality from cancer of the stomach. The interpretation of the significant negative INCM effect may be similar to that in the model set for the unspecified category of lung cancer. Stomach cancer has been,

TABLE XV
Comparison of Ethnic and Nonethnic Effects in the Models of Male Mortality for Four Related Types of Cancer[a]

	Models of male mortality in the U. S.		International
	Nonethnic effects	Strong ethnic effects	pattern
Buc Cav & Ph.	TEMP, PRELEV, POLLUT, CIGS, WINE, DISP	High FRAN, low SCAN, high BRIT	High FRAN, low SCAN
Larynx	TEMP, PRELEV, POLLUT, CIGS, WINE, DISP	High FRAN, low SCAN	High FRAN, low SCAN
Esophagus	–TEMP, PRELEV, POLLUT, CIGS, WINE, DISP, MALT	High OTHEUR, high BRIT	High FRAN, low SCAN
Stomach	–TEMP, PRELEV, –INCM, –CIGS, WINE, –DISP, MALT	High OTHEUR	High OTHEUR

[a] As indicated by the subset models and ridge trace.

according to Macdonald (29), a generalized diagnosis for many types of digestive cancer, a catch-all rubric for primary cancers that should have had a more specific diagnosis, and thus it would be recorded as cause of death more frequently in states with a poorer medical infrastructure, i.e., those with lower income levels.

The strong positive ethnic effect OTHEUR is matched by the high ranks of the Other European countries in male mortality from cancer of the stomach. The model effect in the U. S. is confirmed in Haenszel's article, where excess risk is shown for men from Poland, Russia, Czechoslovakia, and Germany. However he found that the risk for men from Italy was low whereas males in Italy ranked fifth in the international data. In Table XIV it can be seen that the very significant SLAV effect is the basis for the OTHEUR effect, and that there is a positive ITAL effect in the model, matching the moderately high rank of Italy in Segi.

Males in the British countries have middle ranks in this mortality, coinciding with the null BRIT effect in the model. The low rank of males in France does not have a counterpart in the null model effect of FRAN. The null SCAN effect is matched by the middle rank of males in Norway, but males in Sweden and Denmark rank low.

The ridge trace indicates that the most important effect, negative TEMP, is unstable, decreasing sharply and continuously, but still maintaining a coefficient weight almost twice the second largest. Of the other important effects in the stabilized pattern, OTHEUR also decreases sharply and continuously, but MALT and SCAN are stable. The WINE effect, which is very important in the chosen subset models and which is also very large in the least squares solution for the full model, decreases to almost zero, as do the negative coefficients of DISP, INCM and CIGS. Thus the ridge analysis presents a different model for cancer of the stomach from those chosen from the 12-variable pool by the BMD and LIN programs. In particular, MALT is shown to be the important component of alcohol consumption with great stability in its effect, while WINE totally loses its strength as a factor. Also the ridge regression drops the unstable negative INCM effect and adds SCAN as a strong and stable ethnic effect. Although this does not match the Segi ranking in mortality it should be noted that Macdonald (30) found the incidence rates of stomach cancer in males in Denmark and Norway considerably higher than those in total males, white and nonwhite, in the ten-cities survey of the United States.

8 *Large Intestine excluding Rectum, Males–M153 (ICD 153)*

6 VAR, BMD and LIN

$$\begin{aligned} Y(M153) = {} & 14.762 - \overset{***}{1.243}\ \text{TEMP} + \overset{***}{1.461}\ \text{PRELEV} + \overset{*}{1.073}\ \text{POLLUT} \\ & + \overset{*}{1.158}\ \text{INCM} + .753\ \text{CIGS} \end{aligned}$$

8 VAR, BMD and LIN

$$\begin{aligned} Y(M153) = {} & 14.762 - \overset{**}{.888}\ \text{TEMP} + \overset{***}{1.520}\ \text{PRELEV} + \overset{*}{.934}\ \text{POLLUT} \\ & + \overset{*}{.665}\ \text{CIGS} + \overset{***}{1.652}\ \text{MALT} \end{aligned}$$

10 VAR, LIN

$$\begin{aligned} Y(M153) = {} & 14.762 - \overset{*}{.701}\ \text{TEMP} + \overset{***}{1.427}\ \text{PRELEV} + .624\ \text{POLLUT} \\ & + .420\ \text{CIGS} + \overset{*}{.991}\ \text{BRIT} + \overset{**}{1.306}\ \text{OTHEUR} \end{aligned}$$

12 VAR, BMD and LIN

$$\begin{aligned} Y(M153) = {} & 14.762 - .412\ \text{TEMP} + \overset{***}{1.242}\ \text{PRELEV} + \overset{*}{.835}\ \text{POLLUT} \\ & - .818\ \text{INCM} + \overset{*}{.652}\ \text{CIGS} + \overset{*}{.839}\ \text{MALT} - .557\ \text{WINE} \\ & + \overset{**}{1.335}\ \text{BRIT} + \overset{*}{1.206}\ \text{OTHEUR} \end{aligned}$$

9 *Rectum, Males–M154 (ICD 154)*

6 VAR, BMD and LIN

$$Y(M154) = 6.561 - \overset{***}{1.212}\ TEMP + \overset{**}{.683}\ PRELEV + \overset{**}{.692}\ POLLUT + .532\ CIGS + .618\ ALCO$$

8 VAR, LIN

$$Y(M154) = 6.561 - \overset{***}{.927}\ TEMP + \overset{***}{.829}\ PRELEV + \overset{*}{.495}\ POLLUT + \overset{*}{.520}\ CIGS + \overset{**}{.975}\ MALT$$

10 VAR, BMD and LIN

$$Y(M154) = 6.561 - \overset{***}{.759}\ TEMP + \overset{**}{.537}\ PRELEV + \overset{*}{.482}\ POLLUT - \overset{**}{.986}\ INCM + \overset{**}{.579}\ CIGS + \overset{***}{.912}\ BRIT + \overset{***}{1.198}\ OTHEUR$$

12 VAR, BMD and LIN

$$Y(M154) = 6.561 - \overset{***}{.692}\ TEMP + \overset{**}{.592}\ PRELEV + \overset{*}{.456}\ POLLUT - \overset{***}{1.106}\ INCM + \overset{**}{.511}\ CIGS + .472\ MALT + \overset{***}{.917}\ BRIT + \overset{**}{.981}\ OTHEUR$$

The state patterns of male mortality from cancer of the large intestine and of the rectum are highly correlated ($r = .954$), having over 90% of state variation in common, and the mortality models for these two related primary cancer sites are so similar that they are presented together. From the 6-variable pool the mortality models for both cancer sites have significant negative coefficients for TEMP, significant positive coefficients for PRELEV and POLLUT, and positive but not significant coefficients for CIGS. A positive income effect is in the intestinal cancer model while a positive alcohol consumption effect is in the rectal cancer model. For both cancer sites the models chosen from the 8-variable pool are identical in effects with only small differences in coefficient weights, although the difference in average death rate is great. MALT emerges as the important alcohol consumption factor in both types of cancer mortality.

When the ethnic variables are included in the pools, both cancer sites have the same ethnic pattern in their mortality models–highly significant positive coefficients for BRIT and OTHEUR. The importance of MALT is greatly reduced by the inclusion of OTHEUR in both models but it remains as a positive effect. Negative INCM enters the models for both sites after inclusion of and adjustment for the ethnic variables. Overall, high male mortality levels from cancer of the large intestine and from cancer of the rectum are associated with a cold and wet climate at low altitude, a high degree of pollution, and high levels of cigarette smoking and malt consumption. They also occur where the British and Other European ethnic components of the white population are relatively large and the income level is low.

The British countries rank very high in male mortality from cancer of the intestines, Scotland highest, paralleling the significantly positive BRIT effect in the models. However, of the Other European countries in Segi's study only Belgium ranks high, and so the significantly positive OTHEUR effect in the intestinal cancer models is not matched by the foreign experience. The British countries also rank very high in male mortality from cancer of the rectum, as do the Other European countries except Italy, so that the significantly positive effects BRIT and OTHEUR in the rectal cancer models do correspond to the international experience. In Haenszel's study Irish men have the highest risk in both cancer of the intestines and of the rectum, while men from England and Wales rank fifth out of 12 in intestinal cancer mortality and fourth out of ten in rectal cancer mortality, all confirming the very significant positive coefficients for BRIT in the models for both cancer sites.

The positive influence of the ethnic component OTHEUR is shown in Table XIV to be due solely to the Slavic component in intestinal cancer but due to all three components in rectal cancer, and this corroborates Haenszel's finding of an excess in deaths for Russian and Czechoslovakian men in intestinal cancer, and for Czechoslovakian, German, Austrian, and Italian men in rectal cancer. It would appear that the risk of rectal cancer mortality increases considerably for males who migrate from Italy to the United States.

For both cancer sites Segi ranks the males in France in the middle, which is in line with the null FRAN effect in both model sets. Males in Sweden and Norway are ranked low, but those in Denmark very high, their combined rank a middle one, which matches the null SCAN effect in both model sets. Haenszel also shows a low risk in both cancer mortalities for men from Norway and Sweden, so that the null SCAN effect in these models may be the combination of these low risks with a very high risk in Danish males carried over after migration.

The ridge trace of the intestinal cancer mortality pattern shows that of the four largest effects three, PRELEV, BRIT, and OTHEUR, are unstable, decreasing sharply and continuously, but the fourth effect, POLLUT, is a stable one. The coefficients of MALT and CIGS decrease moderately but stabilize as strong factors, while the negative TEMP effect is stable and maintains its strength. The negative WINE and negative INCM effects are highly unstable, the latter becoming positive in the stabilized pattern.

In the ridge trace of the rectal cancer mortality pattern BRIT and OTHEUR have considerably greater weight than PRELEV at the least squares solution, just as they do in the subset models, but decreases in these two ethnic effects, and stability in this climate variable's effect, bring all three to almost identical stabilized coefficient weights. The magnitude of the negative effect TEMP continuously decreases but remains an important factor. The coefficient estimates of the three effects MALT, CIGS, and POLLUT have almost identical and very stable ridge traces. The INCM effect here too shows great instability, going from a very large negative coefficient in the least squares solution to a positive one in stability.

10 *Biliary Passages and Liver Specified as Primary and Unspecified, Males–M155 (ICD 155, Unspecified Part of ICD 156)*

6 VAR, BMD and LIN

$$Y(\mathrm{M155}) = 4.886 + .151\ \mathrm{PRELEV} + \overset{**}{.301}\ \mathrm{POLLUT}$$

8 VAR, BMD and LIN

$$Y(\mathrm{M155}) = 4.886 + .198\ \mathrm{PRELEV} + \overset{*}{.260}\ \mathrm{POLLUT} - .252\ \mathrm{INCM} + \overset{*}{.365}\ \mathrm{MALT}$$

10 VAR, LIN

$$Y(\mathrm{M155}) = 4.886 - \overset{*}{.201}\ \mathrm{TEMP} + .118\ \mathrm{PRELEV} + \overset{*}{.302}\ \mathrm{FRAN} - \overset{*}{.451}\ \mathrm{BRIT} - \overset{***}{.571}\ \mathrm{SCAN} + \overset{***}{.666}\ \mathrm{OTHEUR}$$

12 VAR, LIN

$$Y(\mathrm{M155}) = 4.886 - .192\ \mathrm{TEMP} + \overset{*}{.164}\ \mathrm{PRELEV} - \overset{*}{.212}\ \mathrm{CIGS} + \overset{**}{.370}\ \mathrm{MALT} + \overset{*}{.340}\ \mathrm{FRAN} - \overset{*}{.389}\ \mathrm{BRIT} - \overset{***}{.628}\ \mathrm{SCAN} + \overset{**}{.441}\ \mathrm{OTHEUR}$$

The category for cancer of the biliary passages and liver usually is comprised of a combination of the specified primary, the specified secondary, and the unspecified, as well as an inseparable mix of cancer of the gallbladder and cancer of the liver. In recent years there has been more differentiation among these subcategories, with the result that Mason was able to extract those deaths recorded to be from liver cancer specified as secondary, leaving only the unspecified liver cancer deaths mixed with the specified primary liver cancer deaths and the gallbladder cancer deaths. It is unfortunate that this category combines cancer of two primary sites that have different epidemiological patterns and sex incidence. Generally the male-female ratio of liver cancer mortality is greater than one, while it is less than one for cancer of the gallbladder, the exception being in the American Indians. That racial group suffers very high mortality from cancer of the gallbladder, the males experiencing even higher death rates than the females (31). The state patterns of white male and of white female death rates for this mixed cancer category are only weakly associated with each other (r = .443), having less than 20% of their variation in common. These two patterns are also among the very few with less than 50% of their variation in common with any other cancer mortality pattern (Table III). In spite of the conglomerate character of this rubric, in which the relative proportions of deaths from primary cancer of the gallbladder, primary cancer of the liver, and unspecified liver cancer are unknown, pronounced patterns emerge in the models.

In the model from the smallest variable pool POLLUT appears to be the chief factor associated with state variation in male mortality for this combined category of cancer. However, when alcohol consumption is subdivided, MALT comes into the model as the most important factor. The importance of the ethnic variables is apparent upon their entrance into the variable pools, for they increase by more than 25% the amount of state variation in mortality accounted for. A very definite pattern emerges of high death rates associated with high proportions of French and Other European, and low proportions of British and Scandinavian, ethnicity in the white population. In the final model the division of alcohol consumption again brings MALT in strongly, only partially reducing the coefficient of its chief associated ethnic effect, OTHEUR, but maintaining both factors as highly significant positive effects.

Segi combined the international classification rubrics ICD 155 and ICD 156 in his national rankings of liver cancer mortality, thereby including the sizable category of specified secondary liver cancer. In spite of this flaw in comparability, the national rankings parallel the ethnic effects in the U. S. mortality models to a considerable degree. Males in France rank second among the 18 national groups in the comparison, matching the significantly positive FRAN effect in the models. Males in the British countries rank low, paralleling the negative BRIT effect. Norway ranks the lowest in this male mortality while Sweden and Denmark rank in the middle. The combined Scandinavian rank is in the lowest third, concurring with the negative SCAN effect. Finally, males in the countries representing the Other European group rank at the top—Italy highest, Germany third, Austria fourth, Belgium fifth, and Netherlands sixth—corroborating the positive OTHEUR effect. Thus the international pattern of high male mortality rates among the French and Other Europeans and low rates among the British and Scandinavians is repeated in the ethnic effects of the U. S. male mortality models for cancer of the biliary passages and liver.

In the ridge analysis two of the major factors, negative SCAN and MALT, have unstable, continuously decreasing coefficient estimates, while the strongest factor, PRELEV, has a stable coefficient. Although the least squares estimate of the coefficient for POLLUT is negative, after a sharp increase it stabilizes very quickly into a sizable positive effect, whereas it was totally eliminated in the subset models after the ethnic variables entered. On the other hand the ethnic effects OTHEUR, FRAN, and negative BRIT are unstable, decreasing considerably in magnitude and are not as important as in the subset models. The coefficients of CIGS and TEMP, which are negative in the least squares solution as well as in the subset models, stabilize at zero value.

11 Pancreas, Males–M157 (ICD 157)

6 VAR, BMD and LIN; 10 VAR, LIN

$$Y(M157) = 9.389 + \overset{**}{.279}\ \text{PRELEV} - .257\ \text{INCM} + \overset{**}{.469}\ \text{ALCO}$$

8 VAR, BMD and Second LIN

$$Y(M157) = 9.389 + \overset{***}{.384}\ \text{PRELEV} - .142\ \text{POLLUT} + \overset{***}{.376}\ \text{WINE}$$

8 VAR, LIN; 12 VAR, Second LIN

$$Y(M157) = 9.389 + \overset{***}{.305}\ \text{PRELEV} + \overset{***}{.321}\ \text{WINE}$$

12 VAR, LIN

$$Y(M157) = 9.389 + \overset{***}{.370}\ \text{PRELEV} - \overset{*}{.294}\ \text{INCM} + \overset{***}{.433}\ \text{WINE} + .242\ \text{SCAN}$$

The models for male mortality from cancer of the pancreas do not account for much of the variation in death rates, 43% at most, because the largest variable pool does not contain all the necessary factors, the complete 12-variable model explaining only 46.29% of the variation. But a very clear choice is made by the models as to which are the important variables among the 12 included in the largest pool. PRELEV continues to have a strong positive effect, that is, a wet climate at low elevation is associated with high mortality rates. Clearly the most important model effect is positive WINE, with higher male death rates occurring at higher wine consumption levels. Negative income enters two of the models, but not strongly. The BMD model from the 8-variable pool contains negative POLLUT instead of negative INCM, again raising the possibility of interchangeable income effect and pollution effect. Even though INCM and POLLUT are not highly correlated (r = .407) the variation that they have in common may be the variation operating in the models.

From the ethnic variable pools the BMD program chose models that were only the third and fourth best in the LIN program search, so only the best LIN models are shown. The weakly positive SCAN effect in the models is matched by the moderately high combined rank for Scandinavian males—Sweden (fourth), Denmark (fifth), and Norway (eighth). Haenszel ranks men from Norway and Sweden just higher than the U. S. native-white males in this mortality risk, confirming the model effect.

The null effects of the other three ethnic factors implied by their absence from the models are only partially reflected in the international ranking. Males in Scotland rank high while males in England and Wales and Ireland have middle ranks, giving a combined British rank in the middle range, which matches the null BRIT effect in the models. However, Haenszel's finding of very high mortality from cancer of the pancreas in men from England and Wales and from Ireland is not reflected in the models nor in the international ranking. Males in France rank very low in this mortality but there is no matching negative FRAN effect. Similarly, the Other European countries listed in Segi have generally low-ranking male death rates, but no negative OTHEUR effect appears in the models. According to the best subset models for male mortality from cancer of the pancreas the ethnic factors are minimal, while WINE and PRELEV are the dominant factors.

In the ridge trace the coefficient estimates of the two major effects PRELEV and WINE are unstable, decreasing considerably from their least squares values. The positive FRAN effect also decreases but does stabilize as an important factor while the DISP effect reaches the same coefficient estimate as FRAN from a negative original position. The strongly negative INCM effect is very unstable, weakening considerably and continuously. The general instability and weakness of coefficient estimates in the ridge trace reflect, as do the best subset models, the inadequacy of the variable pool to explain the pattern of male mortality from cancer of the pancreas.

12 Kidney, Males–M180 (ICD 180)

6 VAR, BMD and LIN

$$Y(M180) = 3.700 - \overset{***}{.256}\ TEMP + \overset{**}{.124}\ PRELEV + \overset{*}{.167}\ INCM + \overset{*}{.185}\ ALCO$$

8 VAR, BMD and LIN

$$Y(M180) = 3.700 - \overset{***}{.203}\ TEMP + \overset{*}{.105}\ PRELEV + \overset{***}{.253}\ MALT + \overset{**}{.153}\ DISP$$

10 VAR, BMD and LIN

$$Y(M180) = 3.700 - \overset{*}{.112}\ TEMP + \overset{*}{.115}\ PRELEV + .120\ CIGS + \overset{**}{.207}\ ALCO - \overset{*}{.193}\ FRAN + \overset{*}{.189}\ SCAN + \overset{**}{.185}\ OTHEUR$$

12 VAR, LIN

$$Y(M180) = 3.700 - \overset{*}{.113}\ TEMP + \overset{*}{.101}\ PRELEV + .116\ MALT + \overset{***}{.189}\ DISP - .123\ FRAN + \overset{*}{.144}\ SCAN + \overset{*}{.187}\ OTHEUR$$

$$Y(M180) = 3.700 - \overset{**}{.147}\ TEMP + \overset{*}{.109}\ PRELEV + .091\ CIGS + \overset{*}{.131}\ DISP - \overset{*}{.161}\ BRIT + \overset{*}{.184}\ SCAN + \overset{***}{.265}\ OTHEUR$$

The models for male mortality from cancer of the kidney indicate that cold temperatures, high precipitation, and low elevation are major factors in high death rates. Also of great importance is the consumption of malt and of distilled spirits. Cigarette consumption is a positive factor, but not a significant one.

In the models from the ethnic pools the most important effect is a positive OTHEUR with positive SCAN and negative BRIT also significant effects, as well as a negative but weak FRAN effect. Segi does not include this site in his comparisons but reference to the compilation of world cancer incidence rates by the International Union against Cancer reveals that Sweden ranks first and Norway second in kidney cancer in males, paralleling the positive SCAN effect in the models.

Surprisingly, the BMD program chose for this mortality pattern a model from the 12-variable pool that was only the seventh best LIN choice. The two LIN models explain the same amount of variation, have equal C_p values, and include an equal number of factors, but one model gives greater importance to the consumption of distilled spirits and includes MALT and negative FRAN, while the other gives greater importance to a positive Other European effect and includes CIGS and negative BRIT.

In the ridge trace the coefficient estimates of three of the major effects OTHEUR, SCAN, and DISP decrease sharply from their least squares values, and continue a gradual decrease even after general stabilization, but the other two very strong effects, MALT and negative TEMP, are stable, changing little in magnitude. Though they decrease from their least squares values the CIGS and PRELEV effects stabilize as strong factors. The INCM and BRIT effects are very unstable going from negative to positive values of some size, as opposed to their roles in the subset models.

13 Bladder and Other Urinary Organs, Males–M181 (ICD 181)

6 VAR, BMD and LIN

$$Y(M181) = 6.214 - \overset{**}{.342}\ TEMP + \overset{***}{.619}\ PRELEV + \overset{*}{.391}\ INCM + \overset{***}{.806}\ ALCO$$

8 VAR, BMD and LIN

$$Y(M181) = 6.214 - \overset{*}{.307}\ TEMP + \overset{***}{.631}\ PRELEV + .282\ CIGS + \overset{***}{.651}\ MALT + \overset{**}{.448}\ WINE$$

10 VAR, BMD

$$Y(M181) = 6.214 + \overset{***}{.610}\ PRELEV - .245\ POLLUT + \overset{***}{.562}\ ALCO + \overset{***}{.580}\ BRIT + \overset{**}{.448}\ OTHEUR$$

10 VAR, LIN

$$Y(M181) = 6.214 - \overset{*}{.243}\ TEMP + \overset{***}{.532}\ PRELEV - .271\ INCM + \overset{*}{.417}\ ALCO + \overset{*}{.440}\ FRAN + .362\ BRIT + \overset{*}{.420}\ OTHEUR$$

12 VAR, BMD and LIN

$$Y(M181) = 6.214 - .168\ TEMP + \overset{***}{.517}\ PRELEV - .363\ INCM + .331\ MALT + \overset{*}{.263}\ DISP + \overset{*}{.489}\ FRAN + .368\ BRIT + .378\ OTHEUR$$

In the male mortality models for cancer of the bladder, as in those for cancer of the kidney and for the cancers of the digestive system except pancreas, a cold climate is associated with higher death rates. PRELEV is again a significantly positive factor, relating high mortality rates to a wet climate at low elevation. In the nonethnic models alcohol consumption is the most important factor, but it shares its coefficient weight with the positive ethnic effects, FRAN, BRIT, and OTHEUR in the models from the ethnic pools. Both of the models in which ALCO is partitioned include MALT, one showing WINE also to be a significant factor, the other DISP. The models indicate that high levels of all types of alcohol consumption are associated with higher male mortality levels from cancer of the bladder. Cigarette smoking is a factor in one model, but its coefficient is not significant. The effect of INCM changes from positive to negative in this set of models after inclusion of the ethnic variables, all three of which are highly correlated with the income variable (Table V).

Three ethnic factors appear in this set of models, all as positive effects—FRAN, BRIT, and OTHEUR. France ranks in the middle in male mortality from bladder cancer, thus not matching the positive effect of FRAN in the models. However males in England and Wales and in Scotland rank very high (first, third) in bladder cancer mortality, so that the combined rank of the British countries is high in spite of a low rate for males in Ireland. This generally high mortality of men in the British countries is matched by the positive BRIT effect in the models. Sweden and Norway rank low, but Denmark ranks second, so that the combined rank for these countries is a middle one, matched by the null SCAN effect in the models. The death rates from bladder cancer are ranked by Segi for only three of the nations in the Other European group (Italy, Netherlands, and Belgium), but those all rank high, which is in agreement with the positive OTHEUR effect, and with its component effects shown in Table XIV.

According to Haenszel, men from England and Wales had higher death rates than U. S. native whites, supporting the positive BRIT effect, and men from Germany and Russia were also at higher risk, supporting the positive OTHEUR effect. He also found a lower risk in men from Ireland, in line with that country's low international ranking in male bladder cancer mortality.

The ridge trace shows that PRELEV is the most unstable of the major effects, decreasing sharply and continually but nevertheless maintaining the coefficient of greatest weight. In contrast, the stability of the BRIT effect produces a coefficient almost equal to that of PRELEV in the stabilized pattern. The OTHEUR, FRAN, and MALT effects decrease but stabilize as major factors. All the effects of moderate strength, DISP, WINE, CIGS, and negative TEMP, are quite stable with similar coefficient weights. INCM and POLLUT, both negative effects in the subset models and in the least squares solution, have very unstable coefficient estimates, which go from negative to positive.

14 Brain and Other Parts of the Nervous System, Males–M193 (ICD 193)

6 VAR, BMD and LIN; 8 VAR, BMD and Second LIN

$$Y(M193) = 4.293 + .094\,PRELEV + .135\,POLLUT - \overset{**}{.174}\,CIGS$$

10 VAR, BMD

$$Y(M193) = 4.293 + \overset{*}{.180}\,PRELEV + \overset{**}{.252}\,POLLUT - \overset{**}{.178}\,CIGS + \overset{**}{.338}\,SCAN - .245\,OTHEUR$$

10 VAR, LIN

$$Y(M193) = 4.293 + \overset{*}{.156}\,TEMP + \overset{*}{.155}\,PRELEV + \overset{**}{.266}\,POLLUT - \overset{**}{.223}\,FRAN + \overset{***}{.470}\,SCAN - .214\,OTHEUR$$

12 VAR, BMD

$$Y(M193) = 4.293 + .132\,PRELEV + \overset{**}{.237}\,POLLUT - .130\,CIGS - \overset{**}{.281}\,MALT + \overset{***}{.322}\,SCAN$$

The variation in mortality from cancer of the brain and other parts of the nervous system is not as well explained as that of other cancer primaries due to inadequacy of the variable pools. However, two variables emerge as strong positive effects–SCAN and POLLUT. Negative consumption effects alternate in the models with their associated ethnic effects–negative CIGS with negative FRAN and negative MALT with negative OTHEUR. Although the ethnic interpretation is preferable, it cannot be affirmed or rejected since this cancer site is not included in Segi's national rankings. In comparisons of international incidence rates by the International Union against Cancer, two distinct sets of rates are shown for this cancer category. In one set males in Sweden and Norway rank very high, and in the other set Danish males rank second, all three corresponding to the highly significant positive SCAN in the models.

The ridge trace shows the largest effects, POLLUT and SCAN, to be unstable, decreasing sharply, but keeping their top positions of importance. The most stable of the major effects is PRELEV, decreasing only slightly overall. The strongly negative effects in the least squares solution, MALT, FRAN, and DISP, decrease considerably in magnitude but remain negative, but the negative effect OTHEUR becomes positive. The coefficient estimate for CIGS is positive in the least squares solution but stabilizes into a negative value of some size. Thus the negative aspects of the two consumption factors CIGS and MALT which appear in the BMD and LIN models persist in the ridge trace.

15 Lymphosarcoma and Reticulosarcoma, Males–M200 (ICD 200, 202, 205)

6 VAR, BMD and LIN

$$Y(M200) = 4.641 - \overset{**}{.196}\ TEMP + \overset{**}{.237}\ POLLUT + .093\ INCM$$

8 VAR, BMD

$$Y(M200) = 4.641 - \overset{*}{.161}\ TEMP + \overset{**}{.224}\ POLLUT + .138\ MALT$$

8 VAR, LIN

$$Y(M200) = 4.641 - \overset{*}{.166}\ TEMP + .082\ PRELEV + \overset{*}{.171}\ POLLUT + \overset{*}{.167}\ MALT$$

10 and 12 VAR, BMD

$$Y(M200) = 4.641 + .097\ PRELEV + .160\ POLLUT - \overset{*}{.203}\ FRAN + .155\ BRIT + \overset{*}{.225}\ SCAN + .153\ OTHEUR$$

10 and 12 VAR, LIN

$$Y(M200) = 4.641 + \overset{**}{.252}\ POLLUT - \overset{*}{.216}\ INCM + \overset{**}{.284}\ SCAN + .232\ OTHEUR$$

The male mortality model for lymphosarcoma and rèticulosarcoma chosen from the 6-variable pool indicates that high pollution levels and cold temperatures are associated with high death rates. POLLUT is included in all the chosen models, with a positive coefficient that is significant in all but one of them. The division of ALCO brings MALT into the model, but it is dropped after inclusion of the ethnic variables, particularly its close ethnic associate, OTHEUR. All four ethnic variables are in the final BMD model, SCAN significantly positive, FRAN significantly negative, and BRIT and OTHEUR positive, but not significantly. Only two ethnic variables, both positive, are included in the final LIN model, SCAN and OTHEUR. Unfortunately this site is another one not considered by Segi. Haenszel combines deaths from Hodgkin's disease and multiple myeloma with lymphoma, so that his results are not strictly comparable with the models for this category of cancer. Nevertheless, he found that men born in the Other European countries of Austria, Russia, Poland, Italy, and Czechoslovakia showed an excess of deaths from lymphoma, confirming the positive OTHEUR effect, especially its strong Slavic component shown in Table XIV. Males from Norway and Sweden did not show excess risk in his study, and so the positive SCAN effect could not be confirmed.

In the ridge trace the OTHEUR effect is the largest and it is stable. POLLUT and SCAN are unstable, decreasing considerably in magnitude but remain major effects. The PRELEV coefficient decreases gradually but continuously while the BRIT coefficient decreases sharply but stabilizes quickly. However they are both shown to be stronger effects than indicated in the subset models, as are the very stable effects MALT and negative TEMP. The negative INCM effect as usual is highly unstable, becoming weakly positive, as opposed to its significantly negative role in the ethnic models chosen by LIN.

16 Hodgkin's Disease, Males–M201 (ICD 201)

6 VAR, BMD and LIN; 8 VAR, LIN

$$Y(M201) = 2.275 - \overset{**}{.106}\ \text{TEMP} + \overset{*}{.075}\ \text{CIGS}$$

8 VAR, BMD and Second LIN

$$Y(M201) = 2.275 - \overset{**}{.108}\ \text{TEMP} + \overset{*}{.119}\ \text{CIGS} - .060\ \text{DISP}$$

10 VAR, LIN

$$Y(M201) = 2.275 - .059\ \text{TEMP} + .078\ \text{POLLUT} - \overset{**}{.216}\ \text{INCM} + \overset{*}{.117}\ \text{CIGS} + .087\ \text{BRIT} + \overset{*}{.134}\ \text{SCAN}$$

$$Y(M201) = 2.275 + .077\ \text{POLLUT} - \overset{**}{.234}\ \text{INCM} + \overset{**}{.133}\ \text{CIGS} + .087\ \text{BRIT} + \overset{**}{.181}\ \text{SCAN}$$

12 VAR, BMD

$$Y(M201) = 2.275 - \overset{*}{.088}\ \text{TEMP} - .098\ \text{INCM} + .096\ \text{CIGS} - .058\ \text{DISP} + \overset{*}{.140}\ \text{BRIT}$$

12 VAR, LIN

$$Y(M201) = 2.275 - .077\ \text{TEMP} + \overset{**}{.111}\ \text{POLLUT} - \overset{**}{.232}\ \text{INCM} + \overset{**}{.173}\ \text{CIGS} - \overset{*}{.097}\ \text{DISP} + .084\ \text{FRAN} + \overset{**}{.168}\ \text{SCAN}$$

$$Y(M201) = 2.275 + \overset{*}{.093}\ \text{POLLUT} - \overset{**}{.228}\ \text{INCM} + \overset{**}{.185}\ \text{CIGS} - .082\ \text{DISP} + .082\ \text{BRIT} + \overset{**}{.195}\ \text{SCAN}$$

$$Y(M201) = 2.275 + \overset{**}{.110}\ \text{POLLUT} - \overset{**}{.214}\ \text{INCM} + \overset{***}{.217}\ \text{CIGS} - .085\ \text{DISP} + \overset{***}{.234}\ \text{SCAN}$$

The models for male mortality from Hodgkin's disease are similar to those for male mortality from lymphosarcoma in the negative TEMP, positive POLLUT, negative INCM, positive BRIT and positive SCAN effects. However, cigarette consumption, not in the lymphosarcoma models, emerges as a strong and consistent factor in the male mortality pattern for Hodgkin's disease, entering with significant coefficients in every model but one.

From the smallest variable pool both programs chose a two-variable model, which indicates that colder temperatures and higher levels of cigarette consumption are the primary factors in high mortality rates. When ALCO is divided, negative DISP enters the model, but not significantly. Inclusion of the ethnic variables brings BRIT positively and significantly into the BMD model, while both best LIN models bring in BRIT and SCAN positively. Negative INCM and positive POLLUT also enter the models. The models from the largest variable pool combine all the model effects selected from the smaller pools, with the most important factors in high death rates indicated to be low income, high cigarette consumption, high Scandinavian ethnicity, and high levels of pollution.

Neither Segi nor Haenszel treats deaths from Hodgkin's disease as a separate category, precluding comparison of their results with the ethnic effects in the models.

The ridge trace for this mortality is exceptionally stable, realizing a stabilized pattern very early except for two effects, negative INCM and negative DISP, which decrease greatly in magnitude. The effect that is largest in size, negative TEMP, is also the most stable, and the lesser effects, MALT and PRELEV, show stability too. The large positive effects, CIGS and SCAN, decrease sharply from their least squares estimates while the lesser BRIT effect remains stable, so that all three have coefficient weights of similar magnitude in the stabilized pattern.

17 Leukemia and Aleukemia, Males–M204 (ICD 204)

6 and 8 VAR, LIN

$$Y(M204) = 8.735 + \overset{*}{.274}\ INCM - \overset{*}{.265}\ CIGS$$

10 and 12 VAR, BMD and LIN

$$Y(M204) = 8.735 + \overset{*}{.205}\ PRELEV + .217\ INCM - \overset{***}{.587}\ BRIT + \overset{***}{.574}\ SCAN$$

The nonethnic variable pools were completely inadequate for determining a model for leukemia mortality in males, the complete 6-variable and 8-variable equations explaining only slightly over 20% of the variation. The BMD program did not even choose a model from these pools because no one variable met the required F level to enter. The LIN search chose a model that balanced positive income with negative cigarette consumption. It is the ethnic variables that are essential to a model for male leukemia mortality. In addition to positive INCM and positive PRELEV, two highly significant ethnic effects, negative BRIT and positive SCAN, are in the model from the ethnic variable pool. Addition of the ethnic variables to the pools more than doubled the potential amount of variation explained, and quadrupled the amount actually explained by the models (Table IX).

Segi shows that males in England and Wales rank seventeenth out of 20 in leukemia mortality, those in Scotland sixteenth, while the Irish males rank middle to low, the low combined rank of the British countries matching the negative influence of BRIT in the model. On the other hand, males in Denmark rank first, in Sweden second, and in Norway sixth in this mortality, strongly paralleling the positive influence of SCAN in the model. Both null ethnic effects have parallels in Segi's ranking: males in France rank in the middle, and males in the Other European countries rank from high to low, combining into a middle rank.

Since alcohol consumption is not a factor in this mortality pattern the division of ALCO into its three components in the variable pools does not change the models.

The ridge trace for leukemia, as for Hodgkin's disease, is very stable, the coefficient estimates changing little from their least squares solution, except for the two major factors. The SCAN effect, which is much larger than any of the others, and the negative BRIT effect, the second largest, both decrease sharply in magnitude but stabilize while maintaining their importance. The INCM effect has a very different trace from its usual one in the other cancer mortality patterns, because it starts strongly positive and remains so, confirming the association of higher leukemia mortality with higher income levels. The negative CIGS effect also persists in a stable manner.

18 Prostate–M177 (ICD 177)

6 VAR, BMD and Second LIN

$$Y(M177) = 18.040 - \overset{***}{.975}\ TEMP - .262\ INCM$$

8 VAR, BMD and LIN

$$Y(M177) = 18.040 - \overset{***}{.867}\ TEMP - .339\ INCM - .454\ WINE + \overset{*}{.616}\ DISP$$

10 VAR, BMD and LIN

$$Y(M177) = 18.040 - \overset{***}{.853}\ TEMP + \overset{*}{.407}\ PRELEV + \overset{*}{.604}\ SCAN - \overset{**}{.600}\ OTHEUR$$

12 VAR, BMD and LIN

$$Y(M177) = 18.040 - \overset{**}{.630}\ TEMP - \overset{*}{.567}\ INCM - \overset{*}{.493}\ WINE + \overset{**}{.695}\ DISP + .449\ SCAN$$

Negative TEMP is the primary factor in the mortality models for cancer of the prostate. Negative INCM is in most of the models, significantly in the final one. PRELEV does not have its usual importance in this set of models, entering only one, but significantly. Although ALCO is not a model effect, the division into its components indicates that states with high consumption of distilled spirits contrasted with low consumption of wine have higher levels of mortality from prostatic cancer.

SCAN enters the models positively, and this is in accordance with the very high ranks of all three Scandinavian countries in Segi's comparison of prostatic cancer mortality rates—Sweden highest, Norway second, and Denmark fourth. Haenszel confirms the positive SCAN effect with men from Norway standing second and from Sweden fourth in excess mortality risk. While the negative coefficient for OTHEUR is not justified by the middle ranks of most of the Other European countries in Segi's listing except Italy, the latter does rank very low (eighteenth), and it is the negative ITAL effect, which is shown in Table XIV to be the cause of the negative effect of OTHEUR. Haenszel, moreover, places men from Russia and from Italy as lowest in mortality from prostatic cancer, giving further justification for the negative OTHEUR effect.

The ridge regression analysis reveals that the coefficient estimates for all the variables decrease steadily in magnitude from their least squares value until a general stabilization in the pattern. The negative TEMP effect stands alone in its very large size. The SCAN effect is next largest in the stabilized pattern because it does not decrease as sharply as the DISP effect. Other factors that appear in the subset models—negative INCM, negative WINE, negative OTHEUR—as well as two additional effects— negative FRAN and positive BRIT—are shown to have moderate strength in this mortality pattern. However, in checking the international ranking, neither of these ethnic effects has a counterpart in the foreign mortality pattern of prostatic cancer.

III The Models of Female Cancer Mortality

1 *Buccal Cavity and Pharynx, Females–F140 (ICD 140-148)*

6 VAR, LIN

$$Y(F140) = 1.455 + \overset{\ast\ast}{.140}\ \text{TEMP} + .081\ \text{POLLUT} - \overset{\ast\ast}{.180}\ \text{INCM} + \overset{\ast\ast}{.136}\ \text{CIGS}$$

8 VAR, BMD and LIN

$$Y(F140) = 1.455 + .075\ \text{TEMP} + \overset{\ast}{.085}\ \text{POLLUT} + \overset{\ast}{.116}\ \text{CIGS} - \overset{\ast\ast\ast}{.262}\ \text{MALT} + .064\ \text{WINE}$$

10 VAR, BMD

$$Y(F140) = 1.455 + .081\ \text{PRELEV} + \overset{\ast\ast}{.164}\ \text{FRAN} - \overset{\ast\ast}{.149}\ \text{SCAN} - \overset{\ast}{.148}\ \text{OTHEUR}$$

10 VAR, LIN

$$Y(F140) = 1.455 + .094\ \text{POLLUT} + \overset{\ast\ast}{.158}\ \text{FRAN} - \overset{\ast}{.138}\ \text{SCAN} - \overset{\ast}{.197}\ \text{OTHEUR}$$

12 VAR, BMD

$$Y(F140) = 1.455 + .064\ \text{POLLUT} - \overset{\ast\ast\ast}{.231}\ \text{MALT} + \overset{\ast\ast\ast}{.189}\ \text{FRAN} - \overset{\ast\ast}{.136}\ \text{SCAN}$$

12 VAR, LIN

$$Y(F140) = 1.455 + \overset{\ast\ast\ast}{.132}\ \text{POLLUT} - .114\ \text{INCM} + \overset{\ast}{.103}\ \text{CIGS} - \overset{\ast\ast\ast}{.243}\ \text{MALT} + \overset{\ast\ast\ast}{.246}\ \text{FRAN} - \overset{\ast}{.145}\ \text{BRIT}$$

The models of female and of male mortality from cancer of the buccal cavity and pharynx show strong similarities in the factor patterns. In both sets of models POLLUT is a consistent and important effect, and positive FRAN is the principal ethnic factor. Although the positive TEMP effect in the female mortality models is not found in the subset models for males, it was shown to be a moderate and stable factor in the ridge trace of the male mortality pattern. Cigarette consumption enters both sets of models, but it is more important in female mortality. For both males and females WINE is a positive effect, which is replaced by the entry of the ethnic effect FRAN. However, the consumption of distilled spirits is an important factor in male mortality but does not enter any of the female mortality models for this category of cancer. In the female mortality models a significantly negative MALT alternates with a significantly negative OTHEUR, the ethnic variable most closely associated with it. Although the coefficients of MALT are more significant than those for OTHEUR, the ethnic variable is easier to interpret as a negative effect. Moreover, the negative effect of OTHEUR is a factor in the male as well as the female mortality models for this cancer category and it is also consistent with Segi's low ranking of the females in the Other European countries in death rates from this type of cancer. In addition, Haenszel ranks women from Germany lowest in this cancer mortality.

Positive FRAN, which is the strongest ethnic effect in both the male and the female mortality models, matches the top ranking of males in France but contrasts with the low ranking of females there. The implication is that this ethnic effect is not genetic, but results from some pattern of consumption or other activity which is specific to males in France, and applies to both males and females of French background in the United States. Negative SCAN is another consistent ethnic effect in the male and female mortality models for this cancer category, and it also is confirmed by the ranking of the males (very low), but not of the females in Scandinavia, who rank high. Inference again can be made that the ethnic factor is not genetic but involves a change in some custom after migration to the U. S., which brings the female risk level in line with the male. For French women the risk increased, for Scandinavian women it decreased. A British effect is not evident in the male mortality models but enters the final model for female mortality significantly negative, in sharp contrast to the very high ranks of the women living in the British countries, especially in both the Irelands. Haenszel assigns low ranks to women from England and Wales living in the U. S. but the highest rank to women from Ireland. This division within the British group indicates that the very high risk of mortality from cancer of the buccal cavity and pharynx for Irish women continues after migration to the United States, but the high risk for women from England and Wales decreases considerably, producing the negative BRIT effect in the final model.

Low income levels are a factor in the models for females but not for males in this cancer mortality. The greatest difference between the two model sets, however, is the preeminence of the strong factor PRELEV in the mortality models for males, and its almost complete absence in those for females.

The ridge regression analysis shows the coefficient estimates of all the variables except FRAN and negative MALT either to be stable or to stabilize very quickly. The negative MALT effect is very unstable, decreasing sharply and continuously in magnitude, but it remains the most important factor in the stabilized model. It is probable that the negative consumption effect is standing in for another very closely associated factor, which appears to be specifically the German component of the Other European ethnic variable. A very significant negative GERM effect is indicated in Table XIV. The correlation between MALT and the percentage foreign born in Germany is one of the highest between a consumption and an ethnic variable (r = .781), and since females in Germany rank the very lowest in this cancer mortality, the negative MALT effect might actually be a negative German effect. Since the OTHEUR variable comprises several different ethnic groups that are not always similar in their cancer mortality patterns, it is not unlikely that a consumption variable very closely correlated with one of its components may substitute for that specific ethnic effect in the models.

2 *Larynx, Females–F161 (ICD 161)*

6 VAR, BMD and LIN[a]

$$Y(F161) = .233 + .020\ \text{PRELEV} + .024\ \text{POLLUT} - \overset{**}{.052}\ \text{INCM} + .018\ \text{CIGS} + \overset{*}{.037}\ \text{ALCO}$$

8 VAR, LIN

$$Y(F161) = .233 + .020\ \text{PRELEV} + .023\ \text{POLLUT} - .029\ \text{INCM} + \overset{*}{.025}\ \text{CIGS} - .020\ \text{MALT} + \overset{**}{.032}\ \text{WINE}$$

$$Y(F161) = .233 + .022\ \text{PRELEV} + .022\ \text{POLLUT} - \overset{**}{.044}\ \text{INCM} + .022\ \text{CIGS} + \overset{**}{.032}\ \text{WINE}$$

10 VAR, BMD

$$Y(F161) = .233 + .019\ \text{PRELEV} + .015\ \text{POLLUT} - \overset{*}{.044}\ \text{INCM} + .023\ \text{ALCO} + \overset{**}{.042}\ \text{FRAN} - .023\ \text{SCAN}$$

10 VAR, LIN

$$Y(F161) = .233 + \overset{*}{.022}\ \text{PRELEV} + \overset{*}{.029}\ \text{POLLUT} - \overset{*}{.043}\ \text{INCM} + .023\ \text{ALCO} + \overset{**}{.048}\ \text{FRAN} - \overset{*}{.030}\ \text{OTHEUR}$$

12 VAR, BMD and LIN

$$Y(F161) = .233 + .015\ \text{PRELEV} + .019\ \text{POLLUT} - \overset{*}{.046}\ \text{INCM} + \overset{*}{.025}\ \text{DISP} + \overset{**}{.044}\ \text{FRAN} - .021\ \text{SCAN}$$

The models for laryngeal cancer mortality in females are very similar to those for cancer of the buccal cavity and pharynx in females, just as the same two categories of cancer have very similar models for mortality in males. And the concurrences and contrasts between the males' and females' models for cancer of the larynx are similar to those for cancer of the buccal cavity and pharynx. POLLUT is a consistent factor in the mortality models for both sexes, as are WINE and CIGS.

[a] $C_p > p$, model with bias.

The ethnic effects of laryngeal cancer mortality are like those for cancer of the buccal cavity and pharynx in that a strongly positive FRAN and negative SCAN are common to the mortality models of both sexes. The most striking similarity in these two types of cancer mortality is that negative INCM persists in the models for females while it is totally absent in those for males. The chief difference between the two cancer mortalities is that PRELEV is common to both the male and the female mortality models in laryngeal cancer, but appears strongly only in the male mortality models for cancer of the buccal cavity and pharynx. Another difference concerns the consumption factor DISP, which is indicated to be a factor in female mortality as well as male mortality from laryngeal cancer, but only in male mortality from cancer of the buccal cavity and pharynx.

Just as for the men, the ethnic effects of positive FRAN and negative SCAN are confirmed by Segi's high ranks for women in France and low ranks for women in Scandinavia in laryngeal cancer mortality. The women in the Other European countries rank lower than their male counterparts in this type of cancer mortality, those in Germany and Austria ranking very low, and this difference is repeated in the U. S. models, with a negative OTHEUR effect found only in the female mortality model. Table XIV confirms that it is a significantly negative GERM effect that underlies the negative OTHEUR effect. Finally, for cancer of the larynx as for cancer of the buccal cavity and pharynx, the high-ranking death rates of women in the British countries, particularly the top-ranked Irish, do not carry over into the U. S. experience of this ethnic group according to the models.

The ridge traces of the two largest effects, PRELEV and negative SCAN, are very stable. The POLLUT, FRAN, and DISP effects decrease and the WINE effect increases before stabilizing to coefficient estimates of almost the same magnitude. The INCM effect is very unstable but remains definitely negative.

The negative MALT and negative OTHEUR coefficients are quite stable with the consumption effect of consistently greater magnitude than the ethnic effect. The likelihood that the negative MALT effect is again standing in for the Germanic component of the ethnic composite variable OTHEUR is reinforced by the significantly negative GERM effect shown in Table XIV and by the very low ranking of women in Germany and Austria in this cancer mortality. As has been noted previously, the German and Austrian ethnic variables are the two most highly correlated with MALT.

3 Trachea, Bronchus, and Lung, Females–F166 (ICD 162, 163)

6 VAR, BMD and LIN

$$Y(F166) = 5.858 + \overset{***}{.449}\ TEMP + .188\ PRELEV + .277\ CIGS + \overset{**}{.466}\ ALCO$$

8 VAR, BMD and LIN

$$Y(F166) = 5.858 + \overset{**}{.340}\ TEMP + \overset{*}{.216}\ PRELEV + \overset{**}{.345}\ CIGS + \overset{***}{.426}\ WINE$$

10 VAR, BMD and LIN

$$Y(F166) = 5.858 + \overset{*}{.333}\ ALCO + \overset{**}{.620}\ FRAN - .338\ BRIT - \overset{***}{.672}\ SCAN + \overset{*}{.360}\ OTHEUR$$

12 VAR, BMD and Third LIN

$$Y(F166) = 5.858 + .170\ CIGS + \overset{*}{.296}\ WINE + \overset{*}{.499}\ FRAN - .365\ BRIT - \overset{***}{.602}\ SCAN + \overset{**}{.405}\ OTHEUR$$

12 VAR, LIN

$$Y(F166) = 5.858 + \overset{*}{.300}\ WINE + \overset{**}{.588}\ FRAN - .312\ BRIT - \overset{***}{.631}\ SCAN + \overset{**}{.411}\ OTHEUR$$

4 Trachea, and Bronchus and Lung Specified as Primary, Females– F162 (ICD 162)

6 VAR, BMD and LIN; 10 VAR, LIN

$$Y(F162) = 2.028 + \overset{**}{.256}\ TEMP + \overset{**}{.228}\ INCM$$

8 VAR, BMD and LIN

$$Y(F162) = 2.028 + \overset{*}{.215}\ TEMP + \overset{**}{.374}\ INCM - .195\ MALT$$

10 VAR, BMD and Second LIN

$$Y(F162) = 2.028 + \overset{**}{.274}\ TEMP + \overset{**}{.384}\ INCM - .184\ FRAN$$

12 VAR, BMD and LIN

$$Y(F162) = 2.028 + \overset{**}{.245}\ TEMP + \overset{**}{.368}\ INCM + .195\ WINE - \overset{*}{.329}\ FRAN$$

5 *Bronchus and Lung Unspecified as Primary or Secondary, Females–F163 (ICD 163)*

6 VAR, BMD and LIN

$$Y(F163) = 3.392 + .148\ TEMP + .163\ PRELEV - \overset{*}{.372}\ INCM + .284\ CIGS + \overset{**}{.549}\ ALCO$$

8 VAR, BMD and LIN

$$Y(F163) = 3.392 + .168\ TEMP + .190\ PRELEV - \overset{*}{.487}\ INCM + \overset{*}{.363}\ CIGS + \overset{*}{.401}\ MALT + \overset{*}{.292}\ WINE$$

10 VAR, BMD and Second LIN

$$Y(F163) = 3.392 - .231\ INCM + \overset{*}{.467}\ ALCO + \overset{*}{.428}\ FRAN - \overset{***}{.467}\ SCAN$$

12 VAR, BMD and LIN

$$Y(F163) = 3.392 - \overset{*}{.419}\ INCM + \overset{**}{.477}\ MALT + \overset{*}{.255}\ DISP + \overset{**}{.502}\ FRAN - \overset{***}{.554}\ SCAN$$

These three sets of mortality models, which show both the combination of and the division between the specified primary and the unspecified lung cancer deaths reported for females, indicate many similarities between the male and the female mortality patterns, even though there is a large sex difference in the size of the death rates. These similarities are described below.

(1) For both males and females the specified primary models are very different from the unspecified models. The chief dividing factor is income level, with the higher income level states reporting higher specified primary lung cancer death rates and the lower income states higher unspecified lung cancer death rates. The positive and negative income effects cancel each other in the combined category. The reason for this income effect, as described under the mortality models for males, is the likelihood of better medical services and medical recording in the more developed and wealthier states, which is associated with a more frequent specification of primary cancer.

(2) For both sexes the models of the combined category, the one most commonly used in the literature to indicate mortality from lung cancer, resemble more closely the models for the unspecified category, which is to be expected since the latter category is usually the larger one.

(3) The percentage of variation in both male and female death rates explained by the models is much less for the specified primary category than for the unspecified; hence the variable pools are not as relevant to the mortality pattern of greater interest.

(4) In both male and female mortality patterns warmer climate is the most significant factor in the specified primary lung cancer models, but in the unspecified category models the temperature variable enters only the models from the nonethnic variable pools, and nonsignificantly.

(5) For both sexes all three types of alcohol consumption appear as positive factors in the unspecified lung cancer mortality models, but WINE is the only type that enters the specified primary models positively, and its effect is not significant.

(6) CIGS is a factor in the unspecified models for both sexes, but in the specified primary category it enters only once, and nonsignificantly, the male mortality models, and does not appear in those for females.

(7) In the models for both sexes FRAN is a strong positive and SCAN a strong negative ethnic effect in the unspecified category models, but not in the specified primary models. Also for both sexes OTHEUR is a positive effect in the combined category models but not in the specified primary models.

One contrast between males and females in these sets of models is the strength of the climate factor PRELEV in the male, but not in the female, mortality patterns, a sex difference that also exists in the buccal cavity and pharynx and the larynx models. The other sex difference is in the negative effect of the ethnic variable FRAN in the specified primary models for females but not for males.

Only the combined category of specified primary and unspecified is included in Segi's study, and similar relative positions are held by the men and women in each country—those in Britain rank high, those in France and Scandinavia low, and those in the Other European countries from high to low, yielding a combined rank of middle range. Thus, for this category of cancer mortality the ethnic effects in the U. S. are matched only by the Scandinavian experience abroad. It is not surprising to find so little conformation in this category of mortality since its composition depends upon which other cancer primaries are most frequently designated as unspecified (i.e., metastatic) lung cancer. From the similarity between coefficient patterns of the female and of the male mortality models it can be concluded that for the women, as for the men, primary cancers of the buccal cavity and pharynx and of the larynx are recorded as unspecified lung cancer. It should be noted that for females the models for primary lung cancer reflect a significantly negative FRAN effect, which is in agreement with the low rank of women in France. Also the positive effect of OTHEUR is confirmed by Haenszel in his finding of excess mortality risk among women from Russia, Poland, Austria, and Germany for the combined category of lung cancer. The mortality risk of British women in this combined category appears to differ markedly in the U. S. from the high risk level they experience in their native countries, suggesting that an environmental factor is involved.

The ridge traces of the specified primary and the unspecified categories of lung cancer reveal marked differences between the two female mortality patterns in the stability of their coefficient estimates. The INCM effect is consistently and strongly positive in the specified primary pattern and consistently negative in the unspecified category. It decreases sharply in magnitude and then stabilizes in both cases, but it is a more important factor in the specified primary category, second only to the less unstable TEMP effect. POLLUT is a stable and an important effect in the specified primary category, but both the TEMP and the POLLUT effects are highly unstable in the unspecified category, going from negative to positive and never showing any strength. WINE is the only factor of at least moderate strength that the stabilized patterns of these two categories of female mortality have in common, and it is more unstable though more important in the specified primary pattern, decreasing sharply before stabilizing, while it is more stable in the unspecified pattern, increasing in value and stabilizing very quickly. The CIGS coefficient estimates show similar contrasts in the two ridge traces, decreasing sharply and approaching a zero value in the specified primary pattern, but increasing from a zero least squares value to an effect of moderate strength in the unspecified pattern. The two largest effects in the stabilized pattern for the unspecified category, negative SCAN and positive FRAN, are the most unstable, showing the largest decreases in magnitude before stabilizing and then continuing to diminish gradually.

The MALT effect has a different sign in each pattern, negative in the specified primary and positive in the unspecified but it is equally unstable in both, decreasing sharply in magnitude but maintaining moderate strength. It should be noted that half of the variables have coefficients of opposite signs in the stabilized patterns of these two categories–INCM and SCAN are positive; MALT, FRAN, DISP, and PRELEV are negative in the specified primary category; but they all have opposite signs in the unspecified. Therefore it is not surprising that factor effects common to both categories, such as WINE, TEMP, and CIGS, are stronger and more stable in the combined category than they are in the component categories. Otherwise, the ridge trace of the combined category is similar to that of its larger component, the unspecified category.

The similarity between females and males in this set of trachea, bronchus, and lung cancer mortality models is repeated in the ridge regression analysis. The primary dissimilarity between the sexes also appears in the ridge traces, i.e., the PRELEV effect is much more important in the male mortality patterns, where it is a major positive effect in both the specified primary and unspecified categories, while in the female mortality patterns it is of no importance in the specified primary category and of only moderate strength in the unspecified. However, in each case it is a stable effect.

6 *Esophagus, Females–F150 (ICD 150)*

6 VAR, BMD and LIN; 10 VAR, LIN

$$Y(F150) = .940 + .047\ PRELEV + \overset{**}{.103}\ POLLUT - \overset{***}{.145}\ INCM + \overset{***}{.166}\ CIGS$$

8 and 12 VAR, BMD and LIN

$$Y(F150) = .940 - \overset{*}{.064}\ TEMP + \overset{*}{.063}\ PRELEV + \overset{**}{.105}\ POLLUT - \overset{*}{.111}\ INCM + \overset{***}{.176}\ CIGS - \overset{**}{.111}\ MALT + \overset{***}{.125}\ WINE - .077\ DISP$$

10 VAR, BMD

$$Y(F150) = .940 + \overset{***}{.097}\ PRELEV + \overset{***}{.110}\ CIGS - \overset{*}{.065}\ SCAN$$

10 VAR, LIN

$$Y(F150) = .940 + \overset{***}{.139}\ POLLUT - \overset{***}{.177}\ INCM + \overset{***}{.180}\ CIGS$$

The mortality rates from cancer of the esophagus are even lower for females than they are for males, but the state variation in this very small category of mortality still yields interesting models. As in the models for male mortality from cancer of the esophagus the environment associated with higher death rates is defined by positive PRELEV, positive POLLUT, and negative TEMP. The moderately significant negative aspect of the TEMP effect characterizes a transition from the significantly positive effect of TEMP in the models for the respiratory and the upper, exposed cancer sites to the highly significant negative effect of TEMP in the models for the digestive and lower, internal sites. The most striking factor is the persistent effect of CIGS, which appears with highly significant positive coefficients in every model in the set. But just as the smoking effect is much greater than it is in the male models, the alcohol consumption effect is much less, and it is concentrated specifically on the consumption of wine, while MALT and DISP are weakly negative.

The sexes differ completely in ethnic factors with a negative SCAN effect in the female mortality models instead of the strongly positive OTHEUR effect of the male mortality models. Women in Norway and in Sweden rank low in mortality from cancer of the esophagus (eighteenth, sixteenth), and in Denmark they rank in the middle (ninth), resulting in a low combined rank that parallels the negative SCAN effect. The low female death rates from cancer of the esophagus in those Other European countries that are ranked in Segi have no parallel negative OTHEUR effect in the female mortality models. However, Haenszel shows that women from Russia and Czechoslovakia, two countries not listed in Segi, rank the highest in this mortality, so that the risks of all the ethnic components of OTHEUR may range from high to low, combining into a medium level that matches the null effect in the models. The middle rank of women in France conforms to the null effect of FRAN, but the high ranking of women in the British countries has no counterpart BRIT effect in the subset models. However the ridge trace indicates a stable, positive BRIT effect of moderate strength.

The only other effect shown to be stable is PRELEV, which maintains its strength, while the other major positive effects CIGS, POLLUT, and WINE decrease sharply and continuously until they fall below PRELEV in magnitude in the stable pattern. The negative SCAN effect is almost null in the least squares solution, but increases considerably in magnitude, while the negative MALT and negative INCM effects, which are initially very large, decrease in strength until they are less important than SCAN.

The significantly negative TEMP effect in the best subset model diminishes to zero in stabilizing and the negative DISP effect stabilizes to a positive factor of moderate strength in the ridge trace. Since DISP is a strong positive factor in the male mortality from cancer of the esophagus, the ridge regression estimate of a positive coefficient is indicated to be more accurate as well as easier to interpret.

7 *Stomach, Females–F151 (ICD 151)*

6 VAR, BMD and LIN

$$Y(F151) = 7.318 - \overset{***}{1.072}\ TEMP + .290\ POLLUT$$

8 VAR, BMD and LIN

$$Y(F151) = 7.318 - \overset{***}{1.080}\ TEMP + .284\ PRELEV - .332\ CIGS + \overset{*}{.522}\ MALT + \overset{*}{.594}\ WINE - \overset{*}{.576}\ DISP$$

10 VAR, BMD and LIN

$$Y(F151) = 7.318 - \overset{***}{.855}\ TEMP - \overset{**}{.736}\ INCM + \overset{***}{1.087}\ OTHEUR$$

12 VAR, BMD and Second LIN

$$Y(F151) = 7.318 - \overset{***}{.923}\ TEMP - \overset{**}{.803}\ INCM + .326\ MALT + \overset{*}{.467}\ WINE - \overset{*}{.465}\ DISP + \overset{**}{.831}\ OTHEUR$$

12 VAR, LIN

$$Y(F151) = 7.318 - \overset{***}{.985}\ TEMP - \overset{*}{.679}\ INCM + \overset{*}{.496}\ WINE - \overset{*}{.473}\ DISP + \overset{***}{.959}\ OTHEUR$$

The stomach cancer mortality pattern for females, like the mortality pattern for males with which it is highly correlated (r = .961), shows that high death rates are associated with low temperature, low income level, high consumption levels of malt and wine (and low of distilled spirits), and a high percentage of Other European ethnicity. As in the male mortality models, the negative income effect may be due to the use of stomach cancer as a catch-all for recording various types of intestinal cancer deaths, a policy that would be more common in the less developed and less wealthy states. However, negative INCM is a stronger factor in female than in male mortality for most of the respiratory and the digestive cancers, apparently representing an effect over and above the degree of sophistication in medical diagnosis and recording.

Women living in the Other European countries are ranked high by Segi in stomach cancer mortality, matching the significantly positive effect of OTHEUR in the models. Haenszel also ranks the women from Czechoslovakia, Russia, Poland, Germany, Austria, and Italy high, further confirming this ethnic effect.

In female stomach cancer mortality the factors chosen by the ridge regression analysis differ considerably from those chosen by the BMD and LIN programs in ways similar to the results in male stomach cancer mortality. SCAN becomes an important positive factor although its least squares coefficient is slightly negative. MALT also is shown to be an important factor decreasing only slightly over the trace. Although both are unstable and decrease considerably in magnitude, the negative TEMP and positive OTHEUR effects remain the largest in all the models of both male and female mortality. The negative coefficients of DISP and CIGS decrease steadily in magnitude but they remain negative effects of moderate strength in the stable pattern, but the highly unstable negative INCM effect finally goes to zero.

8 *Large Intestine excluding Rectum, Females–F153 (ICD 153)*

6 VAR, BMD and LIN

$$Y(F153) = 15.122 - \overset{***}{1.438}\ \mathrm{TEMP} + \overset{**}{1.010}\ \mathrm{PRELEV} + \overset{***}{1.104}\ \mathrm{POLLUT} + \overset{***}{1.074}\ \mathrm{CIGS}$$

8 VAR, BMD and LIN

$$Y(F153) = 15.122 - \overset{***}{1.084}\ \mathrm{TEMP} + \overset{***}{1.340}\ \mathrm{PRELEV} + \overset{*}{.729}\ \mathrm{POLLUT} + \overset{**}{1.098}\ \mathrm{CIGS} + \overset{**}{1.183}\ \mathrm{MALT} - \overset{*}{.767}\ \mathrm{DISP}$$

10 VAR, BMD and LIN

$$Y(F153) = 15.122 - \overset{**}{1.020}\ \mathrm{TEMP} + \overset{***}{1.083}\ \mathrm{PRELEV} + .630\ \mathrm{CIGS} - .767\ \mathrm{FRAN} + \overset{*}{1.223}\ \mathrm{BRIT} - \overset{*}{.969}\ \mathrm{SCAN} + \overset{***}{1.574}\ \mathrm{OTHEUR}$$

12 VAR, BMD and Second LIN[a]

$$Y(F153) = 15.122 - \overset{**}{.908}\ \mathrm{TEMP} + \overset{***}{1.181}\ \mathrm{PRELEV} + .391\ \mathrm{CIGS} + \overset{*}{.933}\ \mathrm{MALT} - \overset{*}{.687}\ \mathrm{WINE} + \overset{*}{.991}\ \mathrm{BRIT} - \overset{**}{1.078}\ \mathrm{SCAN} + \overset{*}{1.069}\ \mathrm{OTHEUR}$$

12 VAR, Third LIN

$$Y(F153) = 15.122 - \overset{*}{.649}\ \mathrm{TEMP} + \overset{**}{.947}\ \mathrm{PRELEV} + \overset{*}{.811}\ \mathrm{POLLUT} - \overset{*}{1.174}\ \mathrm{INCM} + \overset{**}{.932}\ \mathrm{CIGS} + \overset{*}{1.012}\ \mathrm{MALT} - \overset{*}{.717}\ \mathrm{WINE} + \overset{*}{.915}\ \mathrm{BRIT} + .767\ \mathrm{OTHEUR}$$

[a] $C_p > p$, model with bias.

9 Rectum, Females–F154 (ICD 154)

6 VAR, BMD and LIN[a]

$$Y(F154) = 4.329 - \overset{***}{.591}\,TEMP + \overset{*}{.303}\,PRELEV + \overset{*}{.312}\,POLLUT + .287\,CIGS + .279\,ALCO$$

8 VAR, BMD and LIN[a]

$$Y(F154) = 4.329 - \overset{***}{.562}\,TEMP + \overset{*}{.291}\,PRELEV + \overset{*}{.338}\,POLLUT - \overset{*}{.429}\,INCM + \overset{*}{.357}\,CIGS + \overset{**}{.496}\,MALT + .224\,WINE$$

10 VAR, BMD and Second LIN

$$Y(F154) = 4.329 - \overset{***}{.423}\,TEMP + .134\,PRELEV + \overset{**}{.360}\,POLLUT - \overset{***}{.751}\,INCM + \overset{**}{.417}\,CIGS + \overset{**}{.523}\,BRIT + \overset{**}{.512}\,OTHEUR$$

12 VAR, BMD and Second LIN

$$Y(F154) = 4.329 - \overset{***}{.386}\,TEMP + .165\,PRELEV + \overset{**}{.345}\,POLLUT - \overset{***}{.817}\,INCM + \overset{**}{.380}\,CIGS + .260\,MALT + \overset{**}{.526}\,BRIT + \overset{*}{.393}\,OTHEUR$$

12 VAR, LIN

$$Y(F154) = 4.329 - \overset{***}{.408}\,TEMP + \overset{***}{.451}\,POLLUT - \overset{***}{.853}\,INCM + \overset{***}{.456}\,CIGS + \overset{**}{.533}\,BRIT + \overset{**}{.529}\,OTHEUR$$

Cancer of the large intestine and cancer of the rectum are discussed together because of the high correlation between their state death rates, .954 for male rates and .923 for female rates. In addition there is an equally strong correlation between male and female death rates for each site, .962 for cancer of the large intestine, and .962 for cancer of the rectum. The four sets of models reflect these interrelationships. In all of them high death rates are associated with cold temperature, wet climate, low altitude, high pollution level, high consumption levels of cigarettes and malt (beer), and high proportions of British and Other European ethnicity. All four categories of mortality have a very large percentage of their variation explained by the final models, but more by the male mortality models than by the female (85 vs. 80%). And for both types of cancer mortality the death rate levels show little sex difference, with female mortality rates slightly higher in intestinal cancer and male mortality rates slightly higher in rectal cancer.

Table XVI presents a comparison of factor significance in intestinal and rectal cancer mortality using the best model from each variable pool. It can be

[a] $C_p > p$, model with bias.

TABLE XVI

Comparison of Factor Significance in Intestinal and Rectal Cancer Mortality[a]

	Large Intestine								Rectum							
	Males				Females				Males				Females			
Factor	6V	8V	10V	12V	6V	8V	10V	12V	6V	8V	10V	12V	6V	8V	10V	12V
–TEMP	***	**	*	ns	***	***	**	*	***	***	***	***	***	***	***	***
+PRELEV	***	***	***	***	**	***	***	**	**	***	**	**	*	*	ns	ns
+POLLUT	*	*	ns	*	***	*		*	**	*	*	*	*	*	**	**
–INCM	(+)*			ns				*			**	***		*	***	***
+CIGS	ns	*	ns	*	***	**	ns	**	ns	*	**	**	ns	*	**	**
+MALT	–	***	–	*	–	**	–	*	–	**	–	ns	–	**	–	ns
–WINE	–		–	ns	–		–	*	–		–		–	(+)ns	–	
–DISP	–		–		–	*	–		–		–		–		–	
–FRAN	–	–			–	–	ns		–	–			–	–		
+BRIT	–	–	*	**	–	–	*	*	–	–	***	***	–	–	**	**
–SCAN	–	–			–	–	*		–	–			–	–		
+OTHEUR	–	–	**	*	–	–	***	ns	–	–	***	**	–	–	**	*

[a]Effects in the best model from each variable pool.

–, Not in the variable pool.
ns, In model with nonsignificant coefficient.
*, In model with coefficient significance $.01 < p < .05$.
**, In model with coefficient significance $.001 < p < .01$.
***, In model with coefficient significance $p < .001$.

seen that the environmental factors negative TEMP and positive PRELEV are the most consistently significant effects in the four sets of models. The third environmental factor, POLLUT, is also an important factor, but of less significance, with the exception of female mortality from rectal cancer. Negative INCM is a marginal factor in intestinal cancer mortality, but it is a very significant effect in the rectal cancer models after adjustment for the ethnic factors. The significance of cigarette consumption persists in the models for both sexes for both types of cancer mortality, even after adjustment for the ethnic effects. On the other hand, MALT is a very important factor whose significance decreases when its closely related ethnic variable, OTHEUR, enters the models. This does not mean that MALT is not a factor in the mortality models for these sites, for it appears in all the final models. Evidently a large part of the effect of this component of alcohol consumption operates through the two ethnic variables with which it is most closely correlated, OTHEUR (r = .834) and BRIT (r = .765), but even after adjustment for these significantly positive ethnic factors a positive MALT effect remains in the models.

Two strong ethnic effects that are in all four sets of models are positive OTHEUR and positive BRIT. The latter is corroborated by high ranks in mortality from intestinal and rectal cancer for the women as well as for the men living in the British countries. However the middle to low ranks in intestinal cancer death rates of the women as well as the men living in the Other European countries listed in Segi do not match the positive OTHEUR effect in the models. Haenszel partially confirms this ethnic effect in the female mortality models, as he did for the males, by ranking Russian-born women highest in mortality risk from intestinal cancer. The positive effect of OTHEUR in rectal cancer mortality is matched by the high ranking of women as well as of men in Austria, Belgium, and Germany, and it is confirmed by Haenszel, who places women from Czechoslovakia, Poland, Russia, and Austria above the U. S. native born in this mortality risk.

Two more ethnic effects, negative FRAN and negative SCAN, are found only in the female mortality models for intestinal cancer. These negative ethnic effects do not have a counterpart in the foreign ranking. Women in France rank in the middle, and women in the Scandinavian countries rank from high to low, resulting in a combined rank of middle value. However, Haenszel ranks women from Norway and from Sweden low in intestinal cancer mortality, confirming the negative SCAN effect in the models. The instability and weakness of these two ethnic effects are apparent in the ridge trace where they reduce to almost null in the stabilized patterns of both cancer mortalities. The ridge regression analysis confirms the identical nature of the factor sets in both types of cancer mortality, with differences only in the order of importance of individual effects. The PRELEV effect is more important in intestinal cancer but somewhat less stable than it is in rectal cancer. The negative TEMP effect decreases gradually but continuously in both cancer patterns but it is of relatively more importance in rectal cancer. The coefficients of the five variables POLLUT, MALT, CIGS, BRIT, and OTHEUR approach identity in the stabilized patterns of both cancer mortalities. The POLLUT effect is the most stable one in both patterns but it is exceptionally consistent in intestinal cancer, barely deviating from its least squares estimate. INCM is the most unstable effect in both cancers going from strongly negative to zero or positive.

There is just one substantial difference between the subset models and the stable patterns of the ridge trace—because of its stability the PRELEV effect is given more importance in the ridge regression model.

10 Biliary Passages and Liver Specified as Primary and Unspecified, Females—F155 (ICD 155, Unspecified Part of ICD 156)

6 VAR, BMD and LIN

$$\begin{aligned} Y(F155) = {} & 5.087 - \overset{***}{.473}\ \mathrm{TEMP} - .266\ \mathrm{PRELEV} + \overset{***}{.536}\ \mathrm{POLLUT} \\ & - \overset{*}{.289}\ \mathrm{ALCO} \end{aligned}$$

8 VAR, BMD and Second LIN

$$\begin{aligned} Y(F155) = {} & 5.087 - \overset{**}{.341}\ \mathrm{TEMP} - .165\ \mathrm{PRELEV} + \overset{**}{.429}\ \mathrm{POLLUT} \\ & - \overset{*}{.376}\ \mathrm{INCM} + \overset{***}{.625}\ \mathrm{MALT} - \overset{**}{.407}\ \mathrm{DISP} \end{aligned}$$

10 VAR, BMD and LIN

$$\begin{aligned} Y(F155) = {} & 5.087 - \overset{***}{.460}\ \mathrm{TEMP} - \overset{**}{.312}\ \mathrm{PRELEV} - \overset{***}{.461}\ \mathrm{FRAN} - \overset{***}{.698}\ \mathrm{SCAN} \\ & + \overset{***}{.957}\ \mathrm{OTHEUR} \end{aligned}$$

12 VAR, BMD and LIN

$$\begin{aligned} Y(F155) = {} & 5.087 - \overset{***}{.438}\ \mathrm{TEMP} - \overset{*}{.194}\ \mathrm{PRELEV} - .160\ \mathrm{CIGS} + \overset{***}{.638}\ \mathrm{MALT} \\ & - .222\ \mathrm{DISP} - \overset{*}{.333}\ \mathrm{FRAN} - \overset{***}{.722}\ \mathrm{SCAN} + \overset{***}{.565}\ \mathrm{OTHEUR} \end{aligned}$$

As was stated in the section on the male mortality models for cancer of the biliary passages and liver, this category includes both specified and unspecified primary liver cancer. It also involves two different primary cancers, liver and gallbladder, which differ in their incidence in males and in females. Not only is cancer of the gallbladder more likely to occur in women than in men, but the ratio of gallbladder to liver cancer mortality is usually higher for women than it is for men (31). Thus it is logical to assume that the influence of gallbladder cancer is greater in the female mortality models for this combined category and that liver cancer is predominant in the male mortality models. To the extent of this division, differences between the sets of male and female mortality models will reflect factor differences between mortality from cancer of the liver and of the gallbladder.

This contrast is particularly emphasized by the opposite aspects of the factor PRELEV in both model sets, significantly positive in the male mortality pattern but significantly negative in the female. Thus a low altitude and wet climate are associated with higher male mortality in this category of cancer, but a high altitude and dry climate are associated with higher female mortality. This difference is diminished in the ridge regression analysis, which shows the positive PRELEV effect to be stable and very strong in the stabilized model of male mortality, but the negative PRELEV effect to be unstable and diminish to almost null in the female mortality model. It should be noted that female mortality from cancer of the biliary passages and liver has the only cancer mortality pattern in which PRELEV enters the subset models so consistently and significantly negative, although it does so for several of the noncancer major categories of death (Table XI).

Cold temperature is a much more important factor in high levels of female mortality than of male, according to the subset models, and in the ridge trace, while the TEMP coefficient goes to zero in the stabilized male mortality model, it maintains its importance in spite of decreasing magnitude in the stabilized female mortality model.

In both the male and female mortality models POLLUT is an important effect until the ethnic variables enter, and negative INCM also enters only the nonethnic models in both sets. In the ridge trace the POLLUT effect maintains its strength after adjustment for ethnic effects in the stabilized models for both sexes, and it is especially stable in the female mortality pattern.

The model sets for males and for females have both similarities and differences in their ethnic factors. In both sets negative SCAN and positive OTHEUR are significant ethnic effects, the former partially and the latter strongly paralleled by foreign ranking. Just as with the men, it is the women in Norway who rank very low in this type of mortality while those in Denmark and Sweden rank in the middle. The ranks of women living in the Other European countries are even higher than those of their male counterparts—Germany the highest, Italy second, Austria third, Netherlands fourth, and Belgium sixth, confirming OTHEUR's greater importance in the female mortality models.

OTHEUR is also shown to be a very strong effect in the stabilized pattern, but although the ridge trace confirms the top position of negative SCAN in the male mortality model, it shows this effect to be unstable and diminished to negligible value in the female mortality model. This could happen if Scandinavian males and females were at very low mortality risk in liver cancer but the females suffered a moderate to high mortality risk from cancer of the biliary passages (gallbladder), a large component of the female deaths in this mixed category.

The French effect is significantly positive in male mortality and significantly negative in female, while men in France rank high (second out of 18) but the women rank in the upper middle range (seventh). This effect diminishes in magnitude to a very weak position in the stable model of female mortality. The other sex difference in ethnicity is a significantly negative BRIT effect in the male mortality models, which does not enter the female mortality models, although women in the British countries rank even lower than their male counterparts in this combined category of cancer deaths.

The important but unknown ratio of gallbladder to liver cancer deaths combined with the unknown proportion of unspecified liver cancer involved in each death rate prevent a better comparison between male and female mortality patterns and between their model effects and foreign ranking.[a]

11 Pancreas, Females–F157 (ICD 157)

6 VAR, BMD and LIN

$$Y(F157) = 5.670 - \overset{*}{.123}\ \mathrm{TEMP} + \overset{*}{.149}\ \mathrm{POLLUT} - \overset{*}{.190}\ \mathrm{INCM} + \overset{***}{.305}\ \mathrm{ALCO}$$

8 VAR, BMD and LIN

$$Y(F157) = 5.670 - \overset{**}{.180}\ \mathrm{TEMP} + \overset{**}{.163}\ \mathrm{POLLUT} - .122\ \mathrm{INCM} + \overset{***}{.241}\ \mathrm{WINE}$$

10 VAR, BMD and Second LIN

$$Y(F157) = 5.670 + \overset{**}{.184}\ \mathrm{POLLUT} - \overset{*}{.278}\ \mathrm{INCM} + \overset{***}{.311}\ \mathrm{ALCO} + \overset{*}{.181}\ \mathrm{SCAN}$$

12 VAR, LIN

$$Y(F157) = 5.670 - \overset{*}{.143}\ \mathrm{TEMP} + .121\ \mathrm{POLLUT} - \overset{*}{.225}\ \mathrm{INCM} + \overset{**}{.231}\ \mathrm{WINE} + .167\ \mathrm{OTHEUR}$$

The variable pools are as inadequate for determining models of female mortality from cancer of the pancreas as they were for male mortality, since no model explains as much as 50% of the variation in the mortality pattern of either sex. However, the highly significant positive coefficients for WINE in both the male and the female mortality models should point to this type of alcohol consumption as a strong factor in this cancer mortality. The ridge trace shows the WINE effect, though unstable, to maintain its major importance in the stabilized mortality models for both sexes. The alcohol consumption factor, DISP, does not appear in the subset models for male mortality and weakly enters one of the

[a]More detailed discussion of liver and gallbladder model effects is found in Chapter 8.

female mortality models, but its importance is brought out by the ridge regression analysis. It is an exceptionally stable and very strong positive effect in the stabilized model of female mortality from cancer of the pancreas. The only other effects the male and female mortality models have in common are negative INCM and positive SCAN. The ethnic effect is paralleled by the foreign ranking even more markedly for females than for males, since women in Sweden and Denmark rank first and second, higher than their high-ranked male counterparts. The Scandinavian effect is vitiated in both cases by the low rank of Norway, the women ranking lower than the men. The SCAN effect is unstable in the ridge regression, diminishing to a negligible status in the female as well as the male stabilized mortality models.

The positive effect of OTHEUR, found in the female models but not in the male, is in contrast to the low ranking of women living in the Other European countries listed in Segi, but its validity in the U. S. models is reinforced by Haenszel's ranking of women from Austria first, from Russia third and from Poland seventh, above the U. S. native-born whites. Table XIV shows the weakly positive OTHEUR effect to be the combination of a highly significant positive SLAV effect and a very significant negative GERM effect. Although the magnitude of the OTHEUR effect diminishes in the ridge regression, it remains a very strong factor in the stabilized model.

There are also large differences in the environmental factors indicated in the mortality patterns for both sexes. A highly significant and positive PRELEV consistently enters the models for males, while negative TEMP and positive POLLUT characterize those for females.

12 Kidney, Females–F180 (ICD 180)

6 VAR, BMD and Second LIN

$$Y(F180) = 1.970 - \overset{***}{.232}\ TEMP + .047\ PRELEV$$

8 VAR, LIN

$$Y(F180) = 1.970 - \overset{***}{.147}\ TEMP - \overset{*}{.109}\ CIGS + \overset{**}{.151}\ MALT - \overset{*}{.135}\ WINE + .122\ DISP$$

10 VAR, BMD and LIN

$$Y(F180) = 1.970 - \overset{***}{.186}\ TEMP + .069\ PRELEV - \overset{***}{.237}\ BRIT + \overset{*}{.133}\ SCAN + \overset{**}{.172}\ OTHEUR$$

12 VAR, BMD and LIN

$$Y(F180) = 1.970 - \overset{***}{.149}\ TEMP + \overset{*}{.072}\ PRELEV + .105\ MALT - .100\ FRAN - \overset{*}{.167}\ BRIT + \overset{*}{.133}\ SCAN + .114\ OTHEUR$$

Just as for males the kidney cancer mortality models for females show that cold climate is a highly significant factor in elevated death rates. Positive PRELEV is also an important climate factor in both the male and the female mortality patterns. Alcohol consumption is not as important in female mortality as it is in the male, but the same components, MALT and DISP, are in the models for both sexes. CIGS is a positive factor only for males, and its negative coefficient, along with that of WINE, in the female mortality models from the non-ethnic variable pools probably represents the statistical effort to account for variation that is actually due to the ethnic variables. These negative consumption effects leave the models when the ethnic variables enter them. The negative CIGS effect goes to zero in the ridge trace but the negative WINE effect is very stable, maintaining its importance in the stabilized model.

The ethnic effects in the models for females are the same as those for males, but of differing significance. The factors of low French and British ethnicity and high Scandinavian and Other European ethnicity are associated with higher female, as well as male, death rates from cancer of the kidney. Although the OTHEUR effect is not significant in the final model of the female mortality set, in contrast to its high significance in the male mortality models, it shows great strength in the stabilized female mortality model in spite of a sharp drop from its least squares value. It is shown in Table XIV to combine a very strongly positive SLAV effect with very strongly negative GERM and ITAL effects.

Unfortunately neither Segi nor Haenszel includes this type of cancer in his ranking. The IUAC comparison of 60 incidence rates does rank women in Sweden the highest, paralleling the positive Scandinavian effect in the models.

In the ridge trace the major effect, negative TEMP, shows a gradual but continuous decrease in magnitude. The major positive effects OTHEUR, MALT, and SCAN also decline but the SCAN coefficient only minimally. The PRELEV, DISP, and negative BRIT effects decrease sharply, becoming factors of only marginal value. The negative coefficient estimate for FRAN decreases sharply in magnitude while the negative WINE coefficient estimate is very stable, both showing strength in the stabilized pattern.

13 *Bladder and Other Urinary Organs, Females–F181 (ICD 181)*

6 VAR, BMD and LIN

$$\begin{aligned} Y(F181) = {} & 2.247 - \overset{*}{.086}\ \text{TEMP} + \overset{**}{.133}\ \text{PRELEV} + \overset{**}{.163}\ \text{POLLUT} \\ & - \overset{***}{.241}\ \text{INCM} + \overset{**}{.164}\ \text{CIGS} + \overset{***}{.249}\ \text{ALCO} \end{aligned}$$

8 VAR, BMD and LIN

$$\begin{aligned} Y(F181) = {} & 2.247 - .087\ \text{TEMP} + \overset{**}{.134}\ \text{PRELEV} + \overset{**}{.163}\ \text{POLLUT} \\ & - \overset{**}{.242}\ \text{INCM} + \overset{**}{.165}\ \text{CIGS} + .088\ \text{MALT} + .103\ \text{WINE} + .095\ \text{DISP} \end{aligned}$$

10 VAR, BMD and LIN

$$\begin{aligned} Y(F181) = {} & 2.247 - \overset{***}{.159}\ \text{TEMP} + \overset{***}{.174}\ \text{PRELEV} + \overset{***}{.281}\ \text{ALCO} + .105\ \text{BRIT} \\ & - \overset{***}{.277}\ \text{SCAN} \end{aligned}$$

12 VAR, BMD

$$\begin{aligned} Y(F181) = {} & 2.247 - \overset{**}{.146}\ \text{TEMP} + \overset{***}{.167}\ \text{PRELEV} + \overset{*}{.110}\ \text{MALT} + .079\ \text{WINE} \\ & + \overset{*}{.139}\ \text{DISP} + .110\ \text{BRIT} - \overset{***}{.282}\ \text{SCAN} \end{aligned}$$

12 VAR, LIN

$$\begin{aligned} Y(F181) = {} & 2.247 - \overset{*}{.114}\ \text{TEMP} + \overset{**}{.116}\ \text{PRELEV} + .074\ \text{POLLUT} \\ & - .121\ \text{INCM} + \overset{*}{.137}\ \text{MALT} + \overset{***}{.208}\ \text{DISP} + \overset{**}{.158}\ \text{BRIT} - \overset{***}{.245}\ \text{SCAN} \end{aligned}$$

The models chosen from the nonethnic pools for explaining the variation in female mortality from cancer of the bladder use every available variable. A cold and wet climate at low elevation is associated with higher mortality rates for females, just as it is for males. But positive POLLUT is an important effect in female mortality and not in male mortality. Low income levels and high consumption levels of cigarettes and alcohol are important factors for both sexes. When ALCO is divided, all three of its components enter the models with positive coefficients, but the final model emphasizes MALT and DISP as it does in the male mortality set.

With such agreement between the male and female models in the nonethnic variables, it is surprising to note that their only common ethnic effect is positive BRIT. As do the men, the women in Scotland and in England and Wales rank very high (first, third) while those in Ireland rank much lower (eleventh), but their combined rank is still high, matching the positive BRIT effect in the models. Haenszel ranks women from England and Wales fourth and from Ireland sixth in bladder cancer mortality, further confirming the British effect. Negative SCAN, which is a characteristic only of the female mortality models, must be due primarily to its Swedish component since women in Sweden are ranked low by Segi, and women from Sweden are ranked low by Haenszel. Norwegian women are given middle ranking by Segi and by Haenszel, while women in Denmark rank very high.

Ridge regression analysis indicates that, of the major effects, four–PRELEV, POLLUT, CIGS, and WINE–are very stable, and DISP shows only a gradual decrease. However the negative SCAN effect is very unstable, decreasing sharply in magnitude and continuing a gradual diminishment in the stabilized pattern. The negative TEMP and the negative INCM effects are very unstable, the INCM effect going to zero. The MALT, BRIT, and OTHEUR coefficient estimates diminish sharply, then stabilize into values of moderate strength.

14 Brain and Other Parts of the Nervous System, Females–F193 (ICD 193)

6 and 8 VAR, BMD and LIN

$$Y(F193) = 2.835 - \overset{*}{.090}\ TEMP + \overset{**}{.141}\ POLLUT - \overset{**}{.140}\ CIGS$$

10 VAR, LIN

$$Y(F193) = 2.835 + \overset{***}{.237}\ POLLUT - \overset{**}{.161}\ FRAN + \overset{***}{.252}\ SCAN - .127\ OTHEUR$$

12 VAR, BMD and LIN

$$Y(F193) = 2.835 + \overset{***}{.223}\ POLLUT - \overset{**}{.171}\ MALT - \overset{*}{.133}\ FRAN + \overset{***}{.265}\ SCAN$$

The models for female and male mortality from cancer of the brain explain less than 50% of the state variation, but two factors appear in all of them with consistent strength. The significantly positive coefficients of POLLUT indicate a strong association between high pollution levels and high mortality levels from brain cancer. The significantly positive coefficients of SCAN in all the models from the ethnic pools show that Scandinavians are at higher risk from this mortality. Since neither Segi nor Haenszel considers this cancer site, reference is made to the comparison of national incidence rates by the International Union against Cancer. Women in Sweden, Norway, and Denmark are shown to have very high incidence rates of brain cancer, just as do their male counterparts, paralleling the SCAN effect in the mortality models for both sexes.

These two factors are also the major ones in the stabilized pattern of the ridge trace although they are very unstable, decreasing greatly from their extremely high values in the least squares solution of the full model.

The coefficient estimate for negative CIGS follows an unusual path in the ridge trace, positive in its least squares value, then changing rapidly to a strongly negative value, and then gradually decreasing in magnitude. Although this negative smoking effect is difficult to interpret as a major factor in brain cancer mortality, it appears with strength in both the male and female mortality models. The closely related ethnic factor FRAN also enters the models for both sexes as a negative effect of moderate strength.

This is another cancer primary for which the male mortality models contain a strong PRELEV effect not found in the female mortality models. Here the PRELEV coefficient estimate is very stable at a very low magnitude, as is the negative coefficient of TEMP. The OTHEUR effect is very unstable turning from negative, as it is in the subset models, to weakly positive, while the negative MALT effect diminishes sharply in magnitude to a weak value in the stabilized model.

15 Lymphosarcoma and Reticulosarcoma, Females–F200 (ICD 200, 202, 205)

6 and 8 VAR, LIN

$$Y(F200) = 3.108 - \overset{**}{.146}\ TEMP + .094\ POLLUT + \overset{**}{.152}\ INCM$$

10 and 12 VAR, BMD and LIN

$$Y(F200) = 3.108 + \overset{*}{.116}\ POLLUT - \overset{*}{.109}\ FRAN + \overset{***}{.228}\ SCAN + \overset{*}{.157}\ OTHEUR$$

The models for female mortality from lymphosarcoma and reticulosarcoma differ from those for males in the absence of the positive effects PRELEV, MALT, and BRIT. Positive SCAN is the strongest model effect for both sexes. Segi does not include this cancer group in his comparisons, while Haenszel combines it with multiple myeloma and Hodgkin's disease. In his combined category Haenszel shows that foreign-born women from Russia, Poland, and Austria have an excess mortality risk, thereby confirming the positive OTHEUR effect in the models. The importance of the Slavic component of OTHEUR in this type of mortality is shown in Table XIV. This corroboration was similarly shown for the men.

In the ridge regression analysis the coefficient estimate of SCAN decreases sharply and that of OTHEUR somewhat less, both ethnic effects continuing a gradual decrease in the stabilized pattern but remaining the two largest in value. The POLLUT coefficient estimates follow a similar path but at a smaller magnitude. The INCM effect, after a small increase from its least squares value, is very stable and appears a factor to be considered in mortality from lymphosarcoma and reticulosarcoma. The negative TEMP effect is also very stable in its strong position. While both the MALT and FRAN coefficient estimates are negative in the least squares solution, instability in MALT turns it into a strongly positive effect, but instability in FRAN simply decreases the magnitude of its negative effect.

16 Hodgkin's Disease, Females–F201 (ICD 201)

6 VAR, BMD and LIN

$$Y(F201) = 1.290 - \overset{***}{.154}\ TEMP + .062\ PRELEV + \overset{*}{.064}\ POLLUT$$

8 VAR, BMD and LIN

$$Y(F201) = 1.290 - \overset{***}{.120}\ TEMP + \overset{**}{.097}\ PRELEV + \overset{*}{.068}\ MALT$$

10 and 12 VAR, BMD and LIN

$$Y(F201) = 1.290 - \overset{*}{.074}\ TEMP + .053\ PRELEV + \overset{**}{.133}\ POLLUT - \overset{**}{.181}\ INCM + \overset{*}{.090}\ CIGS + \overset{***}{.191}\ SCAN$$

The models for female mortality from Hodgkin's disease chosen by the computer programs from all the variable pools are concentrated into a set of only three distinct ones, whereas eight models emerged for the male mortality pattern. The frequent environmental combination of cold and wet climate at low elevation and high pollution levels is associated with high female mortality rates but only the pollution factor enters the male mortality models. The strong effect of cigarette consumption for males, though not as significant and consistent for females, does enter the final model for female mortality as the only consumption factor. The strongly positive Scandinavian effect is also a factor in both male and female mortality. Unfortunately this cancer primary is another not included in Segi's study, while Haenszel combines it with the much larger lymphosarcoma category.

In Table IX it can be seen that a highly significant positive SCAN effect characterizes the male and female mortality models for cancer of the brain, for lymphosarcoma and reticulosarcoma, for Hodgkin's disease, and for leukemia. Of the four only leukemia mortality is ranked by Segi, and the very high-ranking mortality of the Scandinavians strongly parallels the positive SCAN effect in the models for leukemia. It is possible that the Scandinavians would rank similarly high in comparable types of cancer–lymphosarcoma and reticulosarcoma, Hodgkin's disease, and perhaps brain cancer–to match the SCAN effect, which appears so strongly and consistently in the models of these cancer mortalities.

In the ridge trace negative TEMP is stable and much greater in magnitude than all the other effects, just as it is in the stabilized male mortality model for Hodgkin's disease. The PRELEV effect is stable, as it is in the male mortality pattern, but it is more important in the female model. The other major effect, SCAN, decreases sharply from its least squares value. The remaining effects diminish to values of similarly small magnitude in the stabilized model, the positive POLLUT effect remaining the largest among them.

17 Leukemia and Aleukemia, Females–F204 (ICD 204)

6 and 8 VAR, BMD and LIN

$$Y(F204) = 5.665 + \overset{**}{.237}\ INCM - \overset{**}{.208}\ CIGS$$

10 and 12 VAR, BMD and LIN

$$Y(F204) = 5.665 + \overset{**}{.190}\ POLLUT - \overset{**}{.255}\ BRIT + \overset{***}{.309}\ SCAN$$

The leukemia mortality models for females explain even less of the variation than they do for males, 31.5% compared with 47.3% by the best model in each set, but the ethnic effects that emerge for both sexes are consistent, highly significant, and strongly related to the experience of their male and female counterparts abroad. Segi ranks women in the Scandinavian countries almost as high as their male counterparts–Denmark first for men and second for women, Sweden second for men and third for women, and Norway sixth for men and eighth for women, out of 20. And he ranks women in the British countries as low or lower than their male counterparts–women in Ireland fifteenth, in England and Wales sixteenth, in Scotland seventeenth, and in Northern Ireland nineteenth. Haenszel confirms these ethnic effects in the U. S., ranking women born in Sweden and in Norway third and fourth, and women born in Ireland and in England and Wales ninth and eleventh, out of 12. Therefore the negative BRIT and positive SCAN effects in the models are matched by the foreign experience and corroborated by the Haenszel study.

The nonethnic factors common to both sexes are positive INCM and negative CIGS, while a significantly positive POLLUT effect in the female mortality model replaces the PRELEV effect in the male mortality model.

The ridge regression analysis shows the two major effects in the stabilized pattern to be SCAN and INCM, both having decreased greatly from their very large least squares values. As in the male mortality pattern, the negative CIGS effect is stable and moderately strong even though its interpretation is difficult. The POLLUT effect is also a stable factor of moderate strength in the female mortality pattern, whereas in the ridge trace of the male mortality pattern it decreased from a strongly positive least squares value to a slightly negative one. The ethnic effects negative FRAN and negative BRIT decrease sharply in magnitude while the OTHEUR effect increases, going from negative to positive, all stabilizing at values of moderate strength.

18 Breast, Females–F170 (ICD 170)

6 VAR, BMD and LIN

$$\begin{aligned} Y(F170) &= 23.856 - \overset{***}{1.648}\ \text{TEMP} + \overset{**}{1.017}\ \text{PRELEV} + \overset{*}{.855}\ \text{POLLUT} \\ &\quad + \overset{**}{1.207}\ \text{INCM} + \overset{*}{.870}\ \text{ALCO} \end{aligned}$$

8 VAR, BMD and LIN

$$\begin{aligned} Y(F170) &= 23.856 - \overset{***}{1.572}\ \text{TEMP} + \overset{***}{1.128}\ \text{PRELEV} + \overset{*}{.756}\ \text{POLLUT} \\ &\quad + \overset{*}{.966}\ \text{INCM} + .854\ \text{MALT} + .517\ \text{WINE} \end{aligned}$$

10 VAR, BMD

$$\begin{aligned} Y(F170) &= 23.856 - \overset{***}{1.235}\ \text{TEMP} + \overset{**}{.845}\ \text{PRELEV} + \overset{*}{.666}\ \text{POLLUT} \\ &\quad + .521\ \text{ALCO} + \overset{*}{.820}\ \text{BRIT} + \overset{**}{1.240}\ \text{OTHEUR} \end{aligned}$$

12 VAR, BMD

$$\begin{aligned} Y(F170) &= 23.856 - \overset{***}{1.187}\ \text{TEMP} + \overset{**}{.769}\ \text{PRELEV} + \overset{*}{.695}\ \text{POLLUT} \\ &\quad + .391\ \text{DISP} + \overset{*}{.880}\ \text{BRIT} + \overset{**}{1.369}\ \text{OTHEUR} \end{aligned}$$

12 VAR, LIN

$$\begin{aligned} Y(F170) &= 23.856 - \overset{***}{1.099}\ \text{TEMP} + \overset{**}{.825}\ \text{PRELEV} + \overset{*}{.809}\ \text{POLLUT} \\ &\quad + .382\ \text{DISP} + \overset{*}{.831}\ \text{BRIT} + .348\ \text{SCAN} + \overset{*}{1.166}\ \text{OTHEUR} \end{aligned}$$

19 Ovary, Fallopian Tubes and Broad Ligament–F175 (ICD 175)

6 and 8 VAR, BMD and LIN

$$Y(F175) = 8.077 - \overset{***}{.561}\ \text{TEMP} + \overset{*}{.244}\ \text{PRELEV} + .243\ \text{POLLUT} + \overset{***}{.595}\ \text{INCM}$$

10 VAR, BMD and Second LIN

$$\begin{aligned} Y(F175) &= 8.077 - \overset{**}{.258}\ \text{TEMP} + \overset{*}{.189}\ \text{PRELEV} + .216\ \text{POLLUT} + .175\ \text{INCM} \\ &\quad + \overset{*}{.281}\ \text{CIGS} - \overset{**}{.424}\ \text{FRAN} + \overset{*}{.315}\ \text{SCAN} + \overset{***}{.573}\ \text{OTHEUR} \end{aligned}$$

10 and 12 VAR, LIN

$$\begin{aligned} Y(F175) &= 8.077 - \overset{*}{.248}\ \text{TEMP} + .156\ \text{PRELEV} + \overset{*}{.275}\ \text{POLLUT} + \overset{**}{.331}\ \text{CIGS} \\ &\quad - \overset{**}{.392}\ \text{FRAN} + \overset{**}{.376}\ \text{SCAN} + \overset{***}{.606}\ \text{OTHEUR} \end{aligned}$$

According to the models high mortality rates from cancer of the breast occur in states with colder temperatures, more rain, lower elevation, higher income and pollution levels, and higher alcohol consumption. When ethnic variables are included in the pool, the high positive coefficient for INCM is replaced with high positive coefficients for BRIT and OTHEUR. Segi ranks England and Wales second and Scotland fourth in breast cancer mortality, matching the positive BRIT effect. However, of the Other European group only Netherlands ranks high (first). Haenszel ranks women from England and Wales second and from Ireland third in mortality risk from breast cancer, confirming the BRIT effect in the models. Haenszel, as does Segi, assigns low ranks to women from the Other European countries, and so the positive OTHEUR effect in the models is not confirmed. One of the models includes a positive but not significant SCAN effect. Of the Scandinavian countries only Denmark ranks high in breast cancer mortality, Sweden is in the middle third, and Norway ranks low. The mixed ranking in this group is in line with the weakness of the positive SCAN effect.

The models with the ALCO division in the variable pool simply divide the effect of this variable into positive but nonsignificant coefficients for one or more of each of its components.

For ovarian cancer mortality the models are similar to those for breast cancer, which is to be expected since these two mortality patterns are highly correlated (r = .908). The models for both sites from the nonethnic pools have the same effects with the exception of positive ALCO in the breast cancer model. The ethnic patterns for these two related primary sites have in common the positive effects of SCAN and OTHEUR, but the positive BRIT effect in breast cancer mortality is replaced by a negative FRAN effect in ovarian cancer mortality. The SCAN and FRAN ethnic effects in the ovarian cancer models are matched by Segi's ranking. Women in Denmark and Sweden rank first and second, respectively, paralleling the positive SCAN effect, while French women rank fifteenth out of 16 in the comparison, matching the negative FRAN effect. Although the women in England, Wales, and Scotland rank high in ovarian cancer mortality, those in the Irelands rank low, producing a combined rank of moderate value that is in line with the null BRIT effect in the models. In cancer of the ovary, as in cancer of the breast, the significantly positive coefficient of OTHEUR is not paralleled by the combined foreign ranking, since again only the Netherlands women rank high. Division of the Other European variable yields positive Germanic and Slavic effects, as shown in Table XIV, which compare with the top ranks Haenszel gives to Russian and Austrian women in ovarian cancer mortality. He also ranks women from Norway very high and Swedish women above U. S. native-white women, confirming the positive SCAN effect.

In both the breast and the ovarian cancer mortality models high income levels are an important factor until the ethnic differences are corrected for. The two model sets differ with respect to the smoking factor, with a significantly positive CIGS only in the mortality models for cancer of the ovary.

Ridge regression analysis confirms that breast and ovarian cancer mortality have their two major factors in common, OTHEUR and negative TEMP. The

OTHEUR effect is more stable in the breast cancer mortality pattern than it is in the ovarian cancer mortality pattern, where it decreases sharply, while the negative TEMP effect is very stable in the ovarian cancer pattern but diminishes considerably in magnitude in the breast cancer pattern. Although there are no other effects whose coefficient estimates approach in magnitude those of OTHEUR and negative TEMP in the ovarian cancer pattern, there are several in the breast cancer pattern. These are the POLLUT and PRELEV effects, which decrease very gradually and maintain their strength, and the BRIT effect, which is very stable. Additionally, MALT, SCAN, INCM, and CIGS have sizable coefficients in the stable model of breast cancer mortality. The SCAN effect decreases gradually but continuously while the MALT effect stabilizes quickly after a small increase from its least squares value. The positive coefficient of CIGS is very stable, but the INCM effect goes from negative to positive, although it does stabilize firmly in a positive value of moderate strength. The ridge trace of breast cancer mortality is different from those of most of the other cancer mortalities in that only one of its model effects is negative. In addition to a negative TEMP effect the ovarian cancer mortality pattern includes negative WINE and negative FRAN in its least squares solution, but they both decrease in magnitude to approximately null values. The positive coefficient estimates for SCAN, POLLUT and INCM in ovarian cancer are of considerable size, although they are much smaller than the OTHEUR coefficient, and they are very stable.

It is important to note that three of the four differences between the best subset models of these two cancer mortalities disappear in the ridge regressions. The important positive BRIT effect in the stabilized model of breast cancer is found in the ovarian cancer pattern, only moderate in strength but very stable. Moreover, the very significant negative FRAN effect in the subset models of ovarian cancer mortality is highly unstable in the ridge trace and diminishes to zero. The significant CIGS effect that appears only in the subset models of ovarian cancer is stable and equally strong in the ridge traces of both breast and ovarian cancer mortality. It is only the positive MALT effect that continues to differentiate between the two cancer mortality patterns in the ridge trace, characterizing the stabilized model of breast cancer but not of ovarian cancer mortality.

20 Cervix Uteri–F171 (ICD 171)

6 and 8 VAR, BMD and LIN

$$Y(F171) = 7.942 + \overset{***}{.672}\ \mathrm{POLLUT} - \overset{***}{1.564}\ \mathrm{INCM} + \overset{***}{.911}\ \mathrm{CIGS}$$

10 and 12 VAR, BMD and LIN

$$Y(F171) = 7.942 - \overset{**}{.507}\ \mathrm{TEMP} + \overset{**}{.383}\ \mathrm{CIGS} - \overset{***}{1.677}\ \mathrm{SCAN}$$

21 Corpus and Other Parts of Uterus, and Uterus Unspecified–F172 (ICD 172, 173, 174)

6 VAR, BMD and Second LIN

$$Y(F172) = 5.880 - \overset{**}{.385}\ TEMP + \overset{*}{.313}\ PRELEV + \overset{*}{.298}\ POLLUT + .255\ CIGS - .364\ ALCO$$

8 VAR, LIN

$$Y(F172) = 5.880 - \overset{**}{.384}\ TEMP + \overset{**}{.386}\ PRELEV + .241\ POLLUT + .300\ CIGS - \overset{*}{.412}\ DISP$$

10 VAR, BMD and Second LIN

$$Y(F172) = 5.880 - \overset{***}{.447}\ TEMP + .194\ PRELEV - .267\ ALCO - .289\ FRAN + \overset{**}{.600}\ BRIT - \overset{***}{.769}\ SCAN + \overset{**}{.498}\ OTHEUR$$

12 VAR, BMD and LIN

$$Y(F172) = 5.880 - \overset{***}{.413}\ TEMP + .184\ PRELEV - \overset{***}{.394}\ WINE + \overset{**}{.448}\ BRIT - \overset{***}{.791}\ SCAN + \overset{**}{.467}\ OTHEUR$$

The mortality models for both categories of uterine cancer differ in several factors. Positive PRELEV, which enters significantly the corpus uteri models, as well as the breast and ovary models, does not appear in any of the cervix models. The INCM effect, which was strongly positive in the breast and ovary models, is strongly negative in the cervix models, and is not included in the corpus uteri models. CIGS is a significantly positive factor in the cervix models as it is in the ovarian cancer models. It is positive but not significant in the corpus uteri models, and it is not a factor in the breast models. Alcohol consumption is neither in the cervix nor the ovary models, but enters the breast models positively and the corpus uteri models negatively.

The only ethnic effect in the cervical cancer mortality models is also the most important ethnic effect in those for corpus uteri. The highly significant negative SCAN effect in the models for both types of uterine cancer contrasts with the positive SCAN effect in the breast and ovarian cancer models. Segi ranks mortality from cancer of the cervix and of the corpus uteri together, and in this combined category Sweden and Norway rank very low, sixteenth and seventeenth, respectively, out of 20. Although Denmark ranks high (third), the combined Scandinavian rank is low, matching the negative SCAN effect in the models for both types of uterine cancer.

The positive OTHEUR effect in the corpus uteri models is matched by the high ranking in total uterine cancer mortality of Austria (second), Italy (fourth), and Germany (fifth), with Belgium middle in rank and only The Netherlands low. The positive BRIT effect in the corpus uteri models is not matched by the middle to low ranks of the British countries, but this could be due to the inclusion of cervical cancer in the combined category of uterine cancer used by Segi.

It should be noted that the category of corpus uteri includes cancer deaths not only of the body and other parts of the uterus, but those deaths from any type of uterine cancer unspecified as to primary or secondary site. The models for such heterogeneous mortality rates will include the model effects of those primary cancers that metastasized to the uterus and were recorded as unspecified uterine cancer deaths. Thus the ethnic pattern for this category may be derived from several model sets: negative FRAN from the ovary models, positive BRIT from the breast models, negative SCAN from the cervix models, and positive OTHEUR from both the breast and the ovary models. Since approximately 70% of metastases to the female genital tract originate in the breast, corpus, cervix, or ovary (32), it is likely that the unspecified uterine cancer deaths do reflect the mortality patterns of these cancer primaries.

The ridge trace of the cervical cancer mortality pattern shows that the negative coefficient estimate of SCAN is much greater in magnitude than any of the others and is also the most unstable, decreasing by one fourth of its least squares value. Nevertheless it remains over twice as large as the next largest coefficient in the stable pattern, that of CIGS. The CIGS effect is very stable, increasing and then decreasing very gradually so that its coefficient estimate changes very little from its least squares value. The POLLUT effect has the same stable trace but at a lower magnitude, while the PRELEV effect goes from negative to its positive position in the stable pattern. The negative INCM effect is very stable as is the negative OTHEUR effect after a slight early increase in magnitude, both maintaining their importance in the stabilized model. The chief differences between the best subset models and the ridge regression analysis are that the significant negative TEMP effect in the former diminishes to zero in the latter, while PRELEV and negative OTHEUR, absent from the subset models, appear as factors of moderate strength in the stabilized model.

The ridge trace for mortality from cancer of the corpus uteri shows little similarity to the one for cervical cancer, except that negative SCAN is an unstable effect in both, and PRELEV and POLLUT are also shared factors. The largest effect in the corpus pattern, PRELEV, is the most stable. The negative TEMP effect decreases in magnitude, but stabilizes as a major factor. The BRIT and OTHEUR effects decrease sharply while the POLLUT and CIGS effects turn from negative to positive in the stable pattern. The ridge regression model differs from the best subset model in assigning greatest importance to the PRELEV factor and including POLLUT as a factor of moderate strength.

IV The Male and Female Skin Cancer Mortality Models

1 Malignant Melanoma of Skin, Males–M190 (ICD 190)

6 VAR, BMD

$$Y(M190) = 1.529 + \overset{***}{.251}\ TEMP - .062\ INCM + \overset{*}{.103}\ CIGS$$

6 VAR, LIN

$$Y(M190) = 1.529 + \overset{***}{.251}\ TEMP + \overset{*}{.078}\ PRELEV - .065\ POLLUT + \overset{*}{.073}\ CIGS$$

8 VAR, BMD and Second LIN

$$Y(M190) = 1.529 + \overset{***}{.178}\ TEMP + .041\ PRELEV + \overset{*}{.102}\ CIGS - \overset{***}{.173}\ MALT + .072\ WINE$$

8 VAR, LIN

$$Y(M190) = 1.529 + \overset{***}{.194}\ TEMP + \overset{**}{.112}\ CIGS - \overset{***}{.176}\ MALT + .067\ WINE$$

10 VAR, BMD and Second LIN

$$Y(M190) = 1.529 + \overset{***}{.192}\ TEMP + \overset{*}{.073}\ PRELEV + .052\ CIGS + .106\ FRAN - \overset{***}{.161}\ OTHEUR$$

10 VAR, LIN

$$Y(M190) = 1.529 + \overset{***}{.180}\ TEMP + \overset{*}{.081}\ PRELEV + \overset{**}{.145}\ FRAN - \overset{***}{.165}\ OTHEUR$$

12 VAR, BMD

$$Y(M190) = 1.529 + \overset{***}{.153}\ TEMP + .052\ PRELEV + .083\ CIGS - \overset{***}{.170}\ MALT + \overset{**}{.175}\ FRAN - .114\ BRIT$$

12 VAR, LIN

$$Y(M190) = 1.529 + \overset{***}{.160}\ TEMP + \overset{*}{.080}\ PRELEV + .122\ INCM - \overset{*}{.147}\ MALT + \overset{**}{.131}\ FRAN - \overset{*}{.143}\ OTHEUR$$

2 Malignant Melanoma of Skin, Females–F190 (ICD 190)

6 VAR, BMD and LIN

$$Y(F190) = 1.118 + \overset{***}{.133}\ \text{TEMP} - \overset{***}{.092}\ \text{INCM}$$

10 VAR, BMD and Third LIN

$$Y(F190) = 1.118 + \overset{***}{.104}\ \text{TEMP} + .042\ \text{PRELEV} - .065\ \text{BRIT} - .050\ \text{OTHEUR}$$

10 VAR, LIN

$$Y(F190) = 1.118 + \overset{***}{.107}\ \text{TEMP} + \overset{*}{.047}\ \text{PRELEV} - .046\ \text{CIGS} - \overset{**}{.076}\ \text{OTHEUR}$$

8 and 12 VAR, LIN

$$Y(F190) = 1.118 + \overset{***}{.107}\ \text{TEMP} - \overset{***}{.124}\ \text{MALT}$$

8 and 12 VAR, LIN (tie); 8 VAR, BMD

$$Y(F190) = 1.118 + \overset{***}{.096}\ \text{TEMP} + .028\ \text{PRELEV} - \overset{***}{.125}\ \text{MALT}$$

3 Other Malignant Neoplasms of Skin, Males–M191 (ICD 191)

6 VAR, BMD and LIN

$$Y(M191) = 1.575 + \overset{***}{.269}\ \text{TEMP} + \overset{**}{.159}\ \text{PRELEV} - \overset{*}{.127}\ \text{POLLUT} - \overset{**}{.147}\ \text{ALCO}$$

8 VAR, BMD and LIN

$$Y(M191) = 1.575 + \overset{***}{.272}\ \text{TEMP} + \overset{***}{.189}\ \text{PRELEV} - \overset{**}{.156}\ \text{POLLUT} - \overset{**}{.138}\ \text{DISP}$$

10 VAR, BMD and LIN

$$Y(M191) = 1.575 + \overset{*}{.130}\ \text{TEMP} + \overset{**}{.140}\ \text{PRELEV} - \overset{*}{.111}\ \text{POLLUT} - \overset{*}{.168}\ \text{ALCO} + \overset{**}{.239}\ \text{FRAN} - \overset{*}{.219}\ \text{BRIT} - \overset{*}{.131}\ \text{SCAN}$$

12 VAR, LIN

$$Y(M191) = 1.575 + \overset{*}{.118}\ \text{TEMP} + \overset{***}{.167}\ \text{PRELEV} - \overset{**}{.132}\ \text{POLLUT} - \overset{**}{.152}\ \text{DISP} + \overset{**}{.231}\ \text{FRAN} - \overset{**}{.236}\ \text{BRIT} - \overset{*}{.142}\ \text{SCAN}$$

4 *Other Malignant Neoplasms of Skin, Females–F191 (ICD 191)*

6 VAR, BMD and Second LIN

$$Y(F191) = .731 + .07\overset{**}{1}\ TEMP + .05\overset{*}{2}\ PRELEV - .12\overset{**}{0}\ INCM + .047\ CIGS - .08\overset{*}{7}\ ALCO$$

8 VAR, BMD and LIN

$$Y(F191) = .731 + .050\ TEMP + .05\overset{*}{8}\ PRELEV - .09\overset{*}{1}\ INCM + .057\ CIGS - .084\ MALT - .066\ DISP$$

10 VAR, BMD and LIN

$$Y(F191) = .731 + .046\ PRELEV - .073\ INCM - .11\overset{**}{3}\ ALCO + .13\overset{**}{3}\ FRAN - .086\ BRIT - .09\overset{**}{2}\ SCAN$$

12 VAR, BMD

$$Y(F191) = .731 + .039\ PRELEV - .08\overset{**}{5}\ MALT - .05\overset{*}{4}\ DISP - .11\overset{***}{4}\ SCAN$$

12 VAR, LIN

$$Y(F191) = .731 + .05\overset{*}{0}\ PRELEV - .08\overset{*}{9}\ MALT - .07\overset{*}{4}\ DISP + .09\overset{*}{1}\ FRAN - .083\ BRIT - .08\overset{*}{9}\ SCAN$$

5 *Models from the 4-Variable Pool of TEMP, PRELEV, POLLUT, and INCM:*

4 VAR, BMD and LIN

$$Y(M190) = 1.529 + .22\overset{***}{5}\ TEMP + .053\ PRELEV$$

$$Y(F190) = 1.118 + .13\overset{***}{3}\ TEMP - .09\overset{***}{2}\ INCM$$

$$Y(M191) = 1.575 + .26\overset{***}{7}\ TEMP + .14\overset{*}{5}\ PRELEV - .12\overset{*}{4}\ POLLUT - .13\overset{*}{1}\ INCM$$

$$Y(F191) = .731 + .06\overset{*}{8}\ TEMP + .05\overset{*}{2}\ PRELEV - .15\overset{***}{8}\ INCM$$

Skin cancer mortality is divided by Mason into deaths due to malignant melanoma of the skin and those due to all other malignant neoplasms of the skin, referred to here as "other" skin cancer. As opposed to the other types of cancer, the ratio of mortality to incidence for nonmelanoma skin cancer is very small, and therefore the mortality models for other skin cancer will involve not only the factors of cancer incidence but also factors of mortality. With all the other types of cancer treated in this chapter, an incidence or etiological model is assumed to underlie closely the mortality model. But in the models of mortality from other skin cancer, etiological factors in its incidence such as exposure to the sun (TEMP) are combined with mortality factors such as the presence or lack of medical facilities or of personal resources (INCM).

It is not surprising that TEMP is strongly positive in all four sets of models since exposure to the sun is known to be an important factor in the incidence of both types of skin cancer (33-35). Its significance is consistent throughout the melanoma mortality models, but in the models for other skin cancer, this temperature factor weakens after adjustment for added variables, disappearing entirely from the models for females.

The other climate factor, PRELEV, is a positive and moderately significant effect in three of the models, but in the male mortality models for other skin cancer it is a highly significant positive effect, even stronger than TEMP in the models from the ethnic pools. Also included in this set of mortality models is a significantly negative POLLUT effect, indicating that a nonindustrial or agricultural environment in which much of men's work exposes them to the sun is associated with a higher risk. This effect is not in the female mortality models for the same cancer site, probably because they are less likely to do agricultural or ranch work out of doors.

A positive CIGS effect is in the nonethnic models of male mortality from malignant melanoma, but loses its strength when the ethnic effects, particularly a strongly positive FRAN, enter the models. The consistently negative coefficients of the alcohol consumption variables in all four of these model sets are not interpretable, indicating that these variables may be standing in for important factors that were not included in the variable pools, such as other ethnic variables.

The ethnic effects include positive coefficients for FRAN and negative coefficients for the other three ethnic variables. This does not coincide with the national rankings in Segi, which is to be expected since it is the environmental and economic factors that predominate in the etiology of skin cancer incidence and mortality. In order to concentrate the models on these factors alone, a 4-variable pool consisting of TEMP, PRELEV, POLLUT, and INCM was used to choose a model for each mortality pattern. The models so derived indicate that mortality from malignant melanoma and other skin cancer is higher in warm and wet climates at lower elevations, and at lower income levels. This combination of factors is strongly characteristic of the deep South, where skin cancer death rates for whites are the highest. Figure 1 illustrates this geographic distribution of both types of skin cancer mortality for males, and Figure 2 illustrates it for females.

The ridge regression analysis of these four skin cancer mortality patterns differs little from the best subset models in the factor combinations indicated as most effective in explaining the variation in each set of death rates. The primary factor, TEMP, is shown to be both strong and stable in its effect in three of the

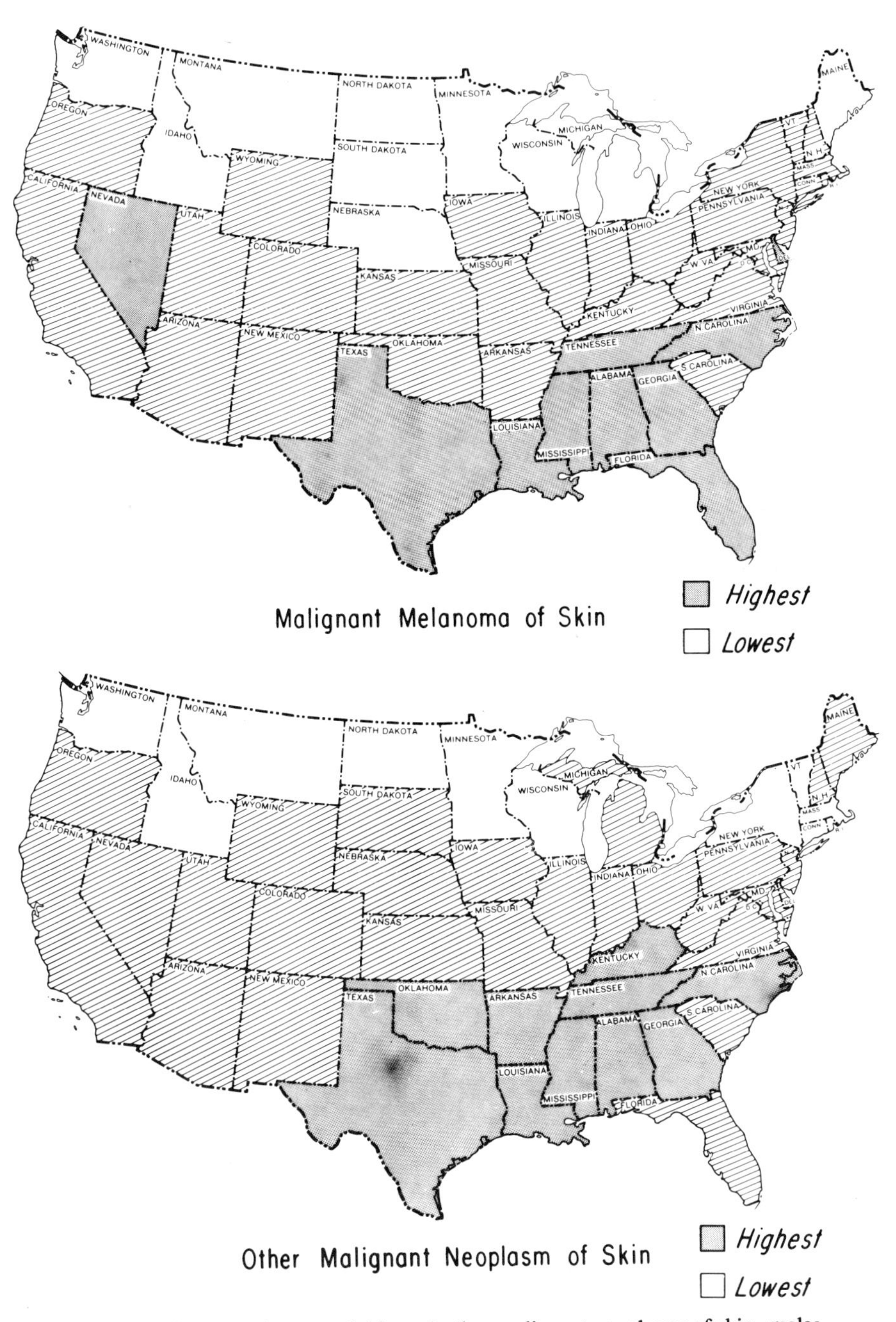

Figure 1. Malignant melanoma of skin and other **malignant neoplasms of skin–males.**

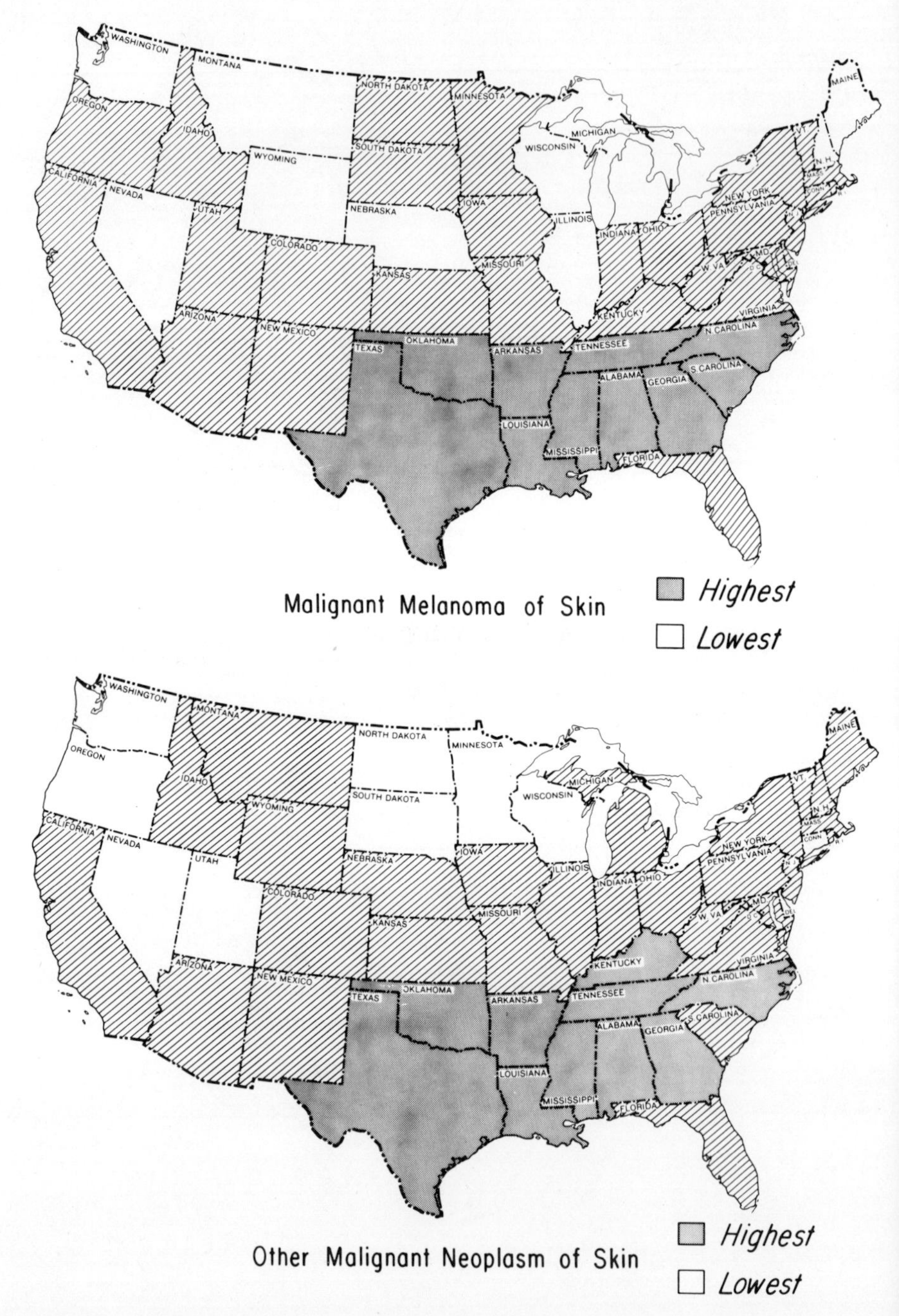

Figure 2. Malignant melanoma of skin and other malignant neoplasms of skin–females.

patterns, while in the fourth, female mortality from other skin cancer, it goes from a negative least squares value to a positive one of moderate strength. This differs from the subset models only in the greater importance given to the TEMP effect in male as well as female other skin cancer mortality. The PRELEV effect is indicated to be stronger in the male than in the female mortality models from both types of skin cancer, both by the best subset model and the ridge trace.

Negative MALT is confirmed as a strong though unstable effect in all the stabilized models of melanoma mortality and of female mortality from other skin cancer, and it is added as a factor in male mortality from other skin cancer, the one model set from which it was excluded in the best subset choices. Although its interpretation is obscure this negative consumption effect is so strongly involved in the skin cancer mortality picture that its meaning or its possible role as an alias should be investigated. The negative alcohol consumption model effects do combine with the environmental factors of high temperature, high precipitation, low elevation, and low pollution levels to characterize the deep South, where levels of alcohol consumption are lowest and skin cancer mortality rates are highest.

The major difference between the best subsets and the ridge regression models lies in the ethnic effects, FRAN and negative BRIT. The ridge trace shows FRAN to be very unstable, going to zero in three of the stabilized mortality patterns and to just moderate strength in the male melanoma mortality model. This contrasts with its strong position in the subset models for male mortality from melanoma and for the mortality of both sexes from other skin cancer. On the other hand, the negative BRIT effect is given greater importance in the stabilized models of melanoma mortality for both sexes, and continues its moderate importance in those for other skin cancer. The ridge trace also confirms the significant negative INCM effect in female mortality from other skin cancer that appears in the subset models from the nonethnic pools. Finally, the CIGS effect that enters the subset models of male melanoma mortality is shown by the ridge trace to be stable and a factor of moderate strength.

V The Male and Female Total Cancer Mortality Models

1 All Malignant Neoplasms, Males–M100 (ICD 140-205)

6 VAR, BMD and Second LIN[a]

$$Y(M100) = 164.81 - 2.19\ TEMP + \overset{***}{12.24}\ PRELEV + 3.49\ INCM + \overset{***}{10.23}\ ALCO$$

6 VAR, Fourth LIN

$$Y(M100) = 164.81 - 2.68\ TEMP + \overset{***}{10.25}\ PRELEV + 2.87\ POLLUT + 3.27\ CIGS + \overset{***}{9.18}\ ALCO$$

8 VAR, BMD and LIN

$$Y(M100) = 164.81 + \overset{***}{12.05}\ PRELEV + 3.26\ CIGS + \overset{***}{8.56}\ MALT + \overset{**}{5.23}\ WINE$$

10 VAR, BMD and Third LIN

$$Y(M100) = 164.81 + \overset{***}{10.31}\ PRELEV - \overset{*}{5.50}\ INCM + 2.54\ CIGS + 4.71\ ALCO + \overset{*}{6.12}\ FRAN + \overset{***}{8.68}\ OTHEUR$$

10 VAR, LIN

$$Y(M100) = 164.81 - 3.08\ TEMP + \overset{***}{10.22}\ PRELEV - 4.21\ INCM + \overset{*}{4.97}\ ALCO + \overset{***}{7.85}\ FRAN - 3.52\ SCAN + \overset{***}{8.62}\ OTHEUR$$

12 VAR, BMD and LIN

$$Y(M100) = 164.81 + \overset{***}{10.98}\ PRELEV - \overset{*}{5.83}\ INCM + 2.85\ CIGS + \overset{*}{5.09}\ MALT + 2.66\ WINE + \overset{*}{6.01}\ FRAN + \overset{*}{6.58}\ OTHEUR$$

[a] $C_p > p$, model with bias.

2 *All Malignant Neoplasms, Females–F100 (ICD 140-205)*

6 VAR, BMD and LIN

$$Y(F100) = 124.37 - \overset{***}{6.28}\ TEMP + \overset{**}{3.47}\ PRELEV + \overset{***}{5.72}\ POLLUT + \overset{***}{3.65}\ CIGS$$

8 VAR, BMD and LIN

$$Y(F100) = 124.37 - \overset{***}{5.06}\ TEMP + \overset{***}{3.99}\ PRELEV + \overset{***}{4.82}\ POLLUT - 2.40\ INCM + \overset{*}{2.90}\ CIGS + \overset{**}{4.78}\ MALT$$

10 VAR, LIN

$$Y(F100) = 124.37 - \overset{***}{6.31}\ TEMP + \overset{***}{3.51}\ PRELEV + 1.87\ POLLUT + \overset{*}{3.07}\ BRIT - \overset{***}{5.35}\ SCAN + \overset{***}{6.39}\ OTHEUR$$

12 VAR, BMD and LIN

$$Y(F100) = 124.37 - \overset{***}{5.90}\ TEMP + \overset{***}{3.98}\ PRELEV + 1.55\ POLLUT + \overset{*}{2.83}\ MALT + 2.55\ BRIT - \overset{***}{5.35}\ SCAN + \overset{*}{4.79}\ OTHEUR$$

The foregoing variety of models that characterize the many different patterns of cancer mortality illustrates that combining all types of malignant neoplasm into a single category in order to derive a total cancer mortality model is akin to adding apples and pears. The cancer mortality models for males will be a combination primarily of the models for trachea, bronchus, and lung, both specified and unspecified as to primary, for prostate, for large intestine and for stomach, all of which together constitute over 50% of male cancer deaths. Cancer of the breast, the large intestine, the ovary, and the uterus, both cervix and corpus, represent over 50% of female cancer mortality. The models for the largest female cancer mortalities are more homogeneous than those for males. This difference is illustrated by the temperature factor. TEMP is a highly significant negative effect in the female mortality models for cancer of the breast, ovary, cervix, corpus uteri, and large intestine. With similarly significant negative coefficients it is a factor in the male mortality models for cancer of the prostate, of the large intestine, and of the stomach, but in the largest category of male cancer deaths–trachea, bronchus, and lung, constituting 22% of male cancer mortality–TEMP enters the models with significantly positive coefficients. The result is that TEMP is a highly significant and consistent negative effect in the female total cancer mortality models, while it barely enters those for the males because its positive and negative effects cancel each other. The other climate variable, PRELEV, is highly significant in all the total cancer mortality models for both males and females, producing easily the largest of the effects in the male mortality models as measured by its coefficients. In the female mortality models the coefficients of PRELEV, though highly significant, are not as large in magnitude as those for (negative) TEMP, (negative) SCAN and OTHEUR, indicating a smaller role in female cancer mortality for this most consistently significant effect in male cancer mortality.

The ridge traces of male and female total cancer mortality confirm the importance of the negative TEMP effect in female mortality and its null effect in the male. The primary importance of PRELEV in male cancer mortality is confirmed, and it is also shown to be the factor of greatest magnitude in the stabilized model of female cancer mortality.

In the best subset models POLLUT appears as a very important effect in female mortality but null in male mortality. In the ridge regression analysis the POLLUT effect is shown to be stable in its very strong role in female mortality, while it goes from negative to strongly positive in male mortality, showing itself to be a much more important factor than was indicated by the best subset models.

The CIGS effect is common to both male and female mortality models in both the best subsets and the ridge regression analysis, but the latter indicates its stability and strength. Of the alcohol consumption factors the MALT effect is strong in the mortality models for both sexes, and WINE is also important in the male mortality model. The ridge trace confirms the importance of these factors and adds DISP as a factor of moderate strength in male mortality.

The ethnic factor, OTHEUR, is a consistent and significantly positive effect in the cancer mortality models of both sexes, and the ridge trace confirms its strength in both mortalities in spite of its instability. In the best subset models the positive FRAN effect is a factor only in male mortality, while positive BRIT and negative SCAN enter only the female mortality models. The strong FRAN factor in male mortality alone is confirmed by the ridge trace, and this is apparently due to the preponderance of the respiratory cancers in total male cancer and the importance of French ethnicity in their mortality patterns.

In the ridge trace BRIT is shown to be strong and very stable not only in the female mortality model but equally in the stabilized model of male mortality. The most surprising difference in the results of the two analytic procedures is that the very significant negative SCAN effect in the best subset model of female mortality and in the least squares solution of the full model, decreases so sharply and continuously in the ridge trace that it becomes null in the stabilized model.

Chapter 4
Comparison of Factors in the Mortality Models of Individual Cancer Sites

I Best Subset Models

It is of interest to observe not only the combinations of factors that influence each type of cancer mortality as indicated by the models, but conversely, which cancer mortalities are influenced by each of the factors. In order to focus on the most important interrelationships between mortality and factor a best model was chosen from the set of models for each type of cancer mortality based on the following considerations, listed in order of their importance: amount of variation explained (R^2); consistency of model effects with other models in the set; identical choice of both the BMD and the LINCUR programs. Two best models were chosen for one cancer site–male mortality from cancer of the trachea, and bronchus and lung specified primary–because two dissimilar models appeared to be equally valid for this very important category of cancer mortality.

Table XVII lists under each variable in the 12-variable pool those cancer primary sites whose best mortality model contains that variable as a positive or negative effect, with or without a significant coefficient. The cancer sites are listed columnarly by the direction and strength of that factor variable in their individual mortality models. At the top are those cancer mortalities most significantly influenced by the positive effect of the factor, and at the bottom those most significantly influenced by its negative effect. When a variable does not enter the best model of a particular cancer mortality, that cancer site is not listed under that variable. Table XVIII summarizes the cancer sites whose best models contain the same factor effect for both male and female mortality.

The factor TEMP separates cancer of the skin and of the trachea, bronchus, and lung from the other cancer primaries, with higher temperature levels associated with higher mortality in the skin and lung cancers, and lower temperature levels associated with higher mortality in almost all of the other cancers.

The factor PRELEV enters most of the models and its effect is positive in all but one. Thus it discriminates among the cancer sites only by degree. The more significant is its coefficient the more closely is a high mortality rate associated

TABLE XVII
Comparison of Cancer Mortalities Influenced by Each Model Effect

Model effect[a]	TEMP		PRELEV		POLLUT	
	Males	Females	Males	Females	Males	Females
+***	Melanoma	Melanoma	Buc Cav & Ph Larynx T, B, & Lung B & L Unspec. Esophagus Lg Intestine Pancreas Bladder Other Skin			Buc Cav & Ph Brain
+**	T, B, & L Spec.	T, B, & L Spec.	Rectum	Bladder Breast Lg Intestine	Buc Cav & Ph Brain Hodgkin's	Esophagus Rectum Hodgkin's Leukemia
+*	T, B, & Lung Other Skin		Liver *et al.* Kidney Leukemia	Esophagus Kidney Ovary Other Skin	Lg Intestine Rectum Larynx T, B, & L Spec.	Lymphosarcoma Breast Lg Intestine
+			T, B, & L Spec. Brain Lymphosarcoma Melanoma	Larynx Rectum Hodgkin's Corpus Ut Melanoma	Esophagus Lymphosarcoma	Larynx Pancreas Bladder Ovary
–	Lg Intestine Liver *et al.* Bladder Hodgkin's					
–*	Kidney	Esophagus Pancreas Hodgkin's Bladder Lg Intestine		Liver *et al.*	B & L Unspec.	
–**	Prostate	Cervix Ut Ovary			Other Skin	
–***	Stomach Rectum	Stomach Rectum Liver *et al.* Kidney Breast Corpus Ut				

Model effect[a]	INCM		CIGS		MALT	
	Males	Females	Males	Females	Males	Females
+***				Esophagus		Liver *et al.*
+**		T, B, & L Spec.	Rectum Hodgkin's	Rectum Cervix Ut Lg Intestine	Liver *et al.*	B & L Unspec.
+*			Lg Intestine	Buc Cav & Ph Ovary Hodgkin's	Lg Intestine	Lg Intestine Bladder
+	T, B, & L Spec. Leukemia	Ovary	T, B, & Lung Melanoma T, B, & L Spec.	T, B, & Lung	Larynx B & L Unspec. Stomach Rectum Kidney Bladder	Stomach Rectum Kidney
–	B & L Unspec. Lg Intestine Bladder	Buc Cav & Ph Bladder	Brain	Liver *et al.*		
–*	Pancreas Prostate	Larynx Lg Intestine B & L Unspec. Esophagus Pancreas	Liver *et al.*			Other Skin
–**	Stomach Hodgkin's	Stomach Hodgkin's			Brain	Brain Esophagus
–***	Rectum	Rectum			Melanoma	Melanoma Buc Cav & Ph

[a] Sign and significance of coefficient in best models, indicated by *a* in Tables VII-X.

TABLE XVII (continued)

Model effect[a]	WINE		DISP		FRAN	
	Males	Females	Males	Females	Males	Females
+***	Pancreas	Esophagus	Esophagus Kidney	Bladder	Buc Cav & Ph Larynx T, B, & Lung B & L Unspec.	Buc Cav & Ph
+**	Stomach	Pancreas	Larynx Prostate		Melanoma Other Skin	Larynx B & L Unspec.
+*		T, B, & Lung Stomach	Buc Cav & Ph Bladder	Larynx B & L Unspec.	Liver *et al.* Bladder	T, B, & Lung Other Skin
+	T, B, & Lung T, B, & L Spec.	T, B, & L Spec.	B & L Unspec.	Breast	Hodgkin's	
–	Lg Intestine			Esophagus Liver *et al.*	Kidney	Kidney
–*	Prostate	Lg Intestine	Stomach Hodgkin's	Stomach Other Skin	Lymphosarcoma	T, B, & L Spec. Liver *et al.* Brain Lymphosarcoma
–**			Other Skin			Ovary
–***		Corpus Ut				

Model effect[a]	BRIT		SCAN		OTHEUR	
	Males	Females	Males	Females	Males	Females
+***	Rectum		Brain Leukemia	Brain Leukemia Lymphosarcoma Hodgkin's	Esophagus Stomach	Liver *et al.* Ovary
+**	Lg Intestine	Rectum Bladder Corpus Ut	Hodgkin's		Rectum Liver *et al.*	T, B, & Lung Stomach Corpus Ut
+*		Lg Intestine Breast	Kidney Lymphosarcoma	Kidney Ovary	Lg Intestine Kidney	Rectum Lymphosarcoma Breast
+	Bladder Lymphosarcoma		Pancreas Prostate T, B, & L Spec.	Breast	B & L Unspec. Bladder Lymphosarcoma	Pancreas Kidney Lg Intestine
–	Melanoma	T, B, & Lung Other Skin	Buc Cav & Ph	Larynx		
–*	Liver *et al.*	Buc Cav & Ph Kidney	Other Skin	Other Skin		
–**	Other Skin	Leukemia	Larynx T, B, & Lung			
–***	Leukemia		B & L Unspec. Liver *et al.*	T, B, & Lung B & L Unspec. Liver *et al.* Bladder Cervix Ut Corpus Ut		

[a] Sign and significance of coefficient in best models, indicated by *a* in Tables VII-X.

TABLE XVIII
Summary of Model Effects Common to Both Male and Female Mortality Models for Individual Cancer Sites[a]

	TEMP	PRELEV	POLLUT	INCM	CIGS	MALT
+	Melanoma T, B, & L Spec.	Larynx Esophagus Lg Intestine Bladder Other Skin Rectum Kidney Melanoma	Buc Cav & Ph Brain Larynx Hodgkin's Rectum Esophagus Lymphosarcoma Lg Intestine	T, B, & L Spec.	Rectum Hodgkin's Lg Intestine T, B, & Lung	Liver *et al.* Lg Intestine B & L Unspec. Stomach Rectum Kidney Bladder
–	Stomach Rectum Liver *et al.* Kidney Lg Intestine Hodgkin's Bladder Sex Sites[b]			Rectum Hodgkin's Stomach Pancreas Bladder B & L Unspec. Lg Intestine	Liver *et al.*	Melanoma Brain

	WINE	DISP	FRAN	BRIT	SCAN	OTHEUR
+	Pancreas Stomach T, B, & Lung T, B, & L Spec.	Larynx Bladder B & L Unspec.	Buc Cav & Ph Larynx T, B, & Lung B & L Unspec. Other Skin	Rectum Lg Intestine Bladder	Brain Leukemia Lymphosarcoma Hodgkin's Kidney	Stomach Rectum Liver *et al.* Lg Intestine Kidney Lymphosarcoma
–	Lg Intestine	Other Skin Stomach	Kidney Lymphosarcoma	Leukemia Other Skin	Liver *et al.* B & L Unspec. T, B, & Lung Larynx Other Skin	

[a] From Table XVI. [b] Breast, ovary, cervix uteri, corpus uteri, prostate.

with a wet climate at low altitude. The one negative exception is the model for female mortality from cancer of the liver and biliary passages, in which the significantly negative effect of PRELEV indicates that higher mortality is associated with a dry climate at high altitude. The women of New Mexico, a state that fits this description, experience the highest mortality from this type of cancer. The cancer models in which the PRELEV effect is most significantly positive are exclusively for male mortality. These include the related group of cancer sites: buccal cavity and pharynx, larynx, and trachea, bronchus, and lung, especially the unspecified category, and esophagus.

The variable that represents population exposure to average levels of combined air pollutants, POLLUT, enters the models as a positive effect with only two exceptions. In one of these, male mortality from skin malignancy other than melanoma, the negative POLLUT effect was considered to represent a farm and ranch environment, one in which males experience greater occupational exposure to the sun. In the second case the negative POLLUT effect in the unspecified category of lung cancer mortality in males could be an indirect expression of the low income level associated with that category, since state levels of income and of pollution are often related to each other.

As proposed in Chapter 3, the income factor, INCM, divides the specified and unspecified categories of lung cancer by reflecting different state levels of medical sophistication. The INCM effect also indicates that a low income level is associated with higher mortality in both sexes from cancer of the large intestine, rectum, stomach, pancreas, and bladder and from Hodgkin's disease. Unfortunately it is not possible to differentiate between individual or general state income level as the acting factor in these mortality patterns.

The cigarette consumption variable, CIGS, appears with greatest significance in female mortality from cancer of the esophagus, and is also significant in female mortality from cancer of the buccal cavity and pharynx. In addition CIGS enters significantly the mortality models for cancer of the cervix and ovary. It is significant for both sexes in mortality from cancer of the large intestine and of the rectum and Hodgkin's disease. This smoking factor also enters the male and female mortality models for cancer of the trachea, bronchus, and lung, and the male models for lung cancer specified primary. CIGS is the model effect most frequently dropped when the variable pools are extended to include ethnic variables, but this does not necessarily rule it out as a factor. Rather, the smoking habits as well as other consumption patterns peculiar to particular ethnic groups could underlie the ethnic effects in the models. Therefore the importance of CIGS as a factor in cancer mortality cannot be gauged solely from the models designated here as "best" since they all were chosen from the ethnic pools. This is also true of the other variables representing factors that are related to ethnicity, such as alcohol consumption, income, and environmental preference.

The alcohol consumption variables differ among themselves in the types of cancer mortality upon which they have their most significant effects. MALT is most important for both males and females in liver cancer mortality and it is also a significant effect for both sexes in mortality from cancer of the large intestine. Malt consumption is also a positive factor for both sexes in cancer of the bladder, stomach, rectum, and kidney and in the unspecified category of cancer of the bronchus and lung.

The factor WINE, like CIGS, is highly significant in female mortality from cancer of the esophagus. It is also a very significant factor for both sexes in mortality from cancer of the pancreas and of the stomach. And wine consumption is a positive factor in the male and female mortality models for the specified primary as well as the combined category of cancer of the trachea, bronchus, and lung.

In male mortality models the consumption of distilled spirits is a significant factor in two separate sets of related cancer primaries: (1) buccal cavity and pharynx, larynx, esophagus; (2) kidney, bladder, prostate. DISP is also a very significant positive effect in the female mortality models for two of these cancer sites–larynx and bladder.

Both the male and the female mortality models for the unspecified lung cancer category contain DISP as a positive effect as they do MALT, in contrast to the specified primary lung cancer models for both sexes, which contain WINE as a positive effect. The strong collinearity among the three components of alcohol consumption produces some odd negative effects in the models. The negative effect of DISP in the stomach cancer models is probably an adjustment to the very strong positive effects of the other two alcohol components in the same models. Similarly the negative effects of MALT and DISP in the female mortality model for cancer of the esophagus could be an adjustment for the extremely high positive significance of WINE in that model.

The ethnic effects in the best models are quite consistent between male and female mortality. French ethnicity is associated with high mortality from cancer of the buccal cavity and pharynx, of the larynx, of the trachea, bronchus, and lung, both unspecified and combined categories, and from skin malignancy other than melanoma; it also implies low mortality from cancer of the kidney and lymphosarcoma. British ethnicity indicates high mortality from cancer of the rectum, of the large intestine, and of the bladder, and low mortality from leukemia and other skin cancer. Scandinavian ethnicity implies high mortality from cancer of the brain and of the kidney, from leukemia, lymphosarcoma, and Hodgkin's disease, and low mortality from cancer of the liver, of the larynx, and of the trachea, bronchus, and lung, both unspecified and combined categories, and from other skin cancer. The ethnicity of the Other European group implies high mortality from cancer of the stomach, the rectum, the liver, the large intestine, and the kidney and from lymphosarcoma. The indication of these best cancer mortality models is that this combination of European ethnics does not experience in the U. S., as a group, low mortality from any type of cancer.

Table XIX compares the ethnic effects in these best models with the relative ranking of those countries in Segi's study that represent immigrant subgroups in the white population of the U. S. Those cancer sites whose mortality data are not available in Segi are marked n.a., as are those for which the rates for Germany are not given, thus reducing the representation of the Other European group below an acceptable minimum. When all the members of an ethnic grouping have middle ranks, their combined rank is indicated as "mid," but when the ranks within a group range from high to low, combining into a middle rank, the notation "mixed" is added.

Of particular interest in Table XIX are those instances in which the positive or negative ethnic effect is paralleled by the relative ranking of its associated European country(ies). A summary of these cases follows:

Positive Effect Is Matched by High Ranking Abroad

FRAN buccal cavity and pharynx, males; larynx, males and females; liver *et al.*, males

BRIT intestine, males and females; rectum, males and females; bladder, males and females; breast, females

SCAN pancreas, males; leukemia, males and females; ovary; prostate

OTHEUR stomach, males and females; liver *et al.*, males and females

Negative Effect Is Matched by Low Ranking Abroad

FRAN ovary

BRIT liver *et al.*, males; leukemia, males and females

SCAN buccal cavity and pharynx, males; larynx, males and females; trachea, bronchus, and lung, males and females; uterus

Also to be noted are those cancer mortality models that involve a strong contradiction between ethnic effect and European experience. Those cases where the model effect implies a high mortality rate but the rank of the associated European country is low, all fall under the FRAN effect–buccal cavity and pharynx, females; trachea, bronchus, and lung, males and females. Those cases where the model effect implies a low mortality rate but the European ranking is high all fall under the BRIT effect–buccal cavity and pharynx, females; trachea, bronchus, and lung, females.

In two types of cancer there is complete consistency in both male and female mortality risk between model ethnic effects and foreign experience. In rectal cancer mortality all eight cells in Table XIX match, reflecting high risk for the British and Other Europeans and average risk for the French and Scandinavians. In leukemia mortality the complete matching reflects low mortality rates for the British, high for the Scandinavians, and average ones for the French and Other Europeans. Laryngeal cancer mortality matches in seven of the cells, indicating

TABLE XIX

Comparison of Ethnic Effects in U. S. Mortality Models[a] with Foreign Ranking in Individual Cancer Sites

Category of mortality	FRAN				BRIT			
	MALES		FEMALES		MALES		FEMALES	
	Effect	Rank	Effect	Rank	Effect	Combined rank	Effect	Combined rank
Buccal cavity and pharynx	Pos.	High	Pos.	Low	Null	Mid exc. Ire. high	Neg.	High
Larynx	Pos.	High	Pos.	High	Null	Mid	Null	High
Trachea, bronchus, and lung	Pos.	Low	Pos.	Low	Null	High exc. Ire. mid	Neg.	High
T, B, & L specified	Null	n.a.	Neg.	n.a.	Null	n.a.	Null	n.a.
B & L unspecified	Pos.	n.a.	Pos.	n.a.	Null	n.a.	Null	n.a.
Esophagus	Null	High	Null	Mid	Null	Mid to High	Null	High
Stomach	Null	Low	Null	Low	Null	Mid	Null	Mid (mixed)
Large intestine	Null	Mid	Null	Mid	Pos.	High	Pos.	High
Rectum	Null	Mid	Null	Mid	Pos.	High exc. Ire. mid	Pos.	High exc. Ire. mid
Biliary passages and liver	Pos.	High	Neg.	Mid	Neg.	Low	Null	Low
Pancreas	Null	Low	Null	Low	Null	Mid to High	Null	Mid to High
Kidney	Neg.	n.a.	Neg.	n.a.	Null	n.a.	Neg.	n.a.
Bladder and other urinary organs	Pos.	Mid	Null	Low	Pos.	High exc. Ires. low	Pos.	High exc. Ires. mid
Brain	Null	n.a.	Neg.	n.a.	Null	n.a.	Null	n.a.
Lymphosarcoma and reticulosarcoma	Neg.	n.a.	Neg.	n.a.	Pos.	n.a.	Null	n.a.
Hodgkin's disease	Pos.	n.a.	Null	n.a.	Null	n.a.	Null	n.a.
Leukemia and aleukemia	Null	Mid	Null	Mid	Neg.	Low exc. Ire. mid	Neg.	Low
Breast			Null	Low			Pos.	High exc. Ire. mid
Ovary			Neg.	Low			Null	High exc. Ires. low
Uterus								
Cervix			Null	Mid			Null	Low exc.
Corpus			Null				Pos.	Scot. mid
Skin								
Melanoma	Pos.	Mid	Null	Mid	Neg.	Mid (mixed)	Null	Mid exc.
Other	Pos.		Pos.		Neg.		Neg.	Ire. high
Prostate	Null	High			Null	Mid		

[a] Best subset model. n.a., Not available or insufficient data in Segi.

Category of mortality	SCAN				OTHEUR			
	MALES		FEMALES		MALES		FEMALES	
	Effect	Combined rank	Effect	Combined rank	Effect	Combined rank	Effect	Combined rank
Buccal cavity and pharynx	Neg.	Low exc. Nor. mid	Null	High	Null	Mid (mixed)	Null	Mid to low
Larynx	Neg.	Low	Neg.	Low	Null	Mid (mixed)	Null	Mid (mixed)
Trachea, bronchus, and lung	Neg.	Low exc. Den. mid	Neg.	Low exc. Den high	Null	Mid (mixed)	Pos.	Mid (mixed)
T, B, & L specified	Pos.	n.a.	Null	n.a.	Null	n.a.	Null	n.a.
B & L unspecified	Neg.	n.a.	Neg.	n.a.	Pos.	n.a.	Null	n.a.
Esophagus	Null	Low	Null	Low exc. Den. mid	Pos.	Mid	Null	Low
Stomach	Null	Low exc. Nor. mid	Null	Low exc. Nor. mid	Pos.	High	Pos.	High
Large intestine	Null	Low exc. Den. high	Null	Mid (mixed)	Pos.	Mid (mixed)	Pos.	Mid (mixed)
Rectum	Null	Mid (mixed)	Null	Mid (mixed)	Pos.	High exc. Italy low	Pos.	High exc. Italy low
Biliary passages and liver	Neg.	Low	Neg.	Mid exc. Nor. low	Pos.	High	Pos.	High
Pancreas	Pos.	High exc. Nor. mid	Null	High exc. Nor. low	Null	Mid to low	Pos.	Mid to low
Kidney	Pos.	n.a.	Pos.	n.a.	Pos.	n.a.	Pos.	n.a.
Bladder and other urinary organs	Null	Low exc. Den. high	Neg.	Mid (mixed)	Pos.	n.a.	Null	n.a.
Brain	Pos.	n.a.	Pos.	n.a.	Null	n.a.	Null	n.a.
Lymphosarcoma and reticulosarcoma	Pos.	n.a.	Pos.	n.a.	Pos.	n.a.	Pos.	n.a.
Hodgkin's disease	Pos.	n.a.	Pos.	n.a.	Null	n.a.	Null	n.a.
Leukemia and aleukemia	Pos.	High	Pos.	High	Null	Mid (mixed)	Null	Mid (mixed)
Breast			Pos.	Mid (mixed)			Pos.	Mid (mixed)
Ovary			Pos.	High exc. Nor. low			Pos.	n.a.
Uterus								
Cervix			Neg.	Low exc. Den. mid			Null	High exc. Neth. low
Corpus			Neg.				Pos.	
Skin								
Melanoma	Null	Mid exc. Nor. high	Null	High exc. Swed. mid	Null	Mid (mixed)	Null	Mid (mixed)
Other	Neg.		Neg.		Null		Null	
Prostate	Pos.	High			Null	Mid (mixed)		

high risk for the French, low for the Scandinavians, and average for Other Europeans and British males. The high risk for women in Britain has no parallel effect in the models. The largest inconsistencies are concentrated in the buccal cavity and pharynx, and the trachea, bronchus, and lung cancer mortalities, especially for females, with the French risk implied to be higher after migration to the U. S. and the British lower.

In observing the relationship between the ethnic model effect OTHEUR and its counterpart foreign mortality levels, it should be noted that the Slavic countries are not included in most of Segi's rankings and therefore only the Germanic countries and Italy are represented in the composite ranking of the Other European group. Thus the Slavic component of OTHEUR, which ongoing analysis stemming from the findings of this study indicates to be the dominant one in cancer mortality (Table XIV), has no appropriate foreign mortality level with which it can be compared, thereby weakening the matching of the OTHEUR effect with the combination of ranks from Segi.

II Ridge Regression Analysis

The ridge regression analysis of the cancer mortality patterns generally confirms the model choices of the BMD and LINCUR programs, while altering considerably the least squares coefficient estimates for the *full* models (those which include every variable in the pool). The main difference between the two analyses is that the stable effects, those whose coefficient estimates change little over their trace in the stabilized patterns, gain in relative importance over those which vary greatly, even though the latter may be largest in magnitude in the least squares solution. Since the stable variables tend to be those which are least correlated with the others and hence least affected by them in the ridge trace, it is POLLUT and PRELEV that gain importance and the urban group of ethnic, consumption and income factors that lose individually. INCM is shown to be an especially unstable effect, decreasing as a factor in all but those mortalities for which there is a specific explanation of income's role, such as the division among states with respect to reporting specified primary or unspecified lung cancer. A large decrease in the magnitude of an ethnic effect when accompanied by stability or increasing magnitude in a consumption effect may indicate that the consumption habit is the basic factor and underlies the ethnic variable's association with the mortality pattern. A summary of the factor effects that are considered to be very strong, strong, and moderately strong, that is, those in the first three columns of Table XII, is given in Table XX to provide a comparison of the ridge regression results with the results of the best subset models given in Tables XVII and XVIII. The statements that follow pertain to these tables.

In the ridge regressions the climate factor, TEMP, more definitively separates the respiratory cancer mortalities from the intestinal and the sex-specific cancers by its positive effect in the former and its negative in the latter. It also involves all the skin cancer mortalities in its positive aspect. In the ridge analysis PRELEV is an even more predominant effect and appears only in its positive aspect. The POLLUT factor is also definitely strengthened, especially in the respiratory, liver, and intestinal cancer mortality patterns. Moreover, it does not enter as a negative effect.

The role of the INCM factor is the most altered in the ridge analysis. Leukemia is added to cancer of the trachea, and bronchus and lung specified to be primary as being influenced by its positive effect, but the negative effects of INCM indicated by the best subset models are greatly decreased in the ridge trace.

The CIGS effect enters more strongly in the ridge patterns because of its comparative stability. In the best subset models its significant coefficient frequently was weakened by the entry of the ethnic variables, especially FRAN. The ridge analysis adds the cancer sites buccal cavity and pharynx, larynx, bronchus and lung unspecified, esophagus, and bladder for both sexes to those already indicated to be influenced by a positive CIGS effect by the best subset models. It also adds two cancer mortalities to the negative CIGS effect column—brain and leukemia—and drops liver.

The MALT factor is very much the same in both the best subsets and the ridge regression analysis. In the latter lymphosarcoma replaces unspecified lung cancer in the positive MALT effect column and other skin cancer replaces brain cancer in the negative. This is one of only two cases where the factor effect is the opposite for males as it is for females. MALT is indicated as a positive factor in male mortality from cancer of the esophagus and a negative factor in female mortality from the same cancer. The WINE factor is much stronger in the ridge analysis, gaining importance in cancer of the buccal cavity and pharynx, of the larynx, of the bronchus and lung unspecified, and of the esophagus and bladder, but not indicating the effect it showed in the best subset models for cancer of the stomach. DISP also gains in the ridge patterns, showing importance in female as well as male mortality from cancer of the esophagus, and it joins WINE as an alcohol consumption factor in mortality from cancer of the pancreas in both sexes. The ridge analysis does not present DISP as a negative effect in female mortality from esophageal cancer or in male or female stomach cancer mortality, as do the best subset models.

The ethnic effects are shown to be very similar in both analyses, with only minor differences. The negative FRAN effect found in the subset models for male mortality from cancer of the kidney and from lymphosarcoma is not indicated by the ridge regression analysis, but the ridge trace does confirm this negative ethnic effect as a factor in brain cancer mortality in both sexes. Esophageal cancer is added to those associated with the positive BRIT effect and

TABLE XX Comparison of Cancer Mortalities Influenced by Each Stabilized Model Effect

	TEMP	PRELEV	POLLUT	INCM	CIGS	MALT
Positive (+)	Males & Females Buc Cav & Ph. T, B, & Lung T, B, & L Spec. Melanoma Other Skin Males Larynx Females	Males & Females Buc Cav & Ph. Larynx T, B, & Lung B & L Unspec. Esophagus Lg. Intestine Rectum Bladder Hodgkin's Dis. Melanoma Other Skin Males T, B, & L Spec. Liver *et al.* Pancreas Kidney Brain Lymphosarcoma Females Breast Ovary Cervix Uteri Corpus Uteri	Males & Females Buc Cav & Ph. Larynx T, B, & Lung T, B, & L Spec. Esophagus Lg. Intestine Rectum Liver *et al.* Brain Lymphosarcoma Males Females Pancreas Bladder Hodgkin's Dis. Leukemia Breast Ovary Cervix Uteri Corpus Uteri	Males & Females T, B, & L Spec. Leukemia Males Lg. Intestine Kidney Females Lymphosarcoma Breast Ovary	Males & Females Buc Cav & Ph. Larynx T, B, & Lung B & L Unspec. Esophagus Lg. Intestine Rectum Bladder Males T, B, & L Spec. Kidney Hodgkin's Dis. Melanoma Females Breast Ovary Cervix Uteri	Males & Females Stomach Lg. Intestine Rectum Liver *et al.* Kidney Bladder Lymphosarcoma Males →Esophagus Hodgkin's Dis. Females T, B, & Lung B & L Unspec. Breast
Negative (−)	Males & Females Stomach Rectum Lg. Intestine Kidney Bladder Lymphosarcoma Hodgkin's Dis. Males Prostate Females Liver *et al.* Pancreas Breast Ovary Corpus Uteri	Males & Females Males Females	Males & Females Males Females	Males & Females Males Pancreas Hodgkin's Dis. Prostate Females Larynx Esophagus Cervix Uteri Other Skin	Males & Females Brain Leukemia Males Females Stomach	Males & Females Melanoma Other Skin Males Brain Females Buc Cav & Ph. Larynx T, B, & L Spec. →Esophagus

	WINE	DISP	FRAN	BRIT	SCAN	OTHEUR
Positive (+)	Males & Females Buc Cav & Ph. Larynx T, B, & Lung T, B, & L Spec. B & L Unspec. Esophagus Pancreas Bladder Males Melanoma Females	Males & Females Larynx B & L Unspec. Esophagus Pancreas Bladder Males Buc Cav & Ph. Kidney Prostate Females T, B, & Lung Breast Ovary	Males & Females Buc Cav & Ph. Larynx T, B, & Lung B & L Unspec. Males T, B, & L Spec. Pancreas Bladder Melanoma Liver *et al.* Females	Males & Females Esophagus Lg. Intestine Rectum Bladder Males Buc Cav & Ph. Kidney Lymphosarcoma Hodgkin's Dis. Prostate Females Larynx Breast Ovary Corpus Uteri	Males & Females Stomach Kidney Brain Lymphosarcoma Hodgkin's Dis. Leukemia Males Prostate Females Breast Ovary	Males & Females Stomach Lg. Intestine Rectum Liver *et al.* Kidney Bladder Lymphosarcoma Leukemia Males →Larynx Esophagus Females T, B, & Lung Pancreas Breast Ovary Corpus Uteri
Negative (−)	Males & Females Males Prostate Females Lg. Intestine Kidney Corpus Uteri	Males & Females Other Skin Males Females Stomach Liver *et al.*	Males & Females Brain Males Prostate Females Kidney Lymphosarcoma Leukemia	Males & Females Leukemia Melanoma Other Skin Males Liver *et al.* Females	Males & Females Buc Cav & Ph. Larynx T, B, & Lung B & L Unspec. Other Skin Males Liver *et al.* Females Esophagus Bladder Cervix Uteri Corpus Uteri	Males & Females Melanoma Males Other Skin Prostate Females Buc Cav & Ph. →Larynx Cervix Uteri

melanoma mortality to the negative BRIT effect, but the negative aspect of the BRIT factor is considerably reduced in the ridge patterns. The SCAN factor is almost identical in ridge regression and best subset models. It is added as a positive effect in stomach cancer mortality, both male and female, by the ridge trace. The effect of OTHEUR is even stronger in the ridge analysis, further confirming its importance in cancer mortality models. Although there appears to be a difference between the two analyses in regard to this ethnic factor, with the ridge trace indicating a negative influence in several cancers while none is shown by the best subset models, the subdivision of OTHEUR produces both positive and negative effects among its component ethnic variables. This division also explains a contradiction in the OTHEUR effect in the ridge trace—positive in male laryngeal cancer mortality and negative in female—by revealing a strong positive Slavic effect in the male subset model and a strong negative Germanic effect in the female (Table XIV).

Chapter 5
Outliers in the Mortality Models for Individual Cancer Sites

I Residual Outliers

A Determination of Outliers among Residuals

Insight into the validity of a regression model can be gained from analysis of its residuals, which in this study are the deviations of observed state death rates from the rates estimated by a model. For each model the residual value for state j is given by

$$Y_j \text{ (residual)} = Y_j \text{ (observed)} - Y_j \text{ (estimated)}$$

where Y_j (observed) is the age-adjusted death rate for state j averaged over a specified time period, and Y_j (estimated) is the estimate of this rate derived as a weighted sum of the factor values (standardized) for state j with the model's coefficient estimates as weights. The set of residuals for any one model is assumed to be normally distributed with an expected value of zero. A positive residual indicates that the observed state death rate is greater than its model estimate and hence underestimated by the model, and a negative residual indicates overestimation of the state death rate by the model.

The residuals that are largest in absolute value for any one model may be simply the maximum and minimum values in the distribution, due to what Anscombe (36) calls inherent variability, or they may be due to measurement error, such as, in this study, incorrect diagnosis or recording of cause of death, or to execution error, such as the inclusion of cases (states) that do not belong to the population of interest. If one state (or D. C.) were characterized by a very high-risk factor that is neither included in the variable pool nor present in the other states, the relationship in that state between its mortality rate and its other factor values would be distorted, and its inclusion with the other states in the regression calculations would similarly distort the overall relationship between factor values and mortality rate described by the coefficient estimates in the model. It is therefore advisable when either measurement or execution error produces a residual of extreme size to omit that case from the calculations. The observation may, however, be a correct one with large inherent variability from the norm and actually a legitimate member of the population of interest. Thus every outsized residual represents an individual situation that should be carefully inspected with respect to its position in the proposed model.

Much has been written about the specification of "outsize" in a residual, some methodology using the apparatus of significance tests to determine which outliers are extreme enough to be rejected. The simplest of these methods uses the standardized residuals, i.e., each residual divided by the root mean square error of the model, and examines those whose value falls in either the positive or the negative 2½% distributional probability tail, thereby implying that any residual whose value is more than two standard deviations from the zero mean value is an outlier. In this study of 49 cases, the 5% tail probability area would be expected to contain two or three (5% of 49) standardized residual values due to inherent variability. More restrictive criteria for designating outliers would involve values falling in the 2%, or the 1% or the .1% tail probability areas, or those which lie more than 3, or even 4, standard deviations away from the mean value.

Studentized residuals, in which the value of each residual is divided by its own standard error, have been considered more appropriate units of analysis. Cook (37) offers procedures for combining the information on the degree of an observation's deviation from the model contained in the Studentized residual with the information on the sensitivity of the coefficient estimates to possible outliers contained in the individual standard errors of the residuals. Calculation of these standard errors requires, at the very least, printouts of the inverse of the covariance matrix by the computer programs, an option given neither by the BMD nor the LINCUR program. If this information had been available, preferably as the standard error of each residual or the standard error of each estimate of the dependent variable, analysis of the residuals could have been more precise and informative.

B Interpretation and Analysis of the Residual Outliers in the Cancer Mortality Models

In this study interest in the large residual values focuses on the reasons why one state's mortality experience is not as well estimated by the model as that of the other states. If it is underestimated, what factor values for that state are too low for its observed death rate, or is some unincluded factor responsible for its high mortality? If it is overestimated, what factor values indicate a much higher death rate than the one observed, and is that state's mortality level consistently overestimated for all categories of cancer? To get this information all the large residuals in a model, that is those whose values fell in the tail areas comprising 5% of the distributional probability, were examined. As was pointed out earlier, with 49 cases at least two are expected to have residual values this large, and so they are not necessarily extreme values or outliers in the usual sense of not belonging to the population under study. To find which of these large residuals were closer to the outlier concept, the position of each with respect to the tail probability areas was determined for the 2, the 1, and the .1% areas. Only one of the 49 cases would be expected to fall in the 2% area, while none would be expected in the smaller end areas, so that, by one convention, those residual values in the 1% or smaller probability areas are the actual outliers in these models. The term outlier, however, is applied less restrictively in this study to all the large residuals under examination, that is, all those falling in the 5% or smaller tail probability areas. These residual outliers were determined for the mortality models from the 12-variable pool for all cancer sites and for the total cancer category, all malignant neoplasms. For comparability and consistency only the models from the largest pool were considered in the inspection of residuals, with one exception—the male mortality models for cancer of the trachea, and bronchus and lung specified to be primary were from both the 10- and the 12-variable pools. Table XXI summarizes the states whose residual values fall in the tail probabilities in the cancer mortality models from the 12-variable pools. The more extreme values are indicated by asterisks.

A state's relative position or rank with respect to the value of each factor and the level of each mortality rate was used to ascertain which of its characteristics was responsible for its conformation to or deviation from a model. Table XXII displays state ranking in the factors of the 12-variable pool. Although actual factor value rather than relative rank would define a state's position more accurately, use of state ranking facilitates the quick comprehension of a state's standing in both the response and the factor variables.

Reference to the coefficient patterns in the best subset models of cancer mortality shown in Tables VII-X, as well as to the chart of residual outliers in Table XXI, will be helpful in understanding the following discussion of each case of outlier underestimation or overestimation.

1 Buccal Cavity and Pharynx (ICD 140-148)

Males—M140 Three states are residual outliers in the male mortality model for cancer of the buccal cavity and pharynx. Two that rank very high in death rates, Connecticut (second) and Massachusetts (fourth), are underestimated, while Florida, ranking moderately high in mortality (sixteenth), is overestimated. Both Connecticut and Massachusetts also rank high in the positive model effects PRELEV, POLLUT, DISP, and FRAN, but their ranking in these factors is not as high as their ranking in mortality rate and therefore the positive contributions of these four effects to the estimates of their death rates are not sufficient to overcome the negative input from the ethnic effect, negative SCAN. Since Connecticut and Massachusetts both rank high in SCAN and the contribution of a high value in a negative factor is strongly negative, the result is to fur-

TABLE XXI Residual Outliers in the Cancer Mortality Models

	Males			Females		
Site	Model	Underestimated	Overestimated	Model	Underestimated	Overestimated
Buccal Cavity & Pharynx	BMD = LIN	CONN MASS	FLA	BMD	TENN	None
				LIN	TENN GA	None
Larynx	BMD	None	FLA	BMD = LIN	DC* VT	COLO* NH
	LIN	None	FLA*			
T, B, & Lung	BMD = LIN	MD	NC	BMD	None	NC* WYO*
T, B, & L Spec.	BMD = LIN	NEBR ALA	CONN	BMD = LIN	NEBR* ALA** CAL*	None
	LIN (10V)	None	CONN			
B & L Unspec.	BMD	None	NEBR	BMD = LIN	OKLA	NEBR*
	LIN	None	DEL			
Esophagus	BMD = LIN	MASS CONN MISS	FLA** DEL	BMD = LIN	GA	None
Stomach	BMD	NM	VT**	BMD	NM ND*	VT**
	LIN	NM	VT**	LIN	NM* ND	VT*
Large Intestine	BMD = LIN	None	FLA**	BMD	NEBR	FLA* MICH WYO
				LIN (3d)	None	FLA**
Rectum	BMD = LIN	None	FLA** MICH	BMD	VT	FLA* MICH WYO
				LIN	VT	FLA MICH WYO*
Liver *et al.*	LIN	None	VT*	BMD = LIN	NM* ILL	None
Pancreas	LIN	LA	FLA**	BMD	None	UTAH FLA**
				LIN	DC	UTAH*
Kidney	LIN	KANS*	FLA ORE WYO	BMD = LIN	ND**	None
	LIN	None	FLA ORE WYO**			
Bladder	BMD = LIN	VT	FLA**	BMD	None	WYO
				LIN	None	None
Brain	BMD	ORE**	None	BMD = LIN	VT*	None
Lymphosarcoma	BMD	VT*	WYO*	BMD = LIN	VT*	ARK
	LIN	VT*	WYO* NEV			
Hodgkin's Disease	BMD	NEBR**	DEL	BMD = LIN	None	WYO*
	LIN	NEBR* MASS	FLA			
	LIN	NEBR	FLA**			
	LIN	MASS	FLA**			

Leukemia	BMD = LIN	DC*	None	BMD = LIN	MONT*	ND
Prostate	BMD = LIN	None	FLA*			
Breast				BMD	None	FLA** W VA*
				LIN	None	FLA** W VA*
Ovary				LIN	NH*	None
Cervix Uteri				BMD = LIN	None	NC
Corpus Uteri				BMD = LIN	OKLA ILL	None
Melanoma	BMD	TEX***	None	LIN	TEX** VT	None
	LIN	TEX**	None			
Other Skin	LIN	None	None	BMD	ALA TENN MONT	None
				LIN	ALA TENN* MONT*	KANS
All Malignant Neoplasms	BMD = LIN	None	FLA***	BMD = LIN	None	FLA* WYO* MICH

No asterisk, $.02 < p < .05$; *, $.01 < p < .02$; **, $.001 < p < .01$; ***, $p < .001$.

TABLE XXII

STATE RANK	TEMP	PRELEV	POLLUT	INCM	CIGS	MALT
1	ARIZ	LA	DC	DC	NEV	WISC
2	FLA	DEL	NY	DEL	NH	MICH
3	LA	FLA	PA	NEV	RI	MD
4	ALA	DC	NJ	CONN	DC	NEV
5	SC	MISS	ILL	NY	DEL	RI
6	MISS	ALA	OHIO	CAL	CONN	NY
7	TEX	RI	DEL	NJ	WYO	NJ
8	ARK	NJ	MICH	ILL	ME	PA
9	OKLA	SC	MD	MICH	NJ	DC
10	GA	MD	KY	WASH	NY	OHIO
11	NC	CONN	RI	WYO	FLA	ILL
12	VA	GA	IND	MASS	VT	DEL
13	TENN	ARK	CONN	MONT	MICH	MONT
14	KANS	MASS	MO	ORE	MONT	CONN
15	MO	NC	MASS	OHIO	ILL	NH
16	KY	ME	SC	RI	OHIO	MINN
17	DEL	KY	TENN	MD	MASS	MASS
18	MD	TENN	VA	PA	COLO	ORE
19	DC	IND	MINN	IND	ARIZ	MO
20	W VA	VA	W VA	NEBR	IND	NEBR
21	PA	MO	CAL	COLO	TEX	WASH
22	IND	ILL	WISC	IOWA	MD	IND
23	UTAH	NY	NEBR	WISC	VA	ARIZ
24	NJ	OHIO	NC	KANS	NC	TEX
25	OHIO	NH	ALA	MO	CAL	COLO
26	IDA	PA	FLA	MINN	ORE	WYO
27	NM	W VA	WASH	TEX	WASH	IDA
28	NEBR	VT	COLO	ARIZ	PA	CAL
29	COLO	MICH	LA	NH	WISC	VT
30	NY	IOWA	TEX	UTAH	NEBR	IOWA
31	CAL	TEX	ME	IDA	KANS	ME
32	CONN	OKLA	ORE	FLA	MINN	LA
33	MASS	WISC	KANS	ND	OKLA	FLA
34	NEV	ORE	IOWA	SD	IDA	ND
35	ILL	MINN	NEV	VA	KY	NM
36	IOWA	KANS	UTAH	ME	IOWA	UTAH
37	ORE	WASH	ARIZ	NM	MO	KY
38	RI	NEBR	VT	OKLA	NM	SD
39	WASH	SD	GA	VT	GA	W VA
40	WISC	ND	MISS	LA	SD	VA
41	SD	CAL	OKLA	W VA	LA	KANS
42	WYO	UTAH	ARK	NC	TENN	TENN
43	VT	WYO	NM	GA	SC	OKLA
44	MONT	MONT	MONT	TENN	W VA	MISS
45	NH	COLO	ND	KY	ND	SC
46	MICH	IDA	SD	SC	ALA	GA
47	MINN	NM	IDA	ALA	MISS	ARK
48	ME	NEV	NH	ARK	ARK	NC
49	ND	ARIZ	WYO	MISS	UTAH	ALA

State Ranking in the Factor Variables

STATE RANK	WINE	DISP	FRAN	BRIT	SCAN	OTHEUR
1	DC	DC	NEV	RI	ND	NY
2	CAL	NEV	DC	MASS	MINN	NJ
3	NEV	NH	RI	NY	WASH	CONN
4	NY	DEL	NY	CONN	SD	ILL
5	NM	VT	CAL	NJ	MONT	PA
6	NJ	FLA	NJ	CAL	ILL	MICH
7	CONN	CONN	CONN	MICH	ORE	WISC
8	VT }	NJ	MASS	NH	WISC	OHIO
9	LA }	CAL	WYO	DC	UTAH	DC
10	RI	ILL	FLA	PA	NEBR	MASS
11	ORE	MASS	LA	MONT	CONN	CAL
12	ARIZ	MD	ILL	WASH	IOWA	MD
13	WASH	NY	MONT	DEL	IDA	FLA
14	MASS	SC	PA	ILL	CAL	RI
15	FLA	WISC	NH	UTAH	WYO	MINN
16	COLO	COLO	DEL	FLA	MASS	DEL
17	MD	MINN	WASH	NEV	NY	NEBR
18	ILL }	WASH	COLO	WYO	NEV	COLO
19	DEL }	RI	MICH	VT	RI	MONT
20	MICH	WYO	MD	ORE	COLO	IND
21	VA	ME	ORE	ME	NJ	WASH
22	PA	LA	ARIZ	OHIO	MICH	MO
23	WISC	VA	VT	COLO	FLA	ND
24	NH	MICH	OHIO	MD	NH	ARIZ
25	OHIO	MONT	IDA	ARIZ	DC	ORE
26	MO	ND	NM	IDA	ARIZ	NH
27	TEX	ARIZ	KANS	MINN	ME	WYO
28	MINN	MO	IND	IOWA	VT	NEV
29	WYO	OHIO	ME	IND	KANS	SD
30	NC	ORE	UTAH	SD	DEL	IOWA
31	SC	NEBR	MO	WISC	PA	W VA
32	OKLA	SD	VA	MO	MD	VT
33	SD	GA	WISC	NEBR	IND	KANS
34	UTAH }	NC	IOWA	VA	OHIO	ME
35	ARK }	NM	MINN	ND	MO	VA
36	GA	PA	TEX	KANS	TEX	UTAH
37	NEBR	KY	W VA	NM	NM	TEX
38	MONT	IDA	NEBR	W VA	VA	IDA
39	ND	TEX	OKLA	TEX	LA	LA
40	IND	OKLA	ND	LA	OKLA	OKLA
41	W VA }	IND	SD	OKLA	ALA	NM
42	ME }	IOWA	ALA	ALA	ARK	GA
43	IDA	UTAH	GA	GA	MISS	ARK
44	TENN	W VA	KY	SC	GA	KY
45	KY	KANS	MISS	KY	W VA	ALA
46	KANS	TENN	SC	NC	TENN	TENN
47	ALA	ALA	ARK	TENN	SC	MISS
48	MISS	ARK	NC	MISS	NC	SC
49	IOWA	MISS	TENN	ARK	KY	NC

ther lower the estimated death rates, increasing the discrepancies with the observed rates.

Florida ranks very high in PRELEV, DISP, and FRAN and its middle ranks in the other two model effects are not sufficient to lower its estimated death rate to the level of its observed one.

Females–F140 Two models were chosen from the 12-variable pool for female mortality from cancer of the buccal cavity and pharynx, one by the BMD program and one by LINCUR. Two states with high mortality rates, Georgia ranking first and Tennessee third, are underestimated outliers–Georgia in the LIN model and Tennessee in both models. The BMD model also underestimates Georgia's death rate with a residual that just misses an outlier position. There are no overestimated outliers in these models. Both states rank very low in the ethnic effect FRAN, which is a very significant positive factor in both models, and both also rank low in the consumption factor CIGS. Georgia additionally ranks low in POLLUT. The positive contributions of both states' low-ranking values in the negative effects INCM, MALT, BRIT, and SCAN are in accord with their high death rates but are insufficient to counteract their low-ranking values in the positive effects FRAN, CIGS, and POLLUT.

2 *Larynx (ICD 161)*

Males–M161 Florida is an overestimated outlier in the male mortality models of cancer of the larynx from both programs. The same variables are in the male mortality model for this cancer site as are in the one for cancer of the buccal cavity and pharynx, yet Connecticut and Massachusetts are not outliers in this case since their mortality rates do not rank quite as high (sixth, eighth, respectively). Because of the importance given to the variable PRELEV in the mortality models for both cancer sites, this positive effect can be considered the chief cause for Florida's overestimation, due to the state's very high rank (third) in that factor.

Females–F161 In the female mortality models for cancer of the larynx, D. C. and Vermont are underestimated outliers while Colorado and New Hampshire are overestimated outliers. D. C., with the highest mortality rate, also ranks very high in the positive effects FRAN (second), DISP (first), POLLUT (first), and PRELEV (fourth). But it also ranks highest in INCM, a negative effect in the model, thereby reducing its estimated death rate. Vermont, second in death rate, ranks high (fifth) in DISP and low (thirty-ninth) in the negative effect INCM, but its low ranking in the positive effects FRAN, PRELEV and POLLUT leads to the underestimation of its high mortality level. Colorado ranks lowest in mortality and New Hampshire forty-third, but their high ranks in the positive effects FRAN and DISP yield estimated death rates that are much higher than their very low observed rates.

3 *Trachea, Bronchus, and Lung (ICD 162, 163)*

Males–M166 The mortality model for cancer of the trachea, bronchus, and lung combining specified as to primary site and unspecified is the only model for males or for females in which Maryland is a residual outlier. Underestimated Maryland has the second highest death rate for this combined lung cancer site, only Louisiana ranking higher. However, Louisiana has the second highest estimated rate while the estimate for Maryland, though high in rank (ninth), is still too low in value. The only factors correctly predicting a high rate for Maryland are PRELEV, in which it ranks high, and negative SCAN, in which it ranks relatively low. The state does not rank sufficiently high in the other positive effects, TEMP, CIGS, WINE, and FRAN, particularly in FRAN, the second most important factor in the model, to match its very high death rate. North Carolina, with a mortality rate that is not extremely low (thirty-seventh), is an overestimated outlier due to its comparatively high rankings in TEMP (eleventh) and PRELEV (fifteenth) and its very low rank (forty-eighth) in the negative effect SCAN.

Females–F166 No states are underestimated outliers in the female mortality model for this combined category of lung cancer, while North Carolina, just as it is in the male models, and Wyoming are overestimated outliers. Wyoming with the next to lowest death rate has high ranks in the positive effects FRAN and CIGS, which push the estimate of its rate too high. North Carolina, ranking very low in female mortality (forty-sixth), has very low scores in the negative effects BRIT and SCAN, which result in the overestimation of its death rate.

4 *Trachea, and Bronchus and Lung Specified as Primary (ICD 162); Bronchus and Lung Unspecified as to Primary or Secondary (ICD 163)*

Males–M162, M163 In the male mortality model for cancer of the trachea, and of the bronchus and lung specified as primary (site M162), high-ranked Alabama (second) and Nebraska (fourth) are underestimated outliers while low-ranked Connecticut (forty-fourth) is an overestimated outlier. There are two models for the unspecified category of lung cancer (site M163) with one residual outlier in each. Nebraska, ranked lowest, is overestimated by the BMD model while twenty-sixth-ranked Delaware, is overestimated by the LIN model. The effects contained in these three models are shown in Table XXIII.

TABLE XXIII
Model Effects in Male Lung Cancer Mortality

Site	Program[a]	Effects								
M162	B = L	+TEMP	+PRELEV		+INCM					
M163	B		+PRELEV	−POLLUT	−INCM	+MALT	+DISP	+FRAN	−SCAN	+OTHEUR
M163	L		+PRELEV	−POLLUT		+MALT		+FRAN	−SCAN	

[a] B, BMD. L, LIN.

Nebraska has middle ranks in the specified primary lung cancer model effects TEMP and INCM and a low rank in PRELEV, ensuring that its very high mortality rate recorded for this category is greatly underestimated. In the same model, Alabama is greatly underestimated, in spite of its very high ranking in TEMP (fourth) and PRELEV (sixth), because of a very low rank (forty-seventh) in INCM. Connecticut is overestimated in this model because its high ranks in INCM (fourth) and PRELEV (eleventh) do not conform to its low recorded mortality rate in the specified primary category.

Nebraska's ranks in all but two of the BMD model effects correctly indicate a low level of male mortality from unspecified lung cancer but they are not extreme enough to predict its bottom-ranking death rate. Its middle ranking in MALT and OTHEUR also raises the estimate over its observed rate enough to produce an outlier residual value. Delaware's high ranks in all of the positive effects in the LIN mortality model for the unspecified category of lung cancer predict a much higher death rate than its observed one of middle rank, but its high ranks in the negative effects INCM (second) and POLLUT (seventh) lower the estimate of its rate by the BMD model sufficiently to avoid an outlier position of overestimation. Since negative INCM is not in the LIN model for this site, the overestimation of Delaware's death rate does produce a residual outlier.

Thus INCM, either as a positive effect in the specified primary lung cancer model, or as a negative effect in the unspecified category model, is an important factor in all the residual outliers of these models.

It should be noted that two other models for male mortality from cancer of the lung specified primary (Table VII) explain more variation than the model from the 12-variable pool discussed above. One of them, the LIN model from the 8-variable pool, is very similar to the 12-VAR model and produces the same residual outliers. However, the other, the LIN model from the 10-variable pool, involves a very different set of factors, specifically POLLUT, CIGS, and SCAN, having only TEMP in common with the other models, and it results in only one residual outlier. Connecticut is again an overestimated outlier, and it is one in this model because its high ranks in the model effects, POLLUT (thirteenth), CIGS (sixth), and SCAN (eleventh), also do not conform to its low recorded mortality rate. No underestimated residual outliers are produced by this model, compared with two in the other models. Thus for male mortality from primary cancer of the lung two very different models emerge as effective candidates in explaining the state mortality patterns.

Females–F162, F163 Just as for the males, Nebraska and Alabama are underestimated outliers in the female mortality models from cancer of the trachea, and bronchus and lung specified primary. However, California is an additional underestimated outlier and there are no overestimated outliers in the female mortality models. All three states rank very high in death rates, Nebraska second, California third, and Alabama fourth, but the underestimation in each case is due to different factors. Nebraska's middle ranks in INCM and in TEMP and low rank in WINE do not conform to its high-ranking recorded death rate in primary lung cancer. Alabama's very low ranking in INCM (forty-seventh) and WINE (forty-seventh) overcome its very high rank (fourth) in TEMP and low rank (forty-second) in the negative effect FRAN to produce a positive (underestimated) residual outlier whose value falls in the 1% tail probability area. In exact contrast California's very high ranking in INCM (sixth) and WINE (second) are offset by its low rank (thirty-first) in TEMP and high rank (fifth) in the negative effect FRAN, resulting in the outlier underestimation of its death rate. California's comparatively low rank in TEMP undoubtedly does not reflect adequately the exposure of its population to warm temperatures since the majority live in the southern part. Both California and Texas extend too far from north to south to be represented by a single temperature value uncorrected for population distribution within the state. A higher value of TEMP could have removed California from an outlier position in this model.

In the model for female mortality from unspecified lung cancer, Oklahoma is an underestimated outlier and Nebraska an overestimated one. Oklahoma, eighth highest in mortality rate, is among the lowest-ranking states in the positive effects MALT, DISP, and FRAN, producing an estimate well below its observed death rate.

Bottom-ranking Nebraska has an overestimated death rate because, although most of its factor values conform to a fairly low mortality rate, none are extreme enough to predict its actual recorded rate, which is the lowest both for males and for females in the unspecified lung cancer category of deaths. It is evident that the very high weighting of specified over unspecified lung cancer deaths for females and for males recorded in Nebraska's medical records must be caused by factors other than those represented in the variable pool.

5 *Esophagus (ICD 150)*

Males–M150 The male mortality model for cancer of the esophagus produces more residual outliers than any other, but only one of these is extreme in value. Massachusetts, Connecticut, and Mississippi are underestimated while Florida and Delaware are overestimated, the residual value for Florida falling in the 1% probability tail area. This model has the following in common with the male mortality model for cancer of the buccal cavity and pharynx: (1) high-ranking Connecticut is an underestimated outlier because of insufficiently high values of PRELEV and POLLUT; (2) high-ranking Massachusetts is an underestimated outlier because of insufficiently high values of PRELEV, POLLUT, and DISP; and (3) Florida is an overestimated outlier because of its high values of PRELEV and DISP. In the model for esophageal cancer Delaware is added to Florida as an overestimated outlier because of high ranking in the same factors, PRELEV and DISP.

Females–F150 Georgia, the only residual outlier in the model for female mortality from cancer of the esophagus, is underestimated. As in the female mortality model for cancer of the buccal cavity and pharynx, its low scores in the positive effects POLLUT and CIGS are primarily responsible.

6 *Stomach (ICD 151)*

Males–M151 The BMD and LIN programs yield two different models from the 12-variable pool for male mortality from stomach cancer. Since the only difference between them is that MALT, the least important variable in the BMD model, is not included in the LIN, it is not surprising that the residual outliers are the same in each model. New Mexico is an underestimated outlier and Vermont an overestimated one. Ranking eighth in mortality, New Mexico's high rank (fifth) in WINE and low rank (thirty-seventh) in the negative INCM effect are not sufficient to overcome its middle rank (twenty-seventh) in the negative TEMP effect and its very low rank (forty-first) in the positive ethnic effect OTHEUR. On the other hand, Vermont's low ranks in the negative effects TEMP (forty-third) and INCM (thirty-ninth) and high rank in WINE (tied for eighth) produce an estimated death rate much higher than its observed one of only middle rank (twenty-seventh).

Females–F151 There are also two stomach cancer mortality models for females. North Dakota and New Mexico are underestimated outliers in both models, while Vermont is an overestimated outlier in both. North Dakota's top rank in mortality is matched by its position as coldest state in the union. In spite of this conformation with the most important effect in the model, low ranks in MALT, WINE, and OTHEUR result in the outlier underestimation of its death rate.

New Mexico ranks even higher (third) in female mortality than in male for this cancer site, and its overestimation is due to the same variable effects that apply to the males since the models for both the sexes are almost identical in factor effects. Also because of this similarity in models Vermont's ranking in the same variable effects produces too high an estimate of its low-ranked (thirty-first) female mortality rate, just as it does for the males. There are especially strong similarities between the sexes in the mortality patterns, in the models, and in the outliers for this type of cancer.

7 *Large Intestine excluding Rectum (ICD 153)*

Males–M153 In the male mortality model for cancer of the large intestine Florida, which ranks twenty-third, is again the only residual outlier. The overestimation of its death rate is due to its very high rank (third) in the positive effect PRELEV combined with the large weight given to this variable in the model. This is reinforced by Florida's high ranking in the positive model effects CIGS, BRIT, and OTHEUR.

Females–F153 Two models are presented for female mortality from cancer of the large intestine. It is interesting to look at the two models and note that one stresses PRELEV and then the ethnic effects, while the model from the other program gives the greatest weight to negative INCM followed by MALT and then PRELEV. Nebraska is an underestimated residual outlier, and Michigan and Wyoming overestimated residual outliers, in the BMD model. Florida is an overestimated residual outlier in both models, very significantly so in the LIN model.

Nebraska's sixteenth-ranked death rate is well predicted by its ranks in OTHEUR (seventeenth) and MALT (twentieth) and by moderately low ranking in the negative effects WINE and TEMP. But its low ranking in the positive effects PRELEV (thirty-eighth), CIGS (thirtieth), and BRIT (thirty-third), and high rank (tenth) in the negative SCAN effect produce outlier underestimation of its mortality.

Florida, with a low recorded death rate ranking thirty-sixth, is overestimated because of its high values of PRELEV, CIGS, BRIT, and OTHEUR in both models and its low INCM level in the second model. Michigan's seventeenth-ranked death rate is strongly overestimated because of its very low rank (forty-sixth) in the negative effect TEMP and its high ranking in MALT, BRIT, and OTHEUR. Wyoming's very low-ranked (forty-fourth) death rate is correctly indicated by its low ranking in PRELEV and POLLUT and high ranking in the negative effect INCM, but its high rank in CIGS and very low rank in the negative effect TEMP combine with middle ranking in the other model effects to raise its estimated rate well over its low observed rate.

8 Rectum (ICD 154)

Males–M154 There are no underestimated outliers in the male mortality models for cancer of the rectum, but Michigan joins Florida as an overestimated outlier. Michigan, thirteenth in mortality rate, is overestimated because of its very low rank in the negative TEMP effect and its high ranking in MALT, BRIT, and OTHEUR. This is exactly the set of factor values that caused the outlier overestimation of Michigan's female mortality rate from cancer of the intestines. Florida's high value for PRELEV is counterbalanced by its high value for the negative TEMP effect, but its high ranking in CIGS, BRIT, and OTHEUR lead to the outlier overestimation of its low-ranking (thirty-first) death rate.

Females–F154 The two models for female mortality from rectal cancer differ in only two effects, PRELEV and MALT, neither with a significant coefficient, and Vermont, ranking third in mortality, is an underestimated residual outlier in both models. Vermont's very high death rate is partially predicted in both models by a moderately high rank (twelfth) in CIGS and low ranks in the negative effects TEMP (forty-third) and INCM (thirty-ninth). Its middle to low ranks in all the other model effects ensure the outlier underestimation of its high mortality level.

Michigan, Wyoming, and Florida are overestimated outliers in both models. Although Michigan is a high mortality state (fifteenth), its even higher ranking in the ethnic effects BRIT (seventh) and OTHEUR (sixth) cause its overestimation. On the other hand Wyoming ranks very low in death rate (forty-seventh) but its ranking in CIGS (seventh) and BRIT (eighteenth) and in the negative effect TEMP (forty-second) ensures the overestimation of its death rate. Florida's high ranks in CIGS, BRIT, and OTHEUR and its moderately low INCM level produce an estimated death rate much higher than its low-ranked (thirty-third) observed rate.

9 *Biliary Passages and Liver (ICD 155, Unspecified Part of ICD 156)*

Males–M155 Vermont, an underestimated outlier in some cancer mortalities, is an overestimated outlier in the model for male mortality from cancer of the liver and biliary passages, a cancer category for which its male death rate ranks very low (forty-eighth). The model implies that a low rate would be expected to occur in a warm climate with a low French and a high Scandinavian ethnicity. Vermont has one of the lowest ranks (forty-third) in TEMP, but middle ranks in the FRAN and SCAN effects (twenty-third and twenty-eighth), which prevent a sufficiently low estimate of its mortality rate.

Females–F155 In the female mortality models for cancer of the liver and biliary passages New Mexico and Illinois are underestimated outliers and no states are overestimated outliers. Both states rank very high in mortality, New Mexico first, Illinois fourth. However, they present an interesting comparison when their ranks in the model effects are examined. New Mexico's low ranking in the negative effects PRELEV, CIGS, DISP, and SCAN conform to its high mortality, but its low ranks in the positive effects MALT and OTHEUR keep its estimated death rate well below the observed rate. In contrast, Illinois' high ranks in MALT and OTHEUR and its low rank in the negative effect TEMP conform to its high mortality, but high ranking in the negative effects SCAN, DISP, FRAN, and CIGS ensure the underestimation of its death rate.

Since this site includes deaths from both liver and gallbladder cancer, its mortality models, especially for females, who experience a greater incidence of gallbladder cancer than males, must combine the factor effects of both cancer primaries. It is possible that the division in this category of cancer mortality is illustrated by the contrasting effects in the two underestimated outliers described above, with New Mexico representing a higher risk in female mortality from gallbladder cancer and Illinois a higher risk from liver cancer. Steiner (38) cites a Los Angeles necropsy series (39) in which among all the ethnic groups only Mexican women had a high incidence of cancer of the gallbladder. In addition, gallbladder disease has been found to be excessive in American Indians (40), especially the Pima of the Southwest (41, 42). And, from a medical textbook (43), "consideration of gallstones is indicated because cholelithiasis is strongly linked with both inflammatory and *malignant* disease of the gallbladder and biliary tract." Indian ethnicity is represented in the white population of New Mexico through Mexican-Americans as well as others of mixed race. Thus that state's outlier position of underestimation could be due to ethnic factors not represented in the variable pool.

The importance of Indian ethnicity could also be applicable to New Mexico's underestimation in the male mortality models for this combination of cancer sites since the American Indian male suffers the highest death rate (crude) from cancer of the gallbladder among all the racial groups in the U. S., males or females (31). It is also only among the American Indians that the male to female ratio for mortality from gallbladder cancer is greater than one (31).

10 Pancreas (ICD 157)

Males–M157 Louisiana, underestimated, and Florida, overestimated, are residual outliers in the male mortality models for cancer of the pancreas. Louisiana's highest-ranking mortality rate conforms to its very high ranks in PRELEV (first) and WINE (eighth) and its low rank in the negative INCM effect (fortieth), but its low rank in SCAN (thirty-ninth) produces the underestimation. Florida's low-ranking death rate (forty-first) is not predicted by any variables in the model. Again its high rank in the important and pervasive model effect PRELEV is the prime factor in the underestimation of its low recorded death rate.

Females–F157 The female mortality models for cancer of the pancreas are the only ones in which Utah is a residual outlier. Ranking lowest in death rate and overestimated by both models, Utah has moderately low scores in the positive model effects POLLUT, WINE, DISP, and OTHEUR, but they are not sufficient when combined with its moderate values for the negative effects TEMP and INCM to estimate correctly so low a death rate.

Florida is overestimated by the BMD model with a residual whose value falls in the 1% probability area of the distribution tails. Its high ranking in the positive effects WINE, DISP, and OTHEUR and low rank in the negative effect INCM completely miss predicting its low-ranking (forty-fourth) death rate. D.C., ranking highest in female mortality from cancer of the pancreas, is an underestimated residual outlier in the LIN model, in spite of its very high ranking in WINE and POLLUT and OTHEUR, because it also ranks highest in the negative effect INCM, thereby reducing its estimate well below the observed death rate.

11 Kidney (ICD 180)

Males–M180 In male mortality from cancer of the kidney there are two LIN models with almost equal credentials. As shown in Table XXIV, in addition to the substitution of MALT for CIGS and of negative FRAN for negative BRIT,

TABLE XXIV
Model Effects in Male Kidney Mortality with Coefficient Ranking

	6	7	5	1	4	3	2
LIN_1	−TEMP	+PRELEV	+MALT	+DISP	−FRAN	+SCAN	+OTHEUR
	4	6	7	5	3	2	1
LIN_2	−TEMP	+PRELEV	+CIGS	+DISP	−BRIT	+SCAN	+OTHEUR

different importance is placed on individual model effects, indicated in the table by coefficient size ranked within each model.

Kansas, ranking nineteenth in death rate, is an underestimated residual outlier in LIN_1 while low-ranking Florida (thirty-fifth), Oregon (thirty-seventh), and Wyoming (thirty-eighth) are overestimated residual outliers in both LIN models. Kansas ranks higher in mortality than is indicated by any of the effects in either model except negative BRIT, in which it ranks low, producing a better estimate in the LIN_2 model. In addition, the inclusion of CIGS rather than MALT increases the estimate as does a weaker coefficient for DISP, an effect in which Kansas ranks very low, thus preventing outlier underestimation in the LIN_2 model. Florida is overestimated by both models in spite of its very high rank in the negative effect TEMP, because of its high or very high ranking in the positive effects PRELEV, DISP, CIGS, and OTHEUR. Oregon and Wyoming are overestimated in both models because of their low ranks in the negative effect TEMP and their high ranks in the positive effect SCAN. In addition Wyoming's high rank in CIGS (seventh) and Oregon's higher than average rank in MALT (eighteenth) contribute further to the overestimation of their rates.

Females–F180 North Dakota has the highest female death rate from cancer of the kidney, just as it does from cancer of the stomach, and it is an underestimated residual outlier in the mortality models for both cancer sites. Its rank as coldest state conforms to this high mortality from both types of cancer. North Dakota also ranks highest in the important effect SCAN and low in the negative effects FRAN and BRIT. However its low-ranking values of MALT, also a factor in the underestimation of its female mortality from stomach cancer, and of PRELEV reduce the estimate of its mortality well below its very high observed level.

12 Bladder and Other Urinary Organs (ICD 181)

Males–M181 High-ranking Vermont (sixth), which was an overestimated residual outlier in the male mortality models for cancer of the stomach and of the liver, is an underestimated one in cancer of the bladder. Its high death rate, though correctly predicted by its high rank in DISP (fifth) and low ranking in the negative effects TEMP and INCM, is underestimated by its lower than average values of the very important effect PRELEV, as well as of MALT and OTHEUR. Florida, ranking twenty-second in mortality, is also an overestimated outlier in the male bladder cancer mortality model. Its very high ranks in the major model effects PRELEV (third), FRAN (tenth), and DISP (sixth) predict a much higher death rate than that recorded for this state.

Females–F181 Two mortality models are chosen for cancer of the bladder in females but they differ only in nonsignificant effects. Wyoming, ranking forty-fifth in mortality, is an overestimated outlier in the BMD model only. Its low score in the negative effect TEMP works toward its overestimation in both models, but this is offset by the inclusion in the LIN model of the positive effect POLLUT, in which it ranks very low (forty-ninth), and the negative effect INCM, in which it ranks high (eleventh).

13 *Brain and Other Parts of the Nervous System (ICD 193)*

Males–M193 Oregon, the only residual outlier, has the highest male death rate from cancer of the brain and it is underestimated by the model. The only effect that predicts its high level of mortality is SCAN, in which it ranks seventh.

Females–F193 High-ranking Vermont (fourth) is the only residual outlier in the female mortality model for cancer of the brain. The underestimation of its high death rate is due to its middle to low ranks in all of the model effects.

14 *Lymphosarcoma and Reticulosarcoma (ICD 200, 202, 205)*

Males–M200 High-ranking Vermont (third) is an underestimated residual outlier in both models of male mortality from lymphosarcoma and reticulosarcoma. Only its low rank (thirty-ninth) in the negative effect INCM in the LIN model conforms to its high death rate. Its low values of the positive effects POLLUT, SCAN, and OTHEUR preclude a good estimate in either model.

Lowest-ranking Wyoming (forty-ninth) is an overestimated residual outlier in both models, and very low-ranking Nevada (forty-eighth) is one in the LIN model, due to these states' higher than average values in the SCAN effect. In the BMD model very high ranks for both states in the negative effect FRAN and low ranks in PRELEV counterbalance their higher than average values for BRIT. However, Nevada escapes an overestimated outlier position in this model because it ranks highest in the negative effect FRAN and next to lowest in PRELEV. Although both Wyoming and Nevada rank very high in the negative effect INCM, it is not enough to prevent the excessive overestimation of their death rates by the LIN model.

Females–F200 Vermont, ranking ninth in female mortality from lymphosarcoma, is also an underestimated residual outlier in the female as it is in the male mortality model. Its middle to low ranks in all the model effects predict a much lower level of mortality than the observed one. Arkansas, with the lowest death rate, is overestimated by the female mortality model, the only instance in which this state appears in a residual outlier position. Although it ranks very low in all three of the positive effects POLLUT, SCAN, and OTHEUR, its very low rank in the negative effect FRAN pushes its estimated death rate well above the observed level. It is apparent that prediction by an inverse type of effect, such as the imputation of a high mortality rate to a population with a small proportion of a low-risk ethnic group (the negative FRAN effect), is detrimental in this case since Arkansas' low ranking in the more direct (positive) effects correctly and sufficiently predicts its low death rate.

15 Hodgkin's Disease (ICD 201)

Males–M201 There are four male mortality models to be considered for Hodgkin's disease, the BMD choice and three ties chosen by LIN, with their effects displayed in Table XXV. The order of importance of each effect within its model as determined by the size of its coefficient is shown above each factor.

Nebraska, ranking third in mortality, is an underestimated residual outlier in three of the models, but Massachusetts, ranking second, replaces it in the LIN_3 model. Differences among the models in ethnic effects determined this outlier pattern between these two states. Nebraska ranks high (tenth) in SCAN but low in FRAN (thirty-eighth) and BRIT (thirty-third), with the result that the LIN_3 model in which the ethnic effects are concentrated on a highly significant SCAN, is the one in which its death rate is not excessively underestimated. In contrast, Massachusetts ranks high in FRAN (eighth) and BRIT (second) and only moderately high in SCAN (sixteenth), so that its death rate is underestimated by that model, which includes only the SCAN ethnic effect. Massachusetts is a residual outlier also in the LIN_1 model, which includes only FRAN and SCAN as ethnic effects, but the presence of BRIT in the other two models keeps the estimate of its death rate sufficiently high.

Delaware ranks lowest in male mortality from Hodgkin's disease. It is an overestimated residual outlier in the BMD model because the SCAN effect, in which Delaware ranks fairly low (thirtieth), is absent. The heavy weight given to this ethnic variable in the three LIN models keeps the estimate of Delaware's death rate sufficiently low to avoid a residual outlier position.

TABLE XXV
Model Effects in Male Mortality from Hodgkin's Disease

	4		2	3	5		1	
BMD	−TEMP		−INCM	+CIGS	−DISP		+BRIT	
	7	4	1	3	5	6		2
LIN_1	−TEMP	+POLLUT	−INCM	+CIGS	−DISP	+FRAN		+SCAN
		4	1	3	5.5		5.5	2
LIN_2		+POLLUT	−INCM	+CIGS	−DISP		+BRIT	+SCAN
		4	3	2	5			1
LIN_3		+POLLUT	−INCM	+CIGS	−DISP			+SCAN

Florida is an overestimated residual outlier in all three LIN models, most extremely in LIN_2 and LIN_3, but not in the BMD model. Its very low recorded mortality, ranking forty-sixth, is best predicted by its very high rank (second) in the negative effect TEMP, and the absence of this variable in the LIN_2 and LIN_3 models leads to heavy overestimation of its mortality level. The inclusion of FRAN, in which Florida ranks high (tenth), ensures the outlier overestimation of its death rate in the LIN_1 model.

Females–F201 The state ranking lowest in female mortality from Hodgkin's disease, Wyoming, is an overestimated outlier in the model. Wyoming's very low ranking in POLLUT (forty-ninth) and PRELEV (forty-third) and high rank in the negative effect INCM (eleventh) are overtaken by its high ranking in CIGS (seventh) and SCAN (fifteenth) and low rank in the negative effect TEMP (forty-second), resulting in the strong overestimation of its very low observed death rate.

16 Leukemia and Aleukemia (ICD 204)

Males–M204 The only outlier in the model for male mortality from leukemia is top-ranked D. C. Its high rank in the negative effect BRIT and middle rank in SCAN, the two most important factors, outweigh its top ranks in the nonsignificant effects PRELEV and INCM to put the underestimation of its death rate in an outlier position.

Females–F204 Montana, ranked second highest in female death rate from leukemia, is an underestimated residual outlier, and low-ranking North Dakota (forty-second) is an overestimated residual outlier in the model for this female mortality. Only the SCAN effect, in which Montana ranks fifth, contributes correctly to the estimate of its high death rate. It is also the SCAN effect, in which North Dakota ranks first, that outweighs that state's low rank in POLLUT to produce an outlier overestimate of its very low death rate.

17 Breast (ICD 170)

Females–F170 Florida and West Virginia are overestimated residual outliers in both the BMD and the LIN models, which differ in only one small effect. Florida has a low-ranking death rate (thirty-fourth), which is greatly overestimated because of the state's very high ranking in PRELEV and DISP and its moderately high ranking in BRIT and OTHEUR. West Virginia's low ranking in the three ethnic model effects and in DISP are not sufficient to overcome its average ranking in the more significant model effects, negative TEMP, PRELEV, and POLLUT, resulting in excessive overestimation of its very low-ranking death rate (forty-fourth).

18 Ovary (ICD 175)

Females–F175 New Hampshire's high-ranking (seventh) death rate from cancer of the ovary is underestimated in the selected model. Only the state's very high rank (second) in CIGS and low rank (forty-fifth) in the negative effect TEMP correctly predict its high death rate, but its position in all the other model effects, particularly its very low rank (forty-eighth) in POLLUT, brings the estimate of its death rate to far below the high observed rate.

19 Cervix Uteri (ICD 171)

Females–F171 North Carolina, ranked sixteenth, is an overestimated outlier in the mortality model for cancer of the cervix uteri. The state's very low rank (forty-eighth) in the negative effect SCAN is not sufficiently offset by its middle rank (twenty-fourth) in CIGS and high rank (eleventh) in the negative effect TEMP to avoid outlier overestimation of its death rate.

20 Corpus and Other Parts of Uterus, and Uterus Unspecified (ICD 172)

Females–F172 Illinois and Oklahoma are residual outliers, both ranking high in death rate and both underestimated, in the mortality model for cancer of the corpus uteri. Illinois, tied for third in mortality level, also ranks very high (fourth) in OTHEUR, moderately high (fourteenth) in BRIT, and low (thirty-fifth) in the negative effect TEMP, but its middle rank (twenty-second) in PRELEV and high ranking in the negative effects SCAN (sixth) and WINE (eighteenth) prevail and produce an outlier underestimate of its very high death rate. Oklahoma's low ranks in the negative effects SCAN (fortieth) and WINE (thirty-second) are outweighed by the combination of its high rank (ninth) in the negative effect TEMP and its low values of BRIT, OTHEUR, and PRELEV, resulting in outlier underestimation of its twelfth-ranking death rate.

21 Prostate (ICD 177)

Males–M177 Florida, recording the lowest death rate in the country from cancer of the prostate, is an overestimated residual outlier in the model. A very high rank (second) in the negative effect TEMP is the only model effect that conforms to the state's very low mortality level. In particular, Florida's high-ranked value for DISP (sixth) ensures that the overestimation of its death rate will be an outlier.

22 Malignant Melanoma of Skin (ICD 190)

Males–M190 Texas, with the highest male mortality rate from malignant melanoma of the skin, is an underestimated residual outlier in both the BMD and the LIN models. Although it ranks high (seventh) in the most important effect in both models, TEMP, its values of FRAN and PRELEV are too low to avoid outlier underestimation in both models. Only low ranks in the negative ethnic effects, BRIT in the BMD model and OTHEUR in the LIN, reinforce the TEMP effect in the correct direction of estimating Texas' very high death rate. Texas is an extreme outlier in the distribution of residuals, falling into the 1% probability tail areas in both models.

Females–F190 Both Texas and Vermont are underestimated residual outliers in the female mortality model for malignant melanoma of the skin. Texas ranks second (tied with Georgia) and Vermont ranks eleventh (tied with California) in death rate. Texas' high rank in TEMP is overcome by its low rank in PRELEV and its middle rank in the negative effect MALT, resulting in an extreme outlier underestimate of its very high death rate. The climate variable PRELEV, like TEMP, cannot represent adequately a very large state such as Texas by a single value; the elevation varies little but the average precipitation varies greatly across the state. Since one of its two largest concentrations of population is in an area of high precipitation, a higher value of PRELEV might better reflect the exposure of the state's population to a wet climate, and would probably remove its underestimated death rate from such extreme outlier positions in both the male and female mortality models for melanoma of the skin.

Vermont is the only northern state among the 15 highest mortality rates and its very low rank (forty-third) in TEMP ensures its underestimation by this model. Its middle ranks in the other two factors also contribute to the underestimation of its high death rate.

23 Other Malignant Neoplasm of the Skin (ICD 191)

Males–M191 There are no residual outliers in the male mortality model for other malignant neoplasms of the skin.

Females–F191 Both models for female mortality from other malignant neoplasms of the skin have the same three underestimated residual outliers, Alabama, Tennessee, and Montana. This is the only one of the four skin cancer model sets in which TEMP does not remain a model effect after the ethnic variables are added. It is possible that if TEMP were in the model Alabama and Tennessee, ranked first and second in mortality, and also very high ranking in TEMP, would not have been so greatly underestimated. Also, if negative INCM had remained in the ethnic models the low income levels of these states could have prevented their residual outlier positions of underestimation. Alabama does rank high (sixth) in PRELEV and Tennessee moderately high (eighteenth), and their low ranks in all the negative effects, MALT, DISP, BRIT, and SCAN contribute to high estimates of their death rates. However the very low ranking of these two states in FRAN (forty-second, forty-ninth) precludes sufficiently high estimates of their death rates. Montana ranks surprisingly high in this type of cancer mortality (thirteenth), and like Vermont in female mortality from malignant melanoma, is the only northern state among those with the highest death rates. Its very low rank (forty-fourth) in PRELEV and high ranks in the negative effects, MALT, BRIT, and SCAN, ensure the underestimation of its high death rate. Only Montana's high rank (thirteenth) in FRAN conforms to its high female mortality from other malignancies of the skin.

Kansas, with a death rate of lower than average rank (thirtieth), is the only overestimated residual outlier in the models for this category of skin cancer. The outlier overestimation of its mortality occurs only in the LIN model and is due to its low ranks in the negative effects MALT, DISP, and BRIT.

Not only is it evident logically, but it is also indicated by the residual outliers in this model, that negative consumption effects are not real factors but stand in for missing factors with which they are closely correlated. Among these may be ethnic variables that are even more specific to a national group than those included in the variable pools. A low consumption of one type of alcohol may characterize such an ethnic group, as well as an occupational preference that increases their risk of skin cancer. Then a negative effect of that alcohol consumption might represent the risk occupation in the models through their ethnic association. It should also be noted here that the negative BRIT and negative SCAN effects in the skin cancer mortality models do not mean that women of British and Scandinavian background are less vulnerable to skin cancer mortality, but that they are less likely to live in a climate that produces skin cancer.

C Summary

The liberal definition of residual outlier used in this study—one whose value falls in the distributional tails comprising 5% of the probability (2½% in each tail)—leads to the expectation of two or three residual outliers among the 49 states in every model, equally divided between underestimated and overestimated state death rates. In Table XXI it can be seen that the only cancer mortality categories for which the model estimation produced more than the expected three residual outliers are male esophagus with five, and male kidney, female larynx, female intestine, female rectum, and female other skin with four each. For the male kidney, female intestine, and female other skin cancer mortality patterns there are alternative models with fewer residual outliers.

Generally there are more overestimated than underestimated outliers in the male cancer mortality models, while the reverse is true for the female cancer mortality models. The most consistently overestimated residual outlier in the male cancer mortality models is Florida, while in the female models Florida and Wyoming are most often in the overestimated outlier position. Neither state appears as an underestimated residual outlier in these cancer mortality models. Vermont is the most frequently underestimated residual outlier in the female cancer mortality models, but no state so emerges in the male models. Vermont also appears as an underestimated residual outlier in the male models, and as an overestimated one in both the male and female models, so that its lack of conformation to the cancer mortality models is generalized.

The persistence of Florida as an overestimated outlier in so many of the mortality models for both males and females suggests that a different policy exists (or existed in the years covered by the data) in that state for recording the residence of those who die there. In Chapter 7 it is shown that the outlier overestimation of Florida's recorded death rates also occurs in the mortality models for causes of death other than cancer and some reasons are suggested for its frequent outlier position of overestimation.

The following 18 states are never residual outliers in the cancer mortality models from the 12-variable pool: Arizona, Idaho, Indiana, Iowa, Kentucky, Maine, Minnesota, Missouri, New Jersey, New York, Ohio, Pennsylvania, Rhode Island, South Carolina, South Dakota, Virginia, Washington, and Wisconsin.

II Outliers in the Influence Space

A A Measure to Screen Potential Outliers

A different approach to detecting extreme or invalid observations lies not in the size of a case's deviation from the derived model but in the distance a case is from the other observations in the p-space of the independent variables. To express this in terms of the data of this study, if a state has a combination of factor values that differ radically from those of the other states, it might disproportionately influence the coefficient estimates in the model. However, this would not be revealed by a large residual value since the odd state's influence could have forced the model closer to its own configuration of factor/mortality relationships. In least squares regression the more extreme factor values have a greater influence in determining the coefficient estimates than do those clustered in midrange. A measure, known as the "weighted squared standardized distance" (WSSD), can be used, according to Daniel and Wood (17) "to spot points which may be controlling the global statistics." This measure is calculated for each state by taking the deviations of that state's factor values from their means, weighting each factor deviation by its associated coefficient in the model under observation, squaring both the deviation and the weight, summing over all factors included in the model, and standardizing by dividing by the variance estimate of the model. The measure for state j is

$$\mathrm{WSSD}_j = \frac{1}{s^2} \sum_{i=1}^{K} [b_i(x_{ij} - \bar{x}_i)]^2$$

where b_i is the coefficient estimate for the ith factor, x_{ij} is state j's value for the ith factor, $\bar{x}_i$ is the mean of the ith factor, K is the number of factor variables brought into the model, and s^2 is the mean squared error of the model. (The factor variables in this study are themselves standardized, so $\bar{x}_i$ equals zero for all i.) Since the influence of an extreme factor value also depends upon the importance of that factor in the model of interest, this measure indicates the relative size of each state's complete contribution to the total effect space or influence space of the model.

The distribution of the WSSD values for each best subset model was plotted, and any values that were so large as to stand apart from the others were noted. Table XXVI lists the states represented by these extreme values in the influence space, bracketing those which were considered to be acting jointly because of

TABLE XXVI

Potential Outliers in the Influence Space of the Best Subset Model for Each Cancer Mortality[a]

Site	Male	Female
Buc Cav & Ph	Nev; $\overline{\text{DC}}$	[$\overline{\text{Ark}}$, $\overline{\text{Nev}}$, $\overline{\text{NC}}$, $\overline{\text{Miss}}$, $\overline{\text{Ala}}$, $\overline{\text{SC}}$, $\overline{\text{DC}}$, $\overline{\text{Ga}}$[b]]
Larynx	Nev; $\overline{\text{DC}}$; Miss	$\overline{\text{DC}}$[b]; Nev; Miss
T, B, & Lung	$\overline{\text{Nev}}$	
T, B, & L Spec.		
B & L Unspec.		
Esophagus	$\overline{\text{DC}}$; Miss[b]	$\overline{\text{DC}}$; Nev; $\overline{\text{Miss}}$; $\underline{\text{Ark}}$
Stomach	$\underline{\text{Miss}}$	Miss
Lg. Intestine	$\underline{\text{Miss}}$	
Rectum	[$\underline{\text{Miss}}$, $\underline{\text{Ark}}$, $\underline{\text{SC}}$, $\underline{\text{Ala}}$] ; DC	[$\underline{\text{Miss}}$, $\underline{\text{Ark}}$, $\underline{\text{SC}}$, $\underline{\text{Ala}}$] ; $\overline{\text{DC}}$
Liver *et al.*	[$\underline{\text{NC}}$, SC]	[($\underline{\text{NC}}$, $\underline{\text{SC}}$); $\underline{\text{Ala}}$, $\underline{\text{Miss}}$, $\underline{\text{Ga}}$, Ark]
Pancreas		
Kidney	$\overline{\text{DC}}$; $\underline{\text{Miss}}$	
Bladder		Miss; $\overline{\text{DC}}$
Brain		
Lymphosarcoma		
Hodgkin's Dis.	[Miss, Ark] ; DC; $\overline{\text{Nev}}$	Miss
Leukemia		
Melanoma		[$\overline{\text{Ala}}$, $\overline{\text{NC}}$, $\overline{\text{Ga}}$, $\overline{\text{SC}}$, $\overline{\text{Miss}}$, $\overline{\text{Ark}}$]
Other Skin	$\underline{\text{DC}}$; $\overline{\text{Miss}}$; Nev	
Prostate	DC; $\underline{\text{Miss}}$	---------
Breast	---------	
Ovary	---------	
Cervix Uteri	---------	
Corpus Uteri	---------	

[a] Underscored states have death rates ranking in the lowest fifth; overbarred states have death rates ranking in the highest fifth.

[b] An outlier in the distribution of residuals.

their similarity in death rate and/or factor value. Each of these states was a potential outlier with respect to its influence in determination of the model rather than with respect to its nonconformity to the model. The degree of influence in each case was tested by examining the model changes that resulted from omitting that state. States were dropped individually or in the pairs shown in brackets in Table XXVI.

It is important to stress here that the subset models were derived without the states representing extreme values in influence space not in order to improve the models but to observe the influence of these exceptional cases on the models. It is usual that if such cases are considered to be outliers representing "bad" points whose influence must be removed, they are dropped. In this study D. C. is one of the three most frequent cases of extreme WSSD values, but its recorded death rates and factor values are probably more accurate than those of most of the states. Rather, D. C. as a totally urban unit represents an extreme point in the factor space which does and should exert strong influence on the chosen model. On the other hand the states of the deep South represent sets of outliers in the influence space and, because of economic and sociological factors, errors in their data are considered to be more likely. However in Table XXVI it can be seen that for some cancer mortalities these states represent not only sets of very low death rates (male and female cancer of the rectum; female cancer of the biliary passages and liver) but also of very high death rates (female cancer of the buccal cavity and pharynx; female melanoma), which are not usually considered to result from recording error.

D. C., Mississippi, and Nevada are those cases most often in outlier positions in the influence space, but only D. C. was shown to have noticeable influence on the subset models, while Nevada and Mississippi exhibited very little.

B Examination of D. C.'s Extreme Values

Because of D. C.'s importance not only as an extreme value in the effect space of several of the cancer mortality models but also as the only representative of a totally urban unit, its specific influence, as evidenced by the model changes that result from its omission, is presented in Table XXVII. The factors that owe their model strength to D. C. are those that are dropped or whose coefficients show marked decreases when D. C. is excluded from the cases. It can be seen that the positive effects of POLLUT, DISP, and FRAN tend to lose their importance, while those of BRIT and WINE and the negative SCAN effect gain when D. C.'s influence is removed. This applies to the models for a group of related mortalities—male cancer of the buccal cavity and pharynx, larynx and esophagus and female cancer of the larynx—and to a lesser degree to the models for male mortality from cancer of the kidney, of the prostate, and from Hodgkin's disease. D. C.'s top ranking in five of these seven cancer mortalities and in the

TABLE XXVII

Changes in Best Subset Models of Cancer Mortality When Extreme Values in Influence Space Are Omitted

Cancer mortality	State's rank in death rate	Model effect added	Model effect with marked increase[a] in coefficient	Model effect dropped	Model effect with marked decrease[a] in coefficient
		(factors strengthened by omission of state)		(factors strengthened by inclusion of state)	
Omission of D. C.					
M-Buc Cav & Ph.	1	BRIT			FRAN (*** to ns)
M-Larynx	1	WINE*, BRIT		POLLUT*, DISP**	FRAN (*** to ns)
F-Larynx	1	BRIT	–SCAN (ns to ***)	POLLUT, DISP*	
M-Esophagus	1	–TEMP, WINE, –SCAN		POLLUT	DISP (*** to ns)
F-Esophagus	8½				
M-Rectum	11				
F-Rectum	10				
M-Kidney	1	CIGS	OTHEUR (* to ***)	MALT	DISP (*** to ns)
F-Bladder	1				
M-Hodgkin's	22½	BRIT		–TEMP, FRAN	
M-Other Skin	41				
M-Prostate	16	PRELEV, –OTHEUR		–WINE*, DISP**	
Omission of Nevada					
M-Buc Cav & Ph.	29				
M-Larynx	15½				
F-Larynx	35	–MALT		PRELEV	
M-T, B, & Lung	9	–POLLUT*, MALT, OTHEUR		CIGS	
M-T, B, & L Spec.	18				
M-B & L Unspec.	9				
F-Esophagus	22				
M-Hodgkin's	7	BRIT		FRAN	
M-Other Skin	23½				

[a] Change of more than one level of significance.
ns, not significant; *, $.01 < p < .05$; **, $.001 < p < .01$; ***, $p < .001$.

Omission of Mississippi					
M-Larynx	31				
F-Larynx	22				
M-Esophagus	33				
F-Esophagus	4			–DISP	
M-Stomach	43				
F-Stomach	35				
M-Lg. Intestine	40				
M-Kidney	49	CIGS, –BRIT	OTHEUR (* to ***)	MALT, –FRAN	DISP (*** to ns)
F-Bladder	37			POLLUT, –INCM	
F-Hodgkin's	36				
M-Other Skin	1	INCM			FRAN (** to ns)
M-Prostate	42				
Omission of Mississippi, Arkansas					
M-Hodgkin's	27, 32			–TEMP, FRAN	
Omission of North Carolina, South Carolina					
M-Liver *et al.*	46½, 33			–TEMP, –CIGS*, FRAN*	
F-Liver *et al.*	46, 48			–CIGS	
Omission of Mississippi, Arkansas, South Carolina, Alabama					
M-Rectum	47, 49, 41, 48			MALT	
F-Rectum	49, 43, 45, 44			PRELEV, MALT	

variables of interest (Table XXII) ensure its strong role in determining the models. The question of the legitimacy of its inclusion, as Hartley recently pointed out (44) is "whether the model is relevant over a full range or a restricted range," and since here relevancy is desired over the whole range of geographic units, from totally urban to totally rural, its exclusion would be misleading.

An evaluation of the validity of D. C.'s contribution might also rest on a pragmatic judgment of the derived models. The loss or weakening of two apparently valid factors in mortality from cancer of the larynx and the esophagus, i.e., levels of pollution and consumption of distilled spirits, when D. C. is omitted would indicate the importance of maintaining it in the derivation. Judgment is not as clear when the changes in ethnic effects are considered. On the one hand the omission of D. C. weakens ethnic effects in the model that were confirmed by foreign ranking, viz., the very significant FRAN effects in male mortality from cancer of the buccal cavity and pharynx and of the larynx, which are matched by the top ranking of males in France in both mortalities. D. C.'s omission also brings BRIT effects into the male mortality models for cancer of the buccal cavity and pharynx and of the larynx, which have no counterpart in higher male death rates in the British countries. These unfavorable changes in the ethnic model effects argue for D. C.'s inclusion. On the other hand, the omission of D. C. brings into the model an ethnic effect that is confirmed by foreign ranking, viz., a positive BRIT effect in female mortality from cancer of the larynx matched by the high ranks of women in Ireland (first), Northern Ireland (second), Scotland (fourth), and England and Wales (sixth), and it greatly strengthens the negative SCAN effect, which is matched by the lowest ranks of women in Sweden and Norway. Thus the model reveals important and apparently valid ethnic factors only when D. C. is dropped. Although on balance no clear-cut decision arises from these differences in model ethnic effects as to the exclusion of D. C., it is of positive value to observe that valid factor information can be gained from the models derived with and without D. C.

When D. C. is omitted from the model for male mortality from laryngeal cancer the WINE effect appears to replace in large part the ethnic effect with which it is most closely associated, FRAN, but D. C.'s omission from the male mortality model for cancer of the kidney removes the MALT effect while strengthening the ethnic variable with which it is most closely associated, OTHEUR. Thus D. C.'s influence favors the ethnic factor in the laryngeal cancer model but favors the alcohol consumption factor in the kidney cancer model. Changes in the mortality model for prostatic cancer when D. C. is dropped involved shifting from significant alcohol consumption effects, DISP, and negative WINE, to a nonsignificant ethnic factor, negative OTHEUR. Although nothing definitive can be determined from these model changes as to the primacy of alcohol consumption or ethnicity in these cancer mortalities, it is evident that inclusion of a totally urban unit such as D. C. does alter the emphasis in particular mortality models between these two types of factors.

Removal of D. C. brings little change to the model of male mortality from Hodgkin's disease, with all the significant effects maintained, and only nonsignificant effects added (BRIT) or dropped (FRAN and negative TEMP). In the remaining models for which D. C. represents an extreme value in the influence space—female mortality from cancer of the esophagus, rectum, and bladder and male mortality from cancer of the rectum and other skin—its removal does not produce any notable changes.

C Other Potential Outliers in Influence Space

Mississippi is a state whose values of factors associated with degree of urbanization rank at the opposite end of the scale from those of D. C. Its death rate also ranks very low in many, but certainly not all, of the categories of cancer mortality. The same procedure for determining D. C.'s role in model derivation was used (Table XXVII), dropping Mississippi from the 49 cases and then deriving the models in whose influence space Mississippi held an extreme value. In male and female mortality from cancer of the rectum a set of four states including Mississippi was dropped and in male mortality from Hodgkin's disease Mississippi and Arkansas were excluded together. The only model showing many changes was that for male mortality from cancer of the kidney. Two nonsignificant effects, MALT and negative FRAN, were dropped while two other nonsignificant effects, CIGS and negative BRIT, were added. However, the most radical changes were in the loss of significance of a very highly significant DISP effect, and in the large increase in significance of a positive OTHEUR effect. Thus the importance of the alcohol consumption factors in male mortality from kidney cancer is considerably reduced when Mississippi is not included, while the Other European ethnic effect becomes much more important and a CIGS effect appears. Since Mississippi ranks lowest in this mortality and very low in all the factors in question its influence is exercised as the lack of a high factor level resulting in the lack of a high level of mortality.

The exclusion of Mississippi engenders minor changes in a few other models as follows: added INCM effect, loss of significance of FRAN effect in male mortality from other skin cancer; loss of nonsignificant negative DISP effect in female mortality from cancer of the esophagus; loss of the nonsignificant effects, POLLUT and negative INCM, in female mortality from cancer of the bladder.

When both Mississippi and Arkansas are excluded as a pair, the model for male mortality from Hodgkin's disease loses the nonsignificant effects FRAN and negative TEMP. Exclusion of the set of four states, Mississippi, Arkansas, South Carolina, and Alabama, results in losing only nonsignificant effects from the rectal cancer mortality models—MALT from the one for males, and MALT and PRELEV from the one for females. Thus the models show a great deal of stability even when a set of states representing extreme values in the influence space is dropped from their derivation.

The exclusion of Nevada from the derivation of those models for which it constitutes an extreme value in influence space results in changes of note in only one model. The male mortality model for the combined category of trachea, bronchus, and lung cancer, both specified primary and unspecified, loses a nonsignificant CIGS effect and gains a significant negative POLLUT effect as well as nonsignificant effects MALT and OTHEUR. Since Nevada does not represent extreme values in the influence space of the models for either of the component mortality patterns, the basis for its special effect in the combined pattern is difficult to trace. Nevada does rank high in death rate for the combined category (ninth) and the unspecified component (ninth), but not the specified primary component (eighteenth). An effort to pinpoint the nature of Nevada's influence by omitting it from the derivation of the models for both component mortalities, i.e., the specified primary and the unspecified lung cancer models, produced no differences in effects. Thus, since Nevada's omission is not warranted from the component mortality models, dropping it from the model of the combined mortality is not indicated.

In the female mortality model for cancer of the larynx the exclusion of Nevada resulted in the loss of PRELEV and the addition of negative MALT, both nonsignificant effects. In the model for male mortality from Hodgkin's disease, FRAN was dropped and BRIT added, also nonsignificant effects.

The omission of low-ranking Arkansas from the model for female mortality from cancer of the esophagus produced no changes in the model effects. Although there were four extreme values in the influence space for this mortality model—Nevada, high-ranking Mississippi and D. C., and low-ranking Arkansas—only one change resulted from excluding any of the four states. This was the loss of the nonsignificant negative DISP effect when Mississippi was omitted. Thus model stability is again shown when states representing extreme values in the influence space are dropped, reducing the likelihood that they are outliers to be discarded.

When the Carolinas were omitted jointly from the mortality models for cancer of the biliary passages and liver several effects were dropped but none added. The male mortality model lost the significant effects FRAN and negative CIGS and the nonsignificant negative TEMP effect. The female mortality model also lost a negative CIGS effect. Several states have extreme values in the influence space of the female mortality model for this combined category of cancer primaries, and they also have very low-ranking death rates, just as do North and South Carolina, but omitting them would deprive the model of most of the lower range of its cases. Similarly, omitting the group of states that represent extreme values in the influence space of the female mortality model for cancer of the buccal cavity and pharynx and that also rank very high in death rate, would deprive the model of its upper range of cases. The same applies to the group of southern states that represent extreme values in the influence space of the female mortality model for melanoma but also constitute the upper range of cases in this type of mortality. Excluding groups such as these from determination of the models simply because they exert strong influence would produce models for only a truncated range of mortality rates.

D Conclusion

Although exclusion of some of the states with extreme values in the influence space resulted in notable change in a few cases, the decision could not be made that they constitute actual outliers which should be dropped from the model derivation. Rather they were considered to represent special but valid cases in each model, and their specific influence was investigated and presented.

It will be seen in Chapter 7 that the same three states that present most of the extreme values in the influence spaces of the cancer mortality models also do so in the set of mortality models for the major categories of death.

Chapter 6
Comparison of Factors in the Mortality Models of Major Categories of Death

I Introduction

In an earlier study (1) at the Anderson Hospital age-adjusted death rates for the major disease categories were calculated and averaged over the 11 years 1949-1959, a period that covers the first half of the 20 years (1950-1969) of Mason and McKay's data. Purely for comparative purposes models were derived for the mortality patterns of these causes of death other than cancer using the same variable pools as for the cancer models. Since these pools were chosen for their combined effects specifically in cancer mortality patterns, it could not be expected that the models derived from such variable pools tailored to the cancer data would behave satisfactorily for other types of mortality patterns. But the nature of this study is essentially comparative, rather than strictly determinative, contrasting a combination of effects that explains statistically the variance of one mortality pattern against a combination that explains the variance of another mortality pattern, always employing the same basic variable pools from which the combinations can be selected. In collating the combinations chosen to explain the variation in mortality due to causes other than cancer, only the models from the 8- and 12-variable pools are shown, i.e., those in which alcohol consumption is divided into its three components. Table XI displays the coefficients in these models of mortality from (nonmalignant) diseases of the circulatory, the respiratory, the digestive and the genito-urinary systems, from infectious and parasitic diseases, from accidental and violent causes, and from all causes including cancer. Diseases of the respiratory system are excepted for flu and asthma, while flu and tuberculosis are omitted from the infectious and parasitic group.

II Nonethnic Factors

Models for total cancer mortality are shown for the rates averaged over both time periods, the full 20-year period for comparability with individual cancer sites and the early 11-year period for comparability with the mortality patterns of other major causes of death. This also permits a comparison over time, since differences between the total cancer mortality models of both periods are due to changes in the relative importance of individual cancer sites occurring in the later years of the longer period, that is, in the 1960s. It is therefore interesting to note that, except for minor differences in the size of the coefficients, but not in their level of significance, the models for the females are identical in both periods. However, in the male mortality models negative TEMP, a significant effect in the early period, does not even enter the models of the complete time period, while CIGS, missing from the early models, enters the 20-year models, but not significantly. A negative income effect, not in the earlier male mortality models, enters one for the full period. Models for the latter half of the 20-year period would have shown these differences more clearly, but the age-adjusted death rates for those years were not averaged separately in Mason and McKay's book.

The decline in importance of cold temperature as a factor in the total cancer mortality model for males reflects the increasing importance of the respiratory cancers, in whose mortality models TEMP is a positive factor. This offsets the negative effect of TEMP in the digestive and genito-urinary cancer mortality models when all cancer deaths are combined into one category.

There are also differences in factor effects among the major categories of mortality. Referring to the cancer mortality model of the earlier time period for comparability with the models of the other major death categories, the variable TEMP appears as an important negative effect only in the mortality models for total cancer and for diseases of the circulatory system. It is a significantly positive factor in the models from the nonethnic pools for infectious and parasitic diseases and for accidental and violent deaths, losing its importance when the ethnic variables are included in the pools. Considering the importance of TEMP as a positive effect in the respiratory cancers, it is interesting that it enters positively, though not significantly, one mortality model of diseases of the respiratory system (other than cancer).

The other climate variable, PRELEV, is an even stronger dividing factor among the major causes of death. Its coefficients are very significantly positive in the mortality models for total cancer and for diseases of the circulatory system, and very significantly negative in those for all the other major categories except diseases of the genito-urinary system, in whose models it is absent. Thus a wet climate at low elevation is associated with higher mortality from cancer and diseases of the circulatory system, while a dry climate at high elevation is associated with higher mortality from diseases of the respiratory and the digestive systems, from infectious and parasitic diseases, and from accidents and violence. The relationship between this factor and urbanization and population density is discussed in Chapters 2 and 9.

POLLUT is a significant positive effect in mortality from diseases of the circulatory, the respiratory, and the genito-urinary systems, in male mortality from diseases of the digestive system, and in female cancer mortality, but in every case it either loses its importance or disappears after adjustment for the ethnic variables. The only important income effect after adjustment for all other variables is a significantly positive coefficient for INCM in both male and female mortality models for diseases of the genito-urinary system.

CIGS and DISP are the weakest of the consumption variables, though their effects may be entering the models through the ethnic factors, which do represent highly differentiated consumption patterns. Although CIGS enters several of the nonethnic models, it is consistently replaced by ethnic factors. Only in the 20-year total cancer mortality pattern for males discussed above does it remain after adjustment for ethnic effects. Consumption of distilled spirits is a factor in male mortality from diseases of the circulatory, of the digestive, and of the genito-urinary systems, and in mortality of both sexes from accidental and violent causes. MALT is an important factor for both male and female mortality patterns in total cancer, in diseases of the digestive system, and in infectious and parasitic diseases, and for female mortality from diseases of the circulatory system and from accidental and violent causes. WINE is a significant positive effect in the mortality of both sexes from diseases of the digestive and of the respiratory systems, and in the male total cancer mortality pattern. The negative effects of MALT and WINE in the mortality models for diseases of the genito-urinary system are probably standing in for associated factors that are not in the variable pools. As has been stated, the variable pools used are specific to cancer mortality patterns and the mortality models for other causes of death are shown for comparison only. As can be seen in Table XI the amount of variation explained (R^2) is over 80% in all of the total cancer mortality models, while this percentage is achieved in only one of the noncancer mortality models.

III Ethnic Factors

In a 1966 volume Segi (45) ranked 30 nations with respect to the age-adjusted death rates for men and for women from causes of death other than cancer. For comparison with the ethnic effects in the U. S. mortality models, the 1956-1957 death rates of 23 of those nations that represent white ethnicity in the United States were reranked within that subset. The results are shown in Table XXVIII and reference to this table is helpful in reading the discussion in this section. A combined rank for a group of countries was calculated by weighting individual national ranks in accordance with their relative proportions in the white population of the U. S. Approximately the upper, the middle, and the lower thirds in ranks were characterized as high, mid, and low, with consideration given to actual value intervals at the breaking points.

In the mortality models for total cancer there is one match between ethnic effect and foreign ranking for males and two for females. The Other European

TABLE XXVIII

Comparison of Ethnic Effects in U. S. Mortality Models[a] with Foreign Ranking in Major Causes of Death

	MALES							
	FRAN		BRIT		SCAN		OTHEUR	
Category of mortality	Effect	Rank	Effect	Combined rank	Effect	Combined rank	Effect	Combined rank
All Malignant Neoplasms	Pos.	Mid	Null	High exc. Ire. mid	Null	Low exc. Den. mid	Pos.	High exc. Italy low
Circulatory System	Null		Pos.		Neg.		Null	
Vascular Lesions affecting Nervous System		Mid		High exc. Ire. low		Mid exc. Den. low		High (mixed)
Heart Diseases		Low		High		Mid exc. Nor. low		Mid
Hypertension without mention of Heart Disease		Mid		High		Low		Mid
Respiratory System	Null		Pos.		Neg.		Null	
Bronchitis		Low		High		Low		Mid
Pneumonia		Mid		Mid		Low		High (mixed)
Digestive System	Pos.		Null		Neg.		Null	
Ulcers		Low		High		Low exc. Swed. mid		Mid
Gastritis		Low		Mid		Low		Mid (mixed)
Cirrhosis		High		Low		Low		High
Genito-Urinary System	Null		Null		Neg.		Null	
Nephritis and Nephrosis		Mid		Mid exc. Ire. high		Low exc. Swed. mid		Mid (mixed)
Infectious and Parasitic Diseases	Pos.		Neg.		Neg.		Neg.	
Accidental and Violent Causes	Pos.		Neg.		Null		Neg.	
Accidents		High		Low exc. Scot. mid		Mid		Mid (mixed)
Suicide		High		Low exc. E & W mid		Mid (mixed)		Mid (mixed)

Category of mortality	FEMALES							
	FRAN		BRIT		SCAN		OTHEUR	
	Effect	Rank	Effect	Combined rank	Effect	Combined rank	Effect	Combined rank
All Malignant Neoplasms	Null	Low	Pos.	Mid exc. Scot. high	Neg.	Low exc. Den. high	Pos.	High exc. Italy low
Circulatory System	Null		Pos.		Neg.		Null	
Vascular Lesions affecting Nervous System		Low		High exc. Ire. mid		Mid exc. Den. low		High (mixed)
Heart Diseases		Low		High exc. E & W mid		Mid exc. Nor. low		Mid (mixed)
Hypertension without mention of Heart Disease		Low		High		Low		Mid
Respiratory System	Neg.		Null		Neg.		Null	
Bronchitis		Low		High		Low		Mid exc. Italy high
Pneumonia		Mid		Mid		Mid exc. Den. low		High (mixed)
Digestive System	Null		Pos.		Neg.		Null	
Ulcers		Low		High		Mid exc. Nor. low		Low
Gastritis		Low		Mid		Low		Mid (mixed)
Cirrhosis		High		Low		Low exc. Den. high		High
Genito-Urinary System	Null		Null		Neg.		Null	
Nephritis and Nephrosis		Mid		Mid (mixed)		Low exc. Swed. mid		Mid (mixed)
Infectious and Parasitic Diseases	Null		Neg.		Neg.		Null	
Accidental and Violent Causes	Pos.		Neg.		Null		Neg.	
Accidents		High		Low exc. Scot. mid		Mid exc. Swed. low		Mid (mixed)
Suicide		Mid		Mid exc. Ire. low		Mid (mixed)		Mid (mixed)

effect is positive for both sexes and the countries of that group included in Segi have a combined rank that is high for both men and women, with Italy a low-ranking exception in both cases. Unfortunately the omission of Russia, Poland, and Lithuania in Segi precludes a full representation of the countries that are counterpart to the ethnic variable OTHEUR. However, it should be noted here that for no major disease category other than cancer is the OTHEUR effect of positive importance nor the ranks of the Other European countries so high. Thus the particular combination of countries represented in OTHEUR is effective in deriving cancer mortality models, as it was designed to be, but not those for other categories of death, in which their common effect is null either because the component ethnic effects are themselves null or are neutralized in the mix.

The other match in the total cancer category is negative SCAN in the female mortality models, which is confirmed by the low ranks of women in Norway and Sweden. However, women in Denmark rank first in cancer mortality, but either their small proportion in the U. S. Scandinavian community or an altered experience after immigration prevents their nullifying the negative SCAN effect in the mortality models. When all malignant neoplasms are combined into a single category of mortality, specific ethnic effects for particular cancer sites are obscured and comparison between U. S. mortality and foreign experience is even more generalized.

Segi gives the national rankings for three subcategories of circulatory system diseases, all of which are presented for comparison with the ethnic effects in the total circulatory system models. For this type of mortality there is clearly a better match between model effect and foreign experience than for cancer mortality. The positive coefficients of BRIT in both the male and the female mortality models correspond to high ranks in all the subcategories for both men and women in the British countries with minimal exception. Similarly, the negative coefficients of SCAN in the mortality models for both sexes correspond to generally low ranks in all three subcategories for both sexes in the Scandinavian countries. The effect of OTHEUR is neutralized by the mixed ranks of the countries it represents, and hence does not enter the models. The null effect of FRAN is matched by the middle ranks in two of the subcategories for males in France. However, the low mortality risk of women in France, indicated by their low ranks in all three subcategories, is not maintained in the U. S. but rises toward the level of their male counterparts. This was also noted in cancer of the buccal cavity and pharynx.

The two subcategories of diseases of the respiratory system ranked by Segi are bronchitis and pneumonia. Here also is found a good match between the ethnic effects in the U. S. and their foreign counterpart ranks. Scandinavian mortality rates in both subcategories are low for both sexes, confirming the negative SCAN effects in the models. The positive BRIT effect for males corresponds to a high male mortality from bronchitis in the British countries, and the negative FRAN effect for females corresponds to a low female mortality from bronchitis in France. Again the null effect of OTHEUR reflects the middle rankings as well as the broad range of ranks for this group.

The three subcategories of diseases of the digestive system with rankings in Segi are not homogeneous with respect to their national characteristics but appear to be competitive in their mortality risks. Both the men and the women in France rank at the very bottom in mortality from ulcers and gastritis, but rank second highest in mortality from cirrhosis, each suffering quadruple the median rate for that sex. This latter risk is matched by the positive FRAN effect in the male mortality model. The FRAN effect may be neutralized in the female mortality model by the low mortality risk for women in France from ulcers and gastritis. In the male mortality models the high mortality risk from cirrhosis evidently outweighs a low mortality risk from ulcers and from gastritis, resulting in a positive FRAN effect, while it is apparently not strong enough in the female mortality models. The men and women living in the British countries both experience a mortality risk that is high from ulcers, middling from gastritis, and low from cirrhosis. In the female mortality models, this high ulcer mortality risk predominates, resulting in a positive BRIT effect, but not in the male mortality models. The negative SCAN effect in the models for both sexes corresponds to the low ranks for both men and women in Scandinavia in mortality from gastritis and cirrhosis, with the exception of the moderately high rank of women in Denmark (tied for seventh out of 23). Although Sweden and Denmark have middle to high ranks in ulcer mortality, Norway ranks very low, thereby maintaining an overall low mortality risk from diseases of the digestive system for the Scandinavian countries.

With Segi's national rankings in mortality from nephritis and nephrosis as the only representative of diseases of the genito-urinary system, the model effects are corroborated. Only negative SCAN appears in the male and the female mortality models, matched by the low ranks of Norway and Denmark in mortality from nephritis and nephrosis, while Sweden ranks in the middle. The other three ethnic effects are null, reflecting the middle or the mixed ranks of the corresponding countries.

Unfortunately the strong ethnic effects in the models of mortality from infectious and parasitic diseases could not be checked because Segi does not include even a subcategory of this set.

The mortality patterns for accidental and violent deaths, included as a contrast to disease mortality, show interesting correspondences between the U. S. models and the national rankings. The positive effect of FRAN in both the male and female mortality models is paralleled by the high ranking of men and women living in France in accidental deaths and the high rank of French men in suicide. In contrast, the negative BRIT effect in the mortality models for both sexes is paralleled by the low ranks of England and Wales and both the Irelands in male and female accidental death rates, and the low ranks of males in Scotland and the Irelands and of females in the Irelands in suicides. No ranks in this death category were high for males or females in any of the British countries. The Scandinavian ranks are mixed in accidental and violent mortality, and the ethnic effect correspondingly null in the models. On the other hand, the ranks of the Other European countries are also mixed in these subcategories, but a negative OTHEUR effect enters both the male and female U. S. mortality models, implying a decrease in risk of accidental and violent death for these ethnic groups after migrating to this country.

IV Deaths from All Causes

Looking at overall mortality, Table XI presents the models chosen from all the variable pools for the total category of deaths from all causes covering the years 1949-1959. Stability in the model effects combines with marked similarities and contrasts between male and female mortality to characterize these two sets of models. It should be noted that state variation in male death rates is not quite as well accounted for by the models as is the variation in female rates, indicated by a smaller R^2 for the male mortality models.

POLLUT emerges as the most consistent nonethnic variable in both male and female mortality, higher levels associated with higher overall death rates. The negative effect TEMP indicates in both model sets that colder temperatures are also associated with higher death rates, but this is a very much stronger effect for females than for males. On the other hand the precipitation/elevation factor PRELEV, dominating the cancer models as a positive effect, is a net negative effect in total male mortality and does not enter the models for females. It is thus apparent that the negative effect of PRELEV in mortality models for diseases of the respiratory and the digestive systems, infectious and parasitic diseases, and accidental and violent causes overcomes its positive effect in the male mortality models for cancer and diseases of the circulatory system, and only counterbalances it in the female mortality models. The key to this difference between total male and total female mortality is in the mortality from accidental and violent causes in which the negative effect of PRELEV is much stronger for males than for females, while this category of deaths is proportionately greater for males than for females (9.8 vs. 5.6%).

In both male and female nonethnic mortality models low income and high cigarette consumption are associated with high death rates, but when the ethnic factors are added to the variable pools, both INCM and CIGS are dropped from the models. This is a strong indication that these two factors are accounted for in many models by their ethnic associations. This does not imply that they are not actual factors since they may be the underlying cause of the ethnic effects.

Alcohol consumption is important in male mortality, particularly the consumption of distilled spirits, while malt consumption is the significant component in female mortality.

Easily the most important factor in both male and female mortality is the ethnic effect, negative SCAN. Referring again to Segi, the Scandinavian countries rank at the bottom in mortality from all causes for both the males and the females, paralleling the U.S. experience.

The greatest difference between the male and female mortality models is the importance of the ethnic effect FRAN in the male mortality models with its omission from those for the females, and the similar importance of BRIT in the female mortality models with its omission from those for the males. This French ethnic effect is confirmed in Segi where males in France rank high in mortality, sixth out of the 23 countries ranked, while the female mortality there is of middle rank (fourteenth). The null British effect for males is confirmed by middle ranks in the death rates for men in England and Wales (thirteenth), Northern Ireland (fourteenth), and Ireland (fifteenth), but the men in Scotland rank high (fifth). Women in England and Wales rank even lower (eighteenth) than the men in mortality, but the women in Ireland rank high in mortality (sixth) and join the high-ranking women in Scotland (seventh) to indicate a generally higher ranking in total mortality for British women than for the men. (This does not mean that the death rates of females are higher than those of males in Britain but that they rank relatively higher among women in the 23 countries of interest than British men do among the males.)

The overall mortality levels of men, and also of women, in the other European countries differ too greatly among themselves to be characterized by a common level. Similarly the OTHEUR effect in both male and female total mortality models is neither significant nor consistent within a model set.

V Ridge Regression Analysis

A summary of the relative importance of the model effects for the major categories of death after stabilization of their coefficient estimates using ridge regression techniques is shown in Table XIII. Comparing the 1950-1969 average death rates with the 1949-1959 averages for All Malignant Neoplasms, the PRELEV effect is confirmed to be the major factor in the total category, but a very unstable one in the male mortality patterns. The coefficient estimates of PRELEV display some stability in the female patterns, but those of POLLUT, MALT, BRIT, and CIGS are very stable in female mortality. While there is almost no difference between the two periods in the relative importance of the model effects in the female mortality patterns, there are definite changes for the males. CIGS and WINE gain much more importance in the full period than they had in the earlier half, and FRAN and MALT also gain in importance. All of these factors except MALT have very stable traces of coefficient estimates.

BRIT is shown to be an important stable effect in the male and in the female patterns of total cancer mortality in both periods. Comparing the male with the female mortality patterns, the POLLUT effect appears in the ridge trace to be relatively more important and definitely more stable in the female patterns. The negative TEMP effect is considerably, and the OTHEUR effect slightly, more important in the female mortality patterns, but neither has stable coefficient estimates throughout the ridge trace of either the male or female patterns.

When comparison is made with the model effects of the other major causes of death, the total cancer category shows strongest similarity with the mortality pattern of diseases of the circulatory system. The major effect PRELEV is confirmed to be the major discriminating effect between cancer and circulatory system diseases, in which it is positive, and almost all the other causes of death, in which it is negative. It is positive but unimportant in the genito-urinary diseases category. The positive and negative effects of PRELEV cancel each other when total mortality from all causes of death is considered. In spite of this balance, the coefficient estimates of PRELEV in the various mortality patterns show stability only when it is a positive effect, that is, in mortality from cancer and from diseases of the circulatory system.

The ridge regression analysis mostly confirms the effects in the models chosen by the BMD and LINCUR programs, but the exceptions are worth noting. The ridge trace shows POLLUT to be a much more important factor in total cancer mortality than indicated by the subset models due to increasing coefficient estimates before stabilization in the male mortality patterns, and due to stability of the coefficient estimates in the female mortality patterns. Also due to their stability the BRIT, FRAN, CIGS, WINE, and MALT effects are indicated by the ridge trace to be more important, particularly in the 20-year mortality patterns. DISP is also shown to be a factor in the male cancer mortality pattern for the full period. In mortality from diseases of the circulatory system the CIGS effect is given much greater importance by the ridge trace in both male and female mortality, its negative coefficient in the latter evolving into a positive one of moderate size. The ridge trace for diseases of the digestive system shows the WINE effect to be the primary alcohol consumption factor in the male mortality pattern, rather than an equal division of importance among all three components as in the model chosen from the 12-variable pool. The primacy and stability of the WINE factor is shown for both male and female mortality from diseases of the digestive system. In the mortality patterns for diseases of the genito-urinary system the strong positive INCM effect in the models chosen from the 12-variable pool is shown in the ridge trace to be highly unstable and of little importance in the stable patterns of both male and female mortality. Similarly, the very large MALT effect indicated by the chosen models of mortality from infectious and parasitic diseases is considerably reduced in the stable patterns for both males and females.

Finally, in the male mortality pattern for all causes of death ridge regression analysis gives much more importance to the CIGS effect and much less to the negative PRELEV and the negative TEMP effects than do the models chosen from the 12-variable pool. However, the models for female mortality from all causes are confirmed by the ridge trace, and in particular, the negative TEMP effect is shown to be the major one in the stable pattern.

Chapter 7
Outliers in the Mortality Models for Major Categories of Death

I Residual Outliers

For the major categories of death examination was made of the residual outliers in both the "nonethnic" and the "ethnic" mortality models, i.e., those models chosen from the 8-variable pool and from the 12-variable pool. They are summarized in Table XXIX, and reference to that table will clarify the discussion of individual residual outliers that follows.

A All Malignant Neoplasms (ICD 140-205): 1950-1969

Males

Florida, ranking only twenty-third in male mortality from total cancer, is an extremely overestimated residual outlier in both the nonethnic and the ethnic models, while Delaware, ranking thirteenth, is an overestimated residual outlier only in the model from the nonethnic variable pool. The climate variable PRELEV, in which Florida ranks third, is the most important factor (has the largest coefficient) in both models for this category of mortality, resulting in a high estimate of total male cancer mortality in that state. Also its high ranking in CIGS (eleventh) and WINE (fifteenth) contribute to the overestimation. In the ethnic model Florida's high ranks in FRAN (tenth) and OTHEUR (thirteenth), both important positive factors, combine with its high value of PRELEV to further overestimate its male mortality rate from all malignant neoplasms.

As in the case of Florida, Delaware's high rank (second) in PRELEV is primarily responsible for the overestimation of its total cancer mortality rate in males. In addition, Delaware ranks even higher in the consumption factor CIGS (fifth) than it ranks in mortality. However, when the ethnic variables enter the models, Delaware ceases to be a residual outlier since its ranks in the ethnic effects FRAN (sixteenth) and OTHEUR (sixteenth) are compatible with its mortality level and make up for its high values of PRELEV and CIGS.

Females

Florida is also an overestimated residual outlier in both models of female mortality from all malignant neoplasms. It ranks much lower in total cancer

TABLE XXIX
Residual Outliers in the Models for Major Categories of Death
From the 8- and 12-Variable Pools

Category of death	Males		Females	
	Underestimated	Overestimated	Underestimated	Overestimated
All malignant neoplasms–ICD 140-205 (1950-1969)				
8 VAR	None	FLA** DEL	None	FLA*
12 VAR	None	FLA***	None	FLA* WYO* MICH
All malignant neoplasms–ICD 140-205 (1949-1959)				
8 VAR	None	FLA ORE	None	FLA**
12 VAR	None	FLA** WYO	None	FLA**
Circulatory system–ICD 400-468 (1949-1959)				
8 VAR	None	FLA** NM	NY	FLA*
12 VAR	None	FLA** NM*	None	FLA** MICH*
Respiratory system excluding influenza and asthma–ICD 470-475, 490-527 (1949-1959)				
8 VAR	COLO**	None	COLO** NM**	None
12 VAR	COLO** ARIZ*	None	COLO** NM	None
Digestive system–ICD 530-587 (1949-1959)				
8 VAR	DC** NM*	ORE*	NM***	ORE
12 VAR	DC* NM*	None	NM***	ORE
Genito-urinary system–ICD 590-637 (1949-1959)				
8 VAR	IND	FLA	DEL** IND	MINN
12 VAR	IND DC	None	DEL	TEX
Infectious and parasitic excluding tuberculosis and influenza–ICD 020-138 (1949-1959)				
8 VAR	TEX** KY	None	TEX** NM*** KY	None
12 VAR	TEX* WYO	IDA*	TEX** NM***	None
Accidental and violent causes–ICD E800-E999 (1949-1959)				
8 VAR	NEV**	None	NEV**	ARIZ
12 VAR	MONT	RI*	IND MASS	None
All causes–ICD 001-E999 (1949-1959)				
8 VAR	None	FLA**	NM**	FLA** MINN
12 VAR	None	FLA**	NM*	FLA* MICH*

No asterisk, $.02 < p < .05$; *, $.01 < p < .02$; **, $.001 < p < .01$; ***, $p < .001$.

death rate for females (forty-third) than for males (twenty-third), so that the likelihood of overestimation is even greater in the female mortality models. Again, Florida's high rank in PRELEV ensures overestimation of its mortality, worsened in the nonethnic model by its high value for CIGS and in the ethnic model by its moderately high ranking in BRIT (sixteenth) and OTHEUR (thirteenth). In this category of deaths the reasons for overestimation of Florida's mortality differ between the sexes only in the interchange of its high ranks in the FRAN and BRIT effects.

In the female total cancer mortality models low-ranking Wyoming (forty-sixth) and moderately high-ranking Michigan (fourteenth) are also overestimated residual outliers. Although Wyoming's very low ranks in PRELEV (forty-third) and POLLUT (forty-ninth) are in accordance with its low mortality rate, the latter factor loses its significance in the ethnic models, while Wyoming's ranking in the added ethnic variables, particularly BRIT (eighteenth) and OTHEUR (twenty-seventh), is not low enough to avoid the overestimation of its very low death rate. Michigan's very high ranks in MALT (second) and POLLUT (eighth) are joined in the ethnic models by its very high ranks in OTHEUR (sixth) and BRIT (seventh) to produce the outlier overestimation of its only moderately high death rate.

B All Malignant Neoplasms (ICD 140-205): 1949-1959

Males

When total cancer mortality is considered for only the first decade of the 20-year period (plus the year 1949), Florida and Oregon are overestimated residual outliers in the male mortality model from the nonethnic pool, but after inclusion of the ethnic variables, Wyoming replaces Oregon. Again Florida's high value of PRELEV and the importance of this variable in both the nonethnic and the ethnic models result in outlier overestimation of its reported male death rate, one that ranks twenty-sixth for this earlier period. The addition of FRAN and OTHEUR to the ethnic model increases this overestimation. Oregon's outlier position in the nonethnic model and Wyoming's in the ethnic model reflect the shift of importance, according to size of coefficients, from WINE in the former models to FRAN in the latter. Oregon, ranking thirtieth in this mortality, has a high rank (eleventh) in WINE and a moderate rank (twenty-first) in FRAN, so that the greater significance of WINE in the nonethnic model overestimates the state's male death rate, while a shift of significance to the ethnic variable FRAN brings the estimated rate closer to the observed rate. Wyoming ranks even lower (forty-fourth) in this mortality, so that the shift of significance from WINE, in which it ranks in the middle (twenty-ninth), to FRAN, in which it ranks high (ninth), increases the estimate of its death rate well beyond the observed level, sending it into a residual outlier position in the ethnic model.

Females

For females the same variables are included in the total cancer mortality models of this early time period as are found in those for the full 20-year period. The levels of the variables CIGS and INCM in the nonethnic model and BRIT and OTHEUR in the ethnic model are responsible for Florida's overestimation, with a reported female death rate ranking only forty-eighth. Because of slight differences in the ranking of death rates and changes in the sizes of the coefficients in the models for this earlier period, Michigan and Wyoming are not residual outliers in these models as they are in the models for the full 20-year period.

C Diseases of the Circulatory System (ICD 400-468): 1949-1959

Males

Florida and New Mexico are overestimated residual outliers in both the nonethnic and ethnic variable pool models for mortality from diseases of the circulatory system. Florida's very low-ranking (forty-sixth) death rate is overestimated because of the state's high values in the model effects PRELEV, CIGS, and DISP. New Mexico, with the lowest death rate in this category, is overestimated in spite of its generally low ranking in all the positive model effects. It does have a low rank in SCAN, a negative though nonsignificant effect, which boosts the estimate somewhat. However, it is probable that an ethnic effect not represented in the variable pool, such as Mexican, is responsible for New Mexico's low male mortality from diseases of the circulatory system.

Females

New York, with the highest female mortality rate from diseases of the circulatory system, is an underestimated residual outlier only in the nonethnic model. New York's rank (twenty-third) in the very important PRELEV effect is lower than this model implies it should be. Its high rank (third) in BRIT, a variable in the ethnic model, compensates for its low value of PRELEV, taking it out of the outlier underestimation position. Conversely, the addition of BRIT, in which Michigan ranks seventh, results in the outlier overestimation of its sixteenth-ranking mortality rate in the ethnic model only. Florida, as it is in the male mortality models, is an overestimated outlier in both the nonethnic and the ethnic models. A high value of PRELEV is again primarily responsible for Florida's outlier position of overestimation, but all of its values in the model effects predict a higher female mortality rate than the one reported, the lowest in the nation.

D Diseases of the Respiratory System (ICD 470-475, 490-527): 1949-1959

Males

Colorado, whose male death rate from diseases of the respiratory system is second highest, is an underestimated residual outlier in both models, while Arizona, with the highest death rate, is an underestimated residual outlier only in the ethnic model. The only variable that correctly predicts Colorado's high mortality rate is PRELEV. Although this negative effect is the most important factor in the model and Colorado's rank in it is very low (forty-fifth), it is not enough to offset its scores in the other factors. Arizona becomes an underestimated residual outlier in the ethnic model not only because TEMP, in which Arizona ranks first, is dropped, but because the state's score in the positive ethnic effect BRIT is of middle rank. The most probable reason for the outlier underestimation of the high mortality in these two states is the absence from the pools of a variable reflecting the in-migration of sufferers of respiratory disease seeking a more favorable climate and environment. Colorado and Arizona have been the traditional states for this flight.

Females

The states with the two highest female death rates from respiratory diseases, New Mexico and Colorado, are underestimated residual outliers in both the nonethnic and the ethnic models. These states have low values of POLLUT, a positive factor in the models. In addition, Colorado's ranks in INCM, FRAN, and SCAN, all negative effects in the models, are high and do not predict the very high observed mortality rate. Just as for the males, better estimates of the very high female mortality from respiratory diseases in these states might be obtained if a variable reflecting the in-migration peculiar to these states were included in the pools.

E Diseases of the Digestive System (ICD 530-587): 1949-1959

Males

D. C. and New Mexico rank first and second in male mortality from diseases of the digestive system, and are underestimated residual outliers in both the nonethnic and the ethnic models. D. C.'s high rank (fourth) in the negative effect, PRELEV, and New Mexico's very low rank (forty-third) in the positive effect, POLLUT, ensure that the model estimates will not be as high as the observed death rates of these two highest mortality states. The proportional distribution of deaths among the subcategories of diseases of the digestive system differs markedly from the national norm in these two cases. Cirrhosis constitutes a much larger portion of digestive disease deaths in D. C., while gastritis and gastroenteritis represent a larger portion in New Mexico. Although the estimated death rate for D. C. is one that correctly ranks highest among the estimated rates, its actual value may fall short of the observed rate because, in D. C.'s case, at the top of the scale the *standardized* values of the alcohol consumption variables are not large enough to estimate closely the *absolute* value of the death rate. It should be recalled that only the independent variables have been standardized, and their variances thereby forced to equal 1, while the dependent variables, the age-adjusted death rates, are not standardized, and therefore take on a wide range of values. This is not the situation behind the underestimation of New Mexico's mortality, but rather it is more likely the lack of a variable reflecting the Mexican ethnic effect.

Oregon, ranking forty-second in mortality rate, is an overestimated residual outlier in the nonethnic model, but the addition of the negative effect SCAN in which it ranks high (seventh) decreases the estimate of its death rate in the ethnic model and brings it out of its outlier position of overestimation.

Females

New Mexico, with the highest female mortality rate from diseases of the digestive system, is a heavily underestimated residual outlier in both models. Its low rank in MALT (thirty-fifth), an important model effect, contributes to the underestimation of its death rate. However, just as in the male mortality models, omission of a variable representing the high proportion of Mexican ethnicity in this state may preclude a close estimate of its death rate. It should be noted here that New Mexico is also an underestimated outlier in the male and female mortality models for cancer of the stomach, a malignant disease of the digestive system.

The only model effect that correctly predicts Oregon's very low-ranking death rate (forty-fifth) is the negative ethnic effect SCAN in which that state ranks high (seventh). Its ranking in none of the other model effects reflects its low observed level of female mortality from digestive diseases.

F Diseases of the Genito-Urinary System (ICD 590-637): 1949-1959

Males

The two top-ranking states in male mortality from diseases of the genitourinary system are underestimated residual outliers, D. C. in the model from the ethnic pool and Indiana in both the nonethnic and the ethnic models. D. C.'s high ranking in the positive effects INCM and DISP is counterbalanced by its similarly high ranking in the negative effects, WINE and MALT. Apparently these negative consumption effects stand in for factors that are not included in the variable pools, and this substitution works particularly badly in the case of D. C. But it is D. C.'s only average rank (twenty-fifth) in the most important effect in the ethnic model, negative SCAN, which ensures the outlier underestimation of its very high death rate. None of Indiana's factor values in either of the models agree with the very high level of its mortality. It does rank fairly low (fortieth) in the negative effect WINE and moderately high (twelfth) in POLLUT, neither of which is sufficient to keep the estimates of its death rate from outlier positions of underestimation in both models.

Females

Delaware with the highest female mortality rate from genito-urinary diseases is an underestimated residual outlier in both models because of moderately high ranking in the negative effects MALT (twelfth) and WINE (tied for eighteenth). Indiana, ranking second highest as it does in the male mortality rates, is an underestimated residual outlier only in the nonethnic model. Since the male and female mortality models are very similar, the reasons for Indiana's underestimation are the same in both sets—none of its factor values correctly estimates its very high death rates for both sexes. Some factor or factors in this high risk of mortality from genito-urinary diseases to Indiana's white population are not included in the variable pools.

Minnesota's lowest-ranked mortality rate, although an overestimated residual outlier in the nonethnic model due to the state's ranking in all the model effects, is better estimated in the ethnic model because of the inclusion of the negative effect SCAN, in which the state ranks second. On the other hand the inclusion of SCAN sends Texas, also a low-ranking state (forty-first) in mortality, into an outlier position of overestimation in the ethnic model because of its low rank (thirty-sixth) in the negative SCAN effect.

G Infectious and Parasitic Diseases (ICD 020-138): 1949-1959

Males

Texas ranks highest in male mortality from infectious and parasitic diseases and its death rate is an underestimated residual outlier in both the nonethnic and the ethnic models. Only its high rank (seventh) in TEMP and low ranking in the negative ethnic effects BRIT, SCAN, and OTHEUR conform to its very high observed death rate. Texas is another state with a very large ethnic group (Mexican) not represented in the variable pools and this ethnic factor could be a primary one in its high mortality from this category of disease. Wyoming with the fourth highest mortality rate is an underestimated residual outlier only in the ethnic model, which brings the consumption effect MALT as well as all the ethnic factors into the estimation. Wyoming's high rank in FRAN (ninth) is outweighed by its moderately high ranks in the negative effects BRIT (eighteenth) and SCAN (fifteenth) and its lower than average value of the very significant MALT factor, producing outlier underestimation of its very high death rate.

Kentucky ranking fifth in mortality is an underestimated residual outlier in the nonethnic model because it does not rank sufficiently high (sixteenth) in the very significant positive effect TEMP, but ranks too high (seventeenth) in the very significant negative effect PRELEV, and in addition, has a low rank in CIGS. The ethnic model better estimates Kentucky's high mortality by including three negative ethnic effects in which Kentucky ranks very low, BRIT (forty-fifth), SCAN (forty-ninth), and OTHEUR (forty-fourth), raising the estimated rate out of its position of outlier underestimation in the nonethnic model.

Idaho's very low mortality rate, ranking forty-second, is overestimated because of its very low rank (forty-sixth) in the negative effect PRELEV, a highly significant factor in both models, but it is only in the ethnic model that its overestimation is an outlier because the state's high rank (thirteenth) in the negative effect SCAN cannot counterbalance its low rank (thirty-eighth) in the negative effect OTHEUR and its middle ranks in BRIT and MALT.

Females

In female mortality from infectious and parasitic diseases the two highest-ranking states, New Mexico (first) and Texas (second), are underestimated outliers in both the nonethnic and the ethnic models. New Mexico's low ranking in the negative effects PRELEV, POLLUT, INCM, BRIT, and SCAN is not sufficient to overcome its middle to low ranking in the positive effects TEMP and MALT in order to produce a sufficiently high estimate for its top-ranking mortality. As in the male mortality models Texas' high rank in TEMP and low ranks in the negative effects BRIT and SCAN do not sufficiently overcome its middle ranks in the other model effects to avoid outlier underestimation. The high proportion of the Mexican ethnic group in these two states could be the missing factor in their very high death rates for both males and females in infectious and parasitic diseases.

Since the male and female models are very similar, the reasons for the outlier underestimation of Kentucky's very high female mortality rate in the nonethnic model but not in the ethnic model are the same as for the males.

H Accidental and Violent Causes (ICD E800-E999): 1949-1959

Males

In male mortality from accidental and violent causes the ethnic and the nonethnic models have only one variable in common, the climate factor PRELEV, and therefore each model has completely different states as residual outliers. Nevada, ranking highest in this mortality for males, is an underestimated residual outlier in the nonethnic model due to its comparatively low rank in TEMP (thirty-fourth) and its very high rank (third) in the negative effect WINE. Nevada's top rank in the very significant ethnic effect FRAN improves the estimate of its mortality in the ethnic model to bring it out of its position of outlier underestimation. Third-ranking Montana is an underestimated residual outlier in the ethnic model because of its too high ranking in the negative factors BRIT (eleventh) and OTHEUR (nineteenth). The state with the lowest mortality rate, Rhode Island, is an overestimated residual outlier in the ethnic model because of its very high ranking in both FRAN (third) and CIGS (third).

Females

Nevada, also ranking highest in female mortality from accidental and violent causes, is again an underestimated residual outlier in the nonethnic model because of its low rank in the very significant factor TEMP. And just as in the case of the males, its top rank in FRAN prevents the outlier underestimation of its high death rate in the ethnic model.

Indiana ranking sixth in female mortality is an underestimated residual outlier in the ethnic model because none of the model effects, except a low-ranking (fortieth) value in the negative effect WINE, conform to its very high death rate.

With a middle-ranking (nineteenth) female death rate Massachusetts is an underestimated residual outlier in the ethnic model because its high rank (eighth) in the positive effect FRAN is outweighed by its high ranks in the negative effects BRIT (second) and OTHEUR (tenth).

Arizona ranks high (ninth) in mortality but it is nevertheless an overestimated residual outlier in the nonethnic model because its ranks in two of the three effects in the model, first in TEMP and forty-ninth in the negative effect PRELEV, predict for it the highest estimated death rate. Its moderate ranking (nineteenth) in the third effect CIGS is not sufficient counterbalance to prevent the outlier overestimation of its death rate.

I All Causes (ICD 001-E999): 1949-1959

Males

Florida, ranking next to lowest (forty-eighth) in male mortality from all causes of death, is an overestimated residual outlier in the models from both the nonethnic and the ethnic variable pools. Its high ranking in the very significantly positive effects DISP (sixth) and FRAN (tenth) and middle ranking in POLLUT (twenty-sixth) and SCAN (twenty-third) overcome its very high ranks in the negative effects TEMP (second) and PRELEV (third) to produce the outlier overestimation of its male mortality rate. Reference to Table XXIX indicates that it is in the diseases of old age such as cancer, heart disease, and stroke that Florida records very low death rates, but these are the categories of death for which its rates are greatly overestimated by the mortality models. From this it can be inferred that it was primarily the deaths of the elderly that may have been underrealized or underreported in Florida for that period. A discrepancy in reported deaths may have been due to the criteria used in that state for assigning out of state residence to recently immigrated retirees who died there. An alternative conclusion is that there is a strong survival factor operating in Florida that is not included in the variable pools.

A third explanation of the persistent outlier overestimation of Florida's death rates, especially in causes of death most related to the elderly, lies in a possible difference in mortality patterns between native Floridians and those who migrated there after surviving to retirement age elsewhere. If an individual's duration of exposure to the factor levels in a state must be considerable before the model effects are operative for him, then the Florida natives would exhibit a death rate closer to the model estimates based on Florida's factor levels. At the same time the subpopulation of migrant retirees from other states might experience lower death rates, thereby diluting the higher native mortality rates, for the following two reasons: (1) exposure of the migrants to lower factor levels in the states of their longest residence; (2) proclivity of the migrants to survive longer than the general population since they represent those who had already survived to retirement age.

Females

In female mortality from all causes Florida, with the lowest death rate, is also an overestimated residual outlier in both the nonethnic and the ethnic models. Its average recorded death rate of 561.2 per 100,000 for this 11-year period is extremely low, the next lowest being Arkansas' average rate of 604.2 per 100,000, further indicating a situation peculiar to Florida in female as well as male mortality.

Minnesota, ranking thirtieth, is an overestimated residual outlier in the female mortality model from the nonethnic variable pool due to higher than average levels of MALT and POLLUT, but the inclusion of the very significant negative effect SCAN reduces its estimated death rate in the ethnic model to a level closer to its observed rate, removing it from the outlier position of overestimation.

Michigan, ranking sixteenth in female mortality, is an overestimated residual outlier in the ethnic model because of its very high rank in the ethnic effect BRIT (seventh). Its high ranks in POLLUT (eighth) and MALT (second) are sufficiently counterbalanced in the nonethnic model by its high rank in INCM (ninth), a negative effect not carried over into the ethnic model.

New Mexico is the only underestimated residual outlier in the female mortality models for deaths from all causes, with its high-ranking (seventh) female death rate excessively underestimated in both the nonethnic and the ethnic models. Its ranking in all the model effects, except for low ranks in the negative effects INCM and SCAN, predict a very low mortality rate for white women in New Mexico. The observed high level of female mortality is therefore due to factors not included in the variable pools. It is probable that the high proportion of Mexican, or Mexican-Indian, ethnicity included in the white population of the state is an important factor. New Mexico's death rates are underestimated residual outliers in both the male and the female mortality models for cancer of the stomach and for nonmalignant diseases of the digestive system. In addition, the state's female death rates from cancer of the liver and biliary passages, from diseases of the respiratory system, and from infectious and parasitic diseases are also underestimated outliers in their respective mortality models, combining to produce the sole outlier underestimate in the model for female mortality from all causes of death.

II Outliers in the Influence Space

In Table XXX it can be seen that the same cases—Nevada, Mississippi, and D. C.—most frequently represent extreme values in the influence space of the subset models for the major categories of death as for the individual cancer mortalities. These three states rank either very high or very low in the factor variables that make up the variable pool used in the model derivation of all the mortality patterns, and therefore any linear combination of their factor values, whether constituting a cancer mortality model or a noncancer mortality model, is also likely to be an extreme value. The persistence of the same states in representing extreme values in the influence space of both the cancer mortality models and the models of the "control" mortality patterns confirms the nature of these cases as points lying in the tail areas of the basic factor space rather than as outliers in specific mortality models from whose derivation they should be excluded. Nevertheless, in order to determine the particular influence of each

TABLE XXX
Potential Outliers in the Influence Space of the Subset Model for Each Major Category of Death[a]

Category of Death	Male	Female
All Malig. Neop. 1950-1969	Nev; Miss	
All Malig. Neop. 1949-1959	Nev; Ariz	ND; ($\underline{\text{SC}}$, $\underline{\text{Ariz}}$, $\underline{\text{NC}}$, Ala, $\underline{\text{Miss}}$)
Dis. of Circulatory System		
Dis. of Respiratory System		
Dis. of Digestive System	$\overline{\text{DC}}^{b}$; $\overline{\text{Nev}}$	
Dis. of Genito-Urinary System	Miss	Miss
Infectious & Parasitic Dis.		
Accidental & Violent Causes	$\overline{\text{Nev}}^{b}$	$\overline{\text{Nev}}^{b}$; $\overline{\text{DC}}$

[a] Underlined states have death rates ranking in the lowest fifth; overbarred states have death rates ranking in the highest fifth.

[b] An outlier in the distribution of residuals.

state that represents an extreme value, the models were rederived omitting each one and then examined for changes. These changes are summarized in Table XXXI.

Just as it did in individual cancer mortality models, in the model of male mortality from all malignant neoplasms (1950-1969) the exclusion of Nevada shifts importance from the ethnic effect FRAN to the alcohol consumption effect WINE and to a BRIT effect. On the other hand, the exclusion of Mississippi from this model produces no changes. When total cancer mortality for the earlier period (1949-1959) is considered with Arizona excluded from the male mortality model, the nonsignificant MALT effect is dropped but the already significant negative TEMP and OTHEUR effects are greatly increased. The exclusion of North Dakota from the female total cancer mortality model for this period adds a nonsignificant negative INCM effect. Neither Arizona nor North Dakota appears as an extreme value in the influence space of the model of any specific type of cancer mortality, but the latter covers a later and longer period (1950-1969).

When Nevada is excluded, the model chosen for male mortality from diseases of the digestive system drops MALT and WINE but strongly increases the significance of the DISP effect, while the omission of D. C. results in the loss of DISP and POLLUT and the addition of OTHEUR. The model involving all the states includes a positive but nonsignificant effect for each of the components of alcohol consumption, but Nevada is necessary to the retention of the MALT and WINE effects, and D. C. to the retention of the DISP effect. Both cases rank very high in this type of mortality, D. C. first and Nevada fourth, and thereby exert considerable influence on the model. The shift of importance among the specific types of alcohol consumption dependent upon the particular influence of individual states does not invalidate any individual component factor, but implies a general alcohol consumption factor in this mortality. However the loss of the POLLUT effect when D. C. is omitted does weaken the validity of a pollution factor.

Nevada ranks highest in both male and female mortality from accidental and violent causes and its omission drops the nonsignificant CIGS effect from the male mortality model and the nonsignificant DISP effect from the female, and eliminates the significance of the negative BRIT effect in the female model. It is interesting that D. C. becomes an underestimated residual outlier in the female mortality model, which has lost the DISP effect, further indication of the importance of the consumption of distilled spirits as a model effect when a totally urban unit such as D. C. is included among the cases.

Mississippi ranks thirteenth in both male and female mortality from diseases of the genito-urinary system and its exclusion from both models produced minimal change, adding only a nonsignificant negative FRAN effect to the male model.

TABLE XXXI

Changes in Subset Models of Major Categories of Death When Extreme Values in Influence Space Are Omitted

Category of death	State omitted	State's rank in death rate	Model effect added (factors strengthened by omission of state)	Model effect with marked increase[a] in coefficient (factors strengthened by omission of state)	Model effect dropped (factors strengthened by inclusion of state)	Model effect with marked decrease[a] in coefficient (factors strengthened by inclusion of state)
M-All Malig. Neop. 1950-69	Nev	18	BRIT**	WINE (ns to **)	FRAN*	
	Miss	29				–INCM (* to ns)
M-All Malig. Neop. 1949-59	Nev	25				
	Ariz	34		–TEMP (* to ***) OTHEUR (* to ***)	MALT	
F-All Malig. Neop. 1949-59	ND	30	–INCM			
M-Dis. of Digestive Sys.	Nev	4		DISP (ns to ***)	MALT WINE	
	DC	1	OTHEUR		POLLUT* DISP	
M-Dis. of Genito-Urinary Sys.	Miss	13	–FRAN			
F-Dis. of Genito-Urinary Sys.	Miss	13				
M-Accidental & Violent	Nev	1			CIGS	
F-Accidental & Violent	Nev	1			DISP	–BRIT (** to ns)
	DC	10			TEMP	

[a] Change of more than one level of significance.

ns, not significant; *, $.01 < p < .05$; **, $.001 < p < .01$; ***, $p < .001$.

The group of states with extreme values in female mortality from all malignant neoplasms (1949-1959)–South Carolina, Arizona, North Carolina, Alabama, and Mississippi–constitutes a large proportion of those with the lowest death rates and thus represents an important set in the total population of states. Rather than exclude them from the model derivation it should simply be noted that their joint position in the model effect space indicates the strong influence that their very low observed death rates exert on the model chosen to explain the total U. S. female cancer mortality pattern of that period.

Chapter 8
Additional Factor Variables: Background Radiation and Mexican Ethnicity

I Background Radiation as a Factor

In Chapter 2 a description is given of the composition of the variable RADIAT, which is used to represent a state population's average yearly exposure to naturally occurring radiation, both cosmic and terrestrial. Derived by Oakley (24) this index is a determination of the average dose equivalents of the neutron and the ionizing components of cosmic radiation and of the radionuclide content of common rocks and soil in the earth's crust. The calculation of each of these three types of natural radiation exposure was done individually, each being determined separately for the urbanized and the unurbanized areas and weighted by the resident populations to obtain the state index. The resulting three indices for each state were added to get the total average dose equivalent per year of exposure to background radiation for the state population. Although the cosmic and terrestrial components are roughly equal in most states, in a few, such as high-ranking Wyoming and low-ranking Florida and Mississippi, the cosmic dose equivalent is almost twice the terrestrial dose. Only Connecticut has a sizable imbalance in the opposite direction, its terrestrial dose equivalent being 25% larger than its cosmic dose. The cosmic and terrestrial state indices, variables RADCOS and RADTER, are not highly correlated, with a correlation coefficient of only .422, or less than 20% common variation. Generally, cosmic radiation is highest in the mountain states and lowest in New England and the Mid-Atlantic Region, while the terrestrial radiation exposure is highest across the north from east to west and lowest in the South Atlantic and Gulf states. The cosmic component RADCOS was calculated essentially as an index of the elevation weighted by population distribution and thus is closely related to the precipitation/elevation variable PRELEV ($r=-.800$). The terrestrial component RADTER combines ground and aerial survey data with census data on housing to adjust for the differences in protective shielding of various building materials. Because of its north-south variation, it is most closely associated (negatively) with the temperature variable TEMP ($r=-.575$) and is similarly related to PRELEV ($r=-.568$). Hence the total radiation variable RADIAT is closely related ($r = -.807$) to

PRELEV[a], and because of this close association with the strongest and most consistent factor effect in the mortality models, additional analysis was undertaken to determine the role radiation might have in the precipitation/elevation model effects.

In its comprehensive report on the effects of populations' exposure to low levels of ionizing radiation, known as the 1972 BEIR report (46), the National Academy of Sciences Advisory Committee on the Biological Effects of Ionizing Radiation collated the results of all the investigations into genetic and somatic effects from human and animal exposure and concluded that the safety dose of 170 mrem/year (millirems per year) from all man-made sources except medical recommended by the Radiation Protection Guide was set "unnecessarily high . . . in an effort to balance societal needs against genetic risks." (46) They calculated that an additional 170 mrem over the naturally occurring average annual dose of approximately 100 mrem would cause an annual increase of .05% in the incidence of cases of serious dominant or X-linked diseases and defects, increasing by fivefold at an equilibrium approached several generations later; an increase in congenital abnormalities and partly genetic diseases of .1% in the first generation and .75% at equilibrium; and an increase of 5% in the general ill health, which is known to be proportional to the mutation rate in genetic damage. In addition to the increased genetic risk the Committee predicted increased somatic risks resulting from an addition to annual background exposure of this designated "safe" dosage of 170 mrem, amounting to approximately 6000 cancer deaths yearly, an increase of about 2% over the spontaneous cancer death rate.

These predictions were based on an assumption of a linear, nonthreshold relationship between dose and effect, by which the observed relationship in the higher dose-response levels of experimental studies is extrapolated back to low-level dosages close to the background level. Since an environment of zero dose level of ionizing radiation does not exist, estimated effects resulting from increments to that null dosage must be purely theoretical. But within the range of state average dose equivalents of background radiation, from 63 to 140 mrem, some variation in state mortality rates could result from the variation in state population exposure if the linear assumption is valid and if the threshold dose falls somewhere within this background range. Since the threshold dose is that absolutely "safe" dose below which no effects are noted, and since cancer mortality, a possible effect, has been incident to man since the earliest records, it is possible that the "spontaneous" incidence of mutations and cancer implies that the threshold dose of ionizing radiation is zero or at least at some level lower than any found on earth. This conforms to one widely held opinion that only

[a]It should be noted that, as opposed to naturally occurring radiation, radioactive fallout is positively related to PRELEV because its deposition on earth is associated with precipitation (see p. 225).

zero is the safe dose for any substance proved to be carcinogenic or mutagenic at high doses. The opposite view is that safe levels of substances occurring in nature, such as trace metals, hormones, sunshine, do exist and in fact are necessary to life even though they are harmful at higher dose levels. The assumption of only a zero dose threshold is linked to the one-shot theory of carcinogens—just one cell damaged by a single dose is sufficient to elicit the response. The assumption of a safe dose somewhere above zero is usually held by those who believe that the natural process of cell repair can withstand exposure below some threshold dose over time, and that irreversible damage occurs from the cumulative effect of exceeding that dose over time. Resolution of these two hypotheses will require the development of a model for the carcinogenic process itself.

Several studies (8, 47, 48) have attempted to relate the variation in state populations' exposure to naturally occurring ionizing radiation to the variation in state cancer death rates, but no positive, and in fact some negative, effects were found. A negative effect would imply that, within the range of state levels of background radiation, higher levels were associated with lower mortality rates and vice versa. In the present study the radiation factor was added to the largest variable pool, new subset models were derived by both the BMD and the LIN programs, and changes in the model effects were observed in order to investigate the role of background radiation in each mortality pattern.

The changes that occurred in the best subset models when RADIAT was added to the pool are summarized in Table XXXII. Since in almost all cases the inclusion of a RADIAT effect in the new model replaced a PRELEV effect (opposite in sign) in the first model, the table divides the cancer mortalities into three groups: those with neither PRELEV nor RADIAT entering either of the models; those for which PRELEV is not replaced by RADIAT but enters the subset models from both the 12-variable and the 13-variable pools; those for which a RADIAT effect enters the subset model chosen from the larger variable pool, and thereby replaces a PRELEV effect in the first model, with the exceptions noted at the bottom of Table XXXII. An increase in R^2 is used as a general indicator of model improvement although it is not in every case due solely to a direct substitution of these two factors but may also result from a change in the whole configuration of model effects accompanying each factor.

The RADIAT effect is positive in only two of the cancer mortality subset models, those for male thyroid cancer mortality and for female mortality from cancer of the biliary passages and liver. The predominantly negative effects of the radiation factor in the cancer models match the consistently positive effects of PRELEV, with which RADIAT is strongly negatively correlated. This generally negative effect is in accordance with the results of the studies cited above, which tried to relate the level of background radiation to leukemia and other cancer mortality (8, 47, 48). Mason and Miller proposed that the absence of a detectable increase in areas with higher than usual background radiation was due

TABLE XXXII
The Radiation Effect in Cancer Mortality[a]

Neither PRELEV nor RADIAT effect in either model		PRELEV effect[b] maintained, model unchanged	
Males	Females	Males	Females
Stomach	B & L Unspec.	Buc Cav & Ph.	Larynx
Prostate	Stomach	Larynx	Lg. Intestine
Hodgkin's Dis.	Pancreas	B & L Unspec.	Rectum
	Cervix Uteri	Esophagus	Breast
	Brain	Lg. Intestine	Ovary
	Lymphosarcoma	Rectum	Corpus Uteri
	Leukemia	Liver *et al.*	Thyroid (–)
		Bladder	
		Other Skin	
RADIAT effect[c] enters model[d]			
Improved model–higher R^2		Poorer model–lower R^2	
Males	Females	Males	Females
T, B, & Lung	T, B, & Lung	Pancreas	Melanoma
T, B, & L Spec.	T, B, & L Spec.	Kidney	Other Skin
Brain	Esophagus	Lymphosarcoma	
Leukemia	Liver *et al.* (+)		
Melanoma	Kidney		
Thyroid (+)	Bladder		
	Hodgkin's Dis.		

[a] Changes in the best subset model when RADIAT is added to the 12-variable pool.
[b] Positive except where indicated negative.
[c] Negative except where indicated positive.
[d] Entry of the RADIAT effect replaces the PRELEV effect of the opposite sign with the following exceptions: thyroid, males, no PRELEV effect in first model; trachea, bronchus, and lung, females, and trachea, bronchus, and lung, specified, females, no PRELEV effect in first model, both negative PRELEV and negative RADIAT effects in second model.

to the rural nature of those areas. This possibility was tested in the present study by adding the urban and population density variables to the pool in order to observe the net effect of RADIAT after adjustment for these two generalized factors in those subset models in which the negative radiation effect is strongest. Those were the mortality models for primary lung cancer in both males and females, and the persistence and strength of the negative radiation effect in both models is discussed in the next section.

II The Effect of Background Radiation in Respiratory Cancer Mortality

The strongest factor-role of RADIAT is as a negative effect in the models for both male and female mortality from cancer of the trachea, bronchus, and lung specified to be primary. A comparison among all the respiratory tract cancer mortalities of the best subset models with and without RADIAT in the variable pool is shown in Table XXXIII. There is a marked improvement in the percentage of variation explained by the models for specified primary lung cancer mortality that include RADIAT—an increase of 8% variation in the male mortality rates and almost 12% in the female rates. Additionally, Connecticut is no longer an overestimated residual outlier in the male mortality models and California is no longer an underestimated residual outlier in the female mortality models when RADIAT is included. However, Delaware takes on a residual outlier position of underestimation in the LIN choice for the female mortality pattern. Connecticut ranks surprisingly high (eleventh) in radiation level (due to its large terrestrial component), so that a significantly negative coefficient for RADIAT considerably lowers the estimate of that state's death rate, thereby removing its residual from an overestimated outlier position. On the other hand California ranks low (thirty-ninth) in RADIAT, so that a negative coefficient raises its estimated death rate, bringing its residual out of an underestimated outlier position. When negative RADIAT enters the model, the weakly positive or null PRELEV effect in the male mortality models for specified primary lung cancer remains null or becomes negative, and the null PRELEV effect in the female mortality model becomes significantly negative. Thus RADIAT does not appear to replace PRELEV in these particular models, but its inclusion indicates that the net effect of PRELEV after adjustment for the radiation effect is a negative one.

The improvement in the subset models for specified primary cancer of the lung is carried into the models for the combined category of specified primary and unspecified lung cancer, with 3% more of the variation in male mortality and 8% more in female mortality explained by the addition of a highly significant negative RADIAT effect. Also, the two outlier residuals in the male mortality model, underestimated Maryland and overestimated North Carolina, are no longer outliers, while North Carolina, Wyoming, and Utah are no longer overestimated outlier residuals in the female mortality models, although Virginia becomes one. In the male mortality model a negative RADIAT effect replaces the very significant positive PRELEV effect. When the negative RADIAT effect enters the female mortality model, the null PRELEV effect becomes significantly negative. In contrast, the models for the larger component of combined lung cancer mortality, i.e., unspecified bronchus and lung, are completely unaffected by the inclusion of RADIAT in the variable pool, remaining the same as the subset models chosen from the 12-variable pool.

Ridge regression analysis confirms the importance of the negative RADIAT effect in the specified primary lung cancer mortality patterns and also in the combined category mortality patterns. Table XXXIV summarizes RADIAT's role as a factor in the ridge regression models, in which the net effect of every

TABLE XXXIII

	Percent R^2 Full eq'n	Percent R^2 Model	TEMP	PRELEV	POLLUT	INCM	CIGS
Trachea, Bronchus, and Lung							
Males							
without RADIAT							
12 VAR BMD = LIN	86.38	84.35	1.68*	3.47***			1.21
with RADIAT							
13 VAR BMD = LIN	89.72	87.32					1.02
Females							
without RADIAT							
12 VAR BMD	72.49	69.99					.17
LIN	72.49	68.67					
with RADIAT							
13 VAR BMD = LIN	78.53	77.70		–.35*			.19
Trachea, Bronchus, and Lung Specified Primary							
Males							
without RADIAT							
12 VAR BMD = LIN	44.26	36.15	2.02***	.82		1.70**	
10 VAR LIN	39.30	37.65	2.39***		1.13*		.88
with RADIAT							
13 VAR BMD	50.41	42.91	1.64**			1.71***	
LIN	50.41	44.08	1.28*	–1.60	1.23*		1.22
2nd LIN	50.41	43.80	1.60**		.23	1.45	.58
Females							
without RADIAT							
12 VAR BMD = LIN	36.33	28.53	.24**			.37**	
with RADIAT							
13 VAR BMD	44.41	40.21	.14	–.25*		.51**	
LIN	44.41	35.66		–.40**	.19	.34*	
Bronchus and Lung Unspecified as to Primary or Secondary							
Males							
without/with RADIAT							
12, 13 VAR							
BMD = 2nd LIN	72.28	71.43		2.40***	–1.78*	–2.01	
LIN	72.28	66.81		2.96***	–1.62*		
Females							
without/with RADIAT							
12, 13 VAR							
BMD = LIN	63.03	59.51				–.42*	
Larynx							
Males							
without/with RADIAT							
12, 13 VAR							
BMD = 2nd LIN	88.00	86.72		.36***	.13*		
LIN	88.00	86.18		.34***	.17**		
Females							
without/with RADIAT							
12, 13 VAR							
BMD = LIN	64.51	61.21		.01	.02	–.05*	

[a]Changes in best subset model when RADIAT is added to the 12-variable pool.

Radiation as a Factor in Respiratory Cancer Mortality[a]

MALT	WINE	DISP	FRAN	BRIT	SCAN	OTHEUR	RADIAT
	1.06		3.47***		−1.61**		
			4.32***		−3.88***	1.31	−3.62***
	.30*		.50*	−.37	−.60***	.41**	
	.30*		.59**	−.31	−.63***	.41**	
	.24		.33*		−.65***	.31*	−.52***
					.99		
							−1.45**
		−.26					−2.19*
		−.41					−1.36**
	.19		−.33*				
−.21	.17		−.29				−.32*
−.32*							−.41**
1.64		1.38	3.22***		−3.50***	2.02	
1.94*			3.59***		−3.11***		
.48**		.25*	.50**		−.55***		
.10		.18**	.35***		−.22**		
		.18**	.38***		−.18**		
		.02*	.04**		−.02		

*, $.01 < p < .05$; **, $.001 < p < .01$; ***, $p < .001$.

variable in the pool approaches a stable value. For both males and females negative RADIAT is indicated to be a very strong though unstable effect in the specified primary and the combined category of lung cancer mortality, and additionally, it is shown to be of moderate strength and stable in the unspecified category. As in the subset models, a strong positive PRELEV effect becomes null in male primary lung cancer mortality and a null PRELEV effect becomes a strong negative one in female primary lung cancer mortality, when the radiation variable is included.

To complete the picture of the radiation effect in respiratory cancer, the mortality models for laryngeal cancer are compared with those for cancer of the trachea, bronchus, and lung. For neither sex does the chosen subset model differ when RADIAT enters the variable pool, but the ridge trace shows that negative RADIAT is a strong effect in the stabilized model of male mortality from laryngeal cancer and a moderate effect in the stabilized model of female laryngeal cancer mortality. However, in neither case does the negative RADIAT effect displace a strong positive PRELEV effect.

From this overall picture of the PRELEV and RADIAT factors in respiratory cancer mortality patterns, it can be seen that negative RADIAT is a very important factor specifically in the male and female mortality patterns for lung cancer specified to be primary. Although the PRELEV effect is either replaced or strongly altered in the subset models for specified primary lung cancer mortality, it remains unchanged as an important factor in the subset models for the unspecified category of lung cancer mortality and for laryngeal cancer mortality. This dichotomy between the two associated factors, PRELEV and RADIAT, in the respiratory cancer mortality subset models is not as marked in the stabilized models since negative RADIAT also appears as a stable factor of moderate strength in the unspecified lung and in the laryngeal cancer mortality patterns for both sexes.

Although the statewide variation in degree of urbanization is well represented by the income, consumption, and ethnic variables, the urban and the population density variables, URBW5N and WDEN50, were added to the variable pool to ensure that the negative RADIAT effect was not standing in for either factor. In the subset model for male mortality from specified primary lung cancer negative RADIAT entered first, then the urban variable, followed by positive TEMP and INCM effects, which caused the urban effect to be dropped due to an *F*-to-remove value below the preset level. This progression does point to the income factor as the primary explanation of the urban effect in this model, the positive income effect representing the influence of state income level in the recording of these lung cancer deaths as specified primary or as unspecified. In the female mortality model it is the population density factor which is brought in first but it too is dropped after the entry of the TEMP and INCM effects. After the negative RADIAT and negative PRELEV effects come into the model the density factor reenters and is followed by a negative urban effect, activity clearly due to the excessive collinearity of the factors within the enlarged variable pool and their joint inability to account for the variation in this mortality pattern. Since less than half the variation in male and in female mortality from lung cancer specified as primary is explained by the models drawn from even the extended variable pools, it is apparent that important factors needed to explain these mortality patterns are missing. It is therefore possible that the negative radiation effect in these models constitutes an attempt to represent the missing factor or factors. All that can be deduced about these factors from the modeling is that they are neither of the two generalized factors, urbanization or population density.

Mason *et al.* (49) compared cancer mortality statistics in counties in Colorado in which uranium mill tailings have been used extensively since 1951 as construction fill material with those in the remainder of the state. They were "unable to detect a significant excess in mortality from lung cancer or leukemia" (49) in those counties, although they did detect significant excesses in cancer of the prostate, pancreas, stomach, and colon. Since they examined death rates through 1967, a latency period of more than 15 years in lung cancer or leukemia would have prevented the true effects from appearing by then. On the other hand, as Mason *et al.* point out, the average concentration of cumulative exposure in the county population had an index of 98.8 working level months compared with a range of 60-4680 for the uranium miners in whom Wagoner *et al.* (50) found lung cancer to be caused by radiation. It would appear that level of exposure is the primary factor in inducing a lung cancer effect—at high occupational levels it is observed, at slightly above naturally occurring levels it is barely detected if it does exist, and within a normal range of naturally occurring levels it may exert a negative (protective) influence, due either to a true effect or to some statistical artificiality. The possible reasons for a statistical quirk in this study's results with respect to the radiation factor have been examined extensively.

III Radiation as a Positive Effect in Other Cancer Mortality

The stronger showing of the RADIAT effect in the ridge regression than in the best subset models of the respiratory cancer mortality patterns also occurs in the other cancer mortality patterns. This can be seen by comparing Table XXXII, which summarizes the changes in the best subset models resulting from the inclusion of RADIAT in the variable pool, and Table XXXIV, which summarizes the strength of RADIAT as a factor in the biased but stabilized models of ridge regression. Although RADIAT does not enter the subset models for male mortality from cancer of the esophagus, large intestine, and bladder, and for female mortality from cancer of the brain and leukemia, it is indicated as a factor of at least moderate strength in the stabilized models of these mortalities.

TABLE XXXIV
Radiation as a Factor[a] in the Stabilized[b] Cancer Mortality Models of the Ridge Trace

	Males		Females	
	Negative	Positive	Negative	Positive
Buc Cav & Ph.	Strong		Strong	
Larynx	Strong		Moderate	
T, B, & Lung	Very Strong		Very Strong	
T, B, & L Spec.	Very Strong		Very Strong	
B & L Unspec.	Moderate		Moderate	
Esophagus	Strong		Strong	
Stomach				
Lg. Intestine	Moderate			
Rectum				
Liver *et al.*				Moderate
Pancreas	Very Strong		Moderate	
Kidney	Moderate		Moderate	
Bladder	Strong		Moderate	
Brain	Strong		Moderate	
Thyroid		Strong		Moderate
Lymphosarcoma	Strong			
Hodgkin's Dis.			Moderate	
Leukemia	Moderate		Moderate	
Melanoma	Strong		Strong	
Other Skin	Strong		Moderate	
Prostate			–	–
Breast	–	–		
Ovary	–	–		
Cervix Uteri	–	–		
Corpus Uteri	–	–		

[a] A moderately strong or very strong effect constitutes a "factor," weak or null effects are designated by blanks.

[b] A very stable effect is indicated by a solid underline, a moderately stable effect by a broken underline.

RADIAT is a positive factor in both the subset and the ridge regression models for the same two types of cancer mortality—male mortality from cancer of the thyroid and female mortality from cancer of the biliary passages and liver. Additionally, it is indicated in the ridge trace to be a positive factor in female mortality from cancer of the thyroid, in concordance with its positive effect in male thyroid cancer mortality.

The positive effect of RADIAT in female mortality from cancer of the biliary passages and liver is not found in the male mortality pattern. This difference parallels the contrasting PRELEV effect in the models from the 12-variable pool, which was negative in the female mortality pattern but positive in the male. Moreover, it reflects the unrelatedness of the male and female mortality patterns in this category of combined cancer primaries, which is due to a higher ratio of liver to gallbladder cancer in males and the reverse in females. Thus it could be inferred that radiation is a positive factor in mortality from cancer of the gallbladder rather than of the liver. To test this, gallbladder cancer death rates for white males and for white females in the single year of 1960 were age-adjusted by the 1960 U. S. population, and subset models were derived by the BMD stepwise regression program from the extended pool, which included RADIAT. As shown in Table XXXV the radiation effect was significantly positive in the female mortality model but missing from the male. This would indicate that a positive radiation effect is specific to gallbladder cancer mortality in females only.

Since the gallbladder mortality rates were based on a single year they were not sufficiently reliable for more in-depth modeling, but it is interesting to note that malt consumption was the most significant factor in the female mortality models, and that it was not only very significant but the only factor in the non-ethnic model for male mortality. In the ethnic model for male mortality the positive MALT effect was replaced by its ethnic counterpart, a very significant positive OTHEUR effect.

The failure of a RADIAT effect to enter the leukemia mortality models may be because this category combines lymphatic, myeloid, monocytic, and acute leukemia while radiation exposure has been shown to be selective in the type of leukemia it initiates. Chronic lymphocytic leukemia, comprising 24% of leukemia deaths in the U. S. population in 1960, was not associated with radiation exposure in either Hiroshima or Nagasaki (46), while myeloid leukemia, which has been induced in irradiated mice (46), accounted for 16.5% of the 1960 leukemia deaths. Unfortunately a breakdown of leukemia mortality rates by state into its components was not available.

The death rates from multiple myeloma were available and, because of recent interest in the effect of low-level radiation on this type of cancer, mortality models were derived using the extended variable pool with RADIAT included. The subset models derived by the BMD and LIN programs were identical, with a negative RADIAT effect in the female mortality model and no radiation effect in the male. As in the leukemia models, the positive SCAN effect was the most significant factor in both male and female mortality (models not shown).

IV Components of Background Radiation

The weak correlation (r = .422) between the two major components of the background radiation index, exposure from cosmic and from terrestrial sources,

TABLE XXXV

Variable pool and program[a]	Percent R^2 Full eq'n	Model	TEMP	PRELEV	POLLUT	INCM	CIGS
M194–Thyroid							
12 VAR BMD = LIN	41.79	36.75				.03	
13 VAR BMD = 8LIN	43.72	41.39	.03				
LIN	43.72	36.97					
14 VAR BMD = LIN	45.20	39.64					
F194–Thyroid							
12, 13 VAR BMD = LIN } 14 VAR LIN	71.08	68.22		−.05***	.05**	−.04	
14 VAR BMD = 15LIN	71.08	62.77					−.04*
M155–Biliary Passages and Liver							
12, 13, 14 VAR LIN	70.76	69.57	−.19	.16*			−.21*
M256–Gallbladder							
12, 13 VAR BMD	41.86	18.74					
12, 13 VAR LIN	41.86	31.92	.15				
14 VAR BMD = LIN	51.06	47.33	.37**	.28**		−.29*	
M455–Liver							
12 VAR BMD = LIN	55.76	50.34	−.33*				
13 VAR BMD = LIN	58.06	53.39	−.41**				
14 VAR BMD = LIN	60.57	56.73	−.48**				
F155–Biliary Passages and Liver							
12 VAR BMD = LIN	75.11	74.31	−.44***	−.19*			−.16
13 VAR BMD	77.24	76.25	−.36**				−.17
LIN	77.24	76.15	−.36**				
14 VAR BMD = LIN	77.54	76.60	−.38**				−.18
F256–Gallbladder							
12 VAR BMD	58.72	46.16				.59*	−.35
LIN	58.72	55.80	−.22			.66**	
13 VAR BMD	62.49	52.72			.27	.37	−.30
LIN	62.49	59.74		.34		.62*	
14 VAR BMD = 3LIN	63.84	61.86			.16	.43	
LIN	63.84	60.26				.53*	
F455–Liver							
12, 13 VAR BMD	45.32	13.14	−.25				
12, 13, 14 VAR LIN	46.43	37.78				−.53*	
14 VAR BMD	46.43	16.70	−.36*				

[a] 13 VAR = 12 VAR + RADIAT; 14 VAR = 12 VAR + RADCOS + RADTER;

Radiation as a Positive Factor in Cancer Mortality

MALT	WINE	DISP	FRAN	BRIT	SCAN	OTHEUR	RADIAT	RADCOS	RADTER
		–.03*				.04	–	–	–
		–.02			.02	.05**	.02	–	–
		–.02				.06***	.01	–	–
		–.02*				.06***	–	.02*	
.05*	–.03**					.06**			
.05**						.04*	–		.03**
.37**			.34*	–.39*	–.63***	.44**			
						.25**		–	–
.25*			–.43**	.49**				–	–
.35**					.39**		–		.42***
			.62**	–.83**	–.77***	.56**	–	–	–
			.64**	–.82**	–.72***	.49**	–.18	–	–
			.53**	–.73**	–.78***	.57**	–		–.28*
.64***		–.22	–.33*		–.72***	.56***	–	–	–
.66***		–.22*	–.34*		–.65***	.53***	.23**	–	–
.61***		–.29**	–.28	–.23	–.58***	.61***	.23	–	–
.66***		–.28*		–.33*	–.57***	.49**	–		.25**
.71**			–.68**				–	–	–
.54**	.65**	–.64**	–.98***				–	–	–
.67**			–.62**				.33*	–	–
.67**	.65**	–.62**	–1.02***				.48*	–	–
.59**	.53*	–.57**	–.81**				–		.36**
.60**	.58**	–.57**	–.88***				–		.32**
					–.38*			–	–
.31	–.64***	.31*	.59**		–.28*				
					–.38**		–		–.17

*, $.01 < p < .05$; **, $.001 < p < .01$; ***, $p < .001$.

indicated sufficient difference in their by-state patterns to warrant testing them separately as potential model effects. Therefore RADIAT was replaced in the variable pool by its components, the yearly average dose equivalent from cosmic sources, RADCOS, and from terrestrial sources, RADTER. Subset models were derived by the BMD program for those mortality patterns in which RADIAT either was indicated or was expected to be a factor of interest: trachea, bronchus, and lung cancer specified primary, bronchus and lung cancer unspecified, diseases of the respiratory system, cancer of the biliary passages and liver, thyroid cancer, Hodgkin's disease, leukemia, and multiple myeloma. The only positive radiation effects were again found in the mortality models for cancer of the thyroid and for cancer of the biliary passages and liver. Table XXXV presents the development of the models for the mortality patterns of thyroid cancer, and of cancer of the biliary passages and liver divided into its two major categories, gallbladder and liver. The subset models shown were derived from the basic variable pools and from extensions of the pools when the total radiation exposure variable RADIAT was added (the 13-variable pool), and when RADIAT was replaced in the pool by its two components, RADCOS and RADTER.

The division of RADIAT brings a positive terrestrial radiation effect into the subset model for female thyroid cancer mortality, whereas previously only the ridge trace had indicated a positive RADIAT effect. While it is the terrestrial component that enters the female mortality model it is the cosmic component that replaces the total radiation effect in the male mortality model.

The two-way division of mortality from cancer of the biliary passages and liver into gallbladder and liver cancer mortality, and of radiation exposure into terrestrial and cosmic sources, provides some important contrasts in model effects. For both males and females RADTER is a highly significant positive effect in the gallbladder cancer mortality models. RADTER enters the liver cancer mortality models as a negative effect, a very highly significant one in male mortality but nonsignificant in female. Apparently the total radiation variable did not enter the male mortality model for cancer of the biliary passages and liver because the positive radiation effect associated with gallbladder cancer and the negative effect associated with liver cancer cancelled each other out. In the female mortality model for the combined category the greater proportion of gallbladder cancer plus the weakness of the negative radiation effect in female liver cancer mortality had permitted a positive radiation factor to enter the model.

Another contrasting factor in gallbladder and liver cancer mortality not evidenced in the models for the combined category is the very significant negative SCAN effect, which is specific only to the liver cancer mortality models for both males and females, while the SCAN effect is significantly positive in the gallbladder cancer mortality model for males. From Table XXXV it can also be seen that the conflicting FRAN effects, positive in the male mortality model for the combined category of cancer of the biliary passages and liver, and negative in the female mortality model, are partly due to differences between the two cancer primaries in this ethnic effect—positive in liver (male), negative in gallbladder (female). It should also be noted that the alcohol consumption effects, especially the very significant positive MALT effect, are stronger in the gallbladder models.

V Radiation as a Factor in the Major Categories of Death

RADIAT enters the best subset models for just a few of the major categories of death, as shown in Table XXXVI. It is a highly significant negative effect in the model for male mortality from diseases of the circulatory system, replacing the moderately significant positive PRELEV effect. Since the other model effects remain the same, the improvement in R^2 from 72.0 to 75.2% reflects the greater effectiveness of RADIAT as a factor. However, the new model produces one more residual outlier, an underestimated rate for West Virginia. Moreover, the very significant positive PRELEV effect in the female mortality models for diseases of the circulatory system does not yield to a RADIAT effect, so that it is unclear which, if either, is the real factor in this category of mortality. This is to be expected in a conglomerate category of mortality, for it is only in the more homogeneous subcategories of deaths that likely factors emerge definitively among the model effects. The models for total cancer mortality illustrate this, for the RADIAT effect does not enter any of them in spite of its interesting appearance in the models of some particular types of cancer mortality.

The models of male and female mortality from nonmalignant diseases of the respiratory system[a] are strongly affected by the radiation variable, as were the male and female mortality models for cancer of the bronchus, trachea, and lung specified as primary, but the RADIAT effect is negative in the lung cancer models and positive in the nonmalignant respiratory disease models. For both male and female mortality from respiratory system disease a very significant positive RADIAT effect replaces a very significant negative PRELEV effect and a nonsignificant positive POLLUT effect. As in the lung cancer models the inclusion of RADIAT produces a definite improvement in the R^2 of the female mortality model—almost 6%—and it also eliminates New Mexico as an underestimated residual outlier. In the male mortality model this substitution is accompanied by other changes—both ethnic effects are dropped and a significantly positive TEMP effect is added—which produce a model with a 5% smaller R^2 and an additional underestimated outlier (three instead of two). Thus the RADIAT factor is not as clearly superior to the PRELEV factor in the male mortality model as it is in the female. In an attempt to pin down these two effects in other respiratory mor-

[a] It should be noted that influenza and asthma have been excluded from this category of respiratory disease and that tuberculosis is under a separate rubric, leaving pneumonia as the chief component (65-75%), then emphysema and bronchitis.

TABLE XXXVI

Radiation Factor in the Major Categories of Death

A. RADIAT Effect in the Subset Model[a]

	Males		Females	
	Negative	Positive	Negative	Positive
All Malignant Neoplasms (1950-1969)	–	–	–	–
All Malignant Neoplasms (1949-1959)	–	–	–	–
Circulatory System (1949-1959)	***	–	–	–
Respiratory System (1949-1959)	–	***	–	***
Digestive System (1949-1959)	–	**	–	*
Genito-Urinary System (1949-1959)	–	–	–	n.s.
Infectious and Parasitic (1949-1959)	–	–	–	–
Accidental and Violent Causes (1949-1959)	–	–	–	–

[a] Significance of coefficients given by n.s., not significant; *, $.01 < p < .05$; **, $.001 < p < .01$; ***, $p < .001$.

B. RADIAT Effect in the Stabilized Model of the Ridge Trace[b]

	Males		Females	
	Negative	Positive	Negative	Positive
All Malignant Neoplasms (1950-1969)	Very Strong		Moderate	
All Malignant Neoplasms (1949-1959)	Strong			
Circulatory System (1949-1959)	Strong			
Respiratory System (1949-1959)		Very Strong		Very Strong
Digestive System (1949-1959)		Strong		Very Strong
Genito-Urinary System (1949-1959)		Moderate		Moderate
Infectious and Parasitic (1949-1959)		Moderate		Very Strong
Accidental and Violent Causes (1949-1959)				Moderate

[b] A very stable effect is indicated by a solid underline, a moderately stable effect by a broken underline.

tality patterns, models were derived for tuberculosis and for influenza. The only significant RADIAT effect entering these models was a positive one in female mortality from influenza, matching the RADIAT effect in the female mortality model from nonmalignant respiratory diseases. It is possible that the positive RADIAT effect in the nonmalignant respiratory disease models represents the negative PRELEV effect with which it is so closely associated. But this cannot be said for the lung cancer models in which a very significant negative RADIAT effect emerged without a precedent positive PRELEV effect of any strength. It was suggested earlier that the negative PRELEV effect in the respiratory disease models probably represents a true association not as an etiological factor but because of the migration of sufferers of respiratory disease to states at high elevation and a dry climate (low values of PRELEV) such as Arizona and Colorado. It is interesting to note here that Arizona was an extremely high residual outlier in the model of male tuberculosis mortality. The gross underestimation of its top-ranking death rate—almost twice the next highest—is undoubtedly due to the lack of a health-migration index in the model.

A significantly positive RADIAT effect enters both the male and female mortality models for diseases of the digestive system, completely replacing the negative PRELEV effect in the male model and partially replacing it in the female model. The replacement produced a minimal improvement in the male mortality model and a 3% increase in the R^2 of the female model. New Mexico was dropped as an underestimated residual outlier in the male model but continued to be a very significantly underestimated residual outlier in the female model. In the following section it is shown that an ethnic factor (Mexican) associated with PRELEV and RADIAT has a more significant effect in the digestive disease mortality models than either of those variables, and its inclusion reduces the size of the RADIAT effect and removes PRELEV completely. Division of the total radiation factor in the variable pool led to the substitution of RADTER for RADIAT in the male mortality model, and of equal RADCOS and RADTER effects for RADIAT in the female mortality model.

The only other subset model for a major category of death which includes RADIAT is that for female mortality from diseases of the genito-urinary system. Nonsignificant positive RADIAT and negative OTHEUR effects replace a moderately significant PRELEV effect, resulting in a 5% increase in R^2 and the elimination of the two residual outliers, underestimated Delaware and overestimated Texas.

Given the very small role of the radiation variable in the subset models for the major categories of death, its strength as a factor in the stabilized models of the ridge regression is unexpected. Like the TEMP and PRELEV effects, the RADIAT effect separates the mortality patterns for total cancer and diseases of the circulatory system from those of the other major categories of death. This is illustrated in Table XXXVI. In the first two categories the TEMP and RADIAT

TABLE XXXVII
Correlations between the Environmental Variables and the Urban/Density Variables[a]

	URBW5N	INCM	DENS50	WDEN50	TEMP	POLLUT	PRELEV	RADIAT
URBW5N	1.000	.769	.516	.545	−.034	.583	.125	−.030
INCM		1.000	.254	.189	−.406	.407	−.158	.201
DENS50			1.000	.755	.144	.822	.746	−.520
WDEN50				1.000	.256	.772	.582	−.402
TEMP					1.000	.171	.354	−.465
POLLUT						1.000	.538	−.383
PRELEV							1.000	−.807
RADIAT								1.000

[a] URBW5N: urban (new definition) white population as percentage of state white population 195
DENS50: total population per square mile land area 1950;
WDEN50: weighted average of area densities with area populations as weights 1950.
See Table I for full definition of variables.

effects are negative and the PRELEV effect positive, while in the remaining categories each effect has the opposite sign, TEMP and RADIAT being positive and PRELEV negative. Although this dichotomy might imply that the radiation variable simply presents an additional way of expressing the urban/rural division between the mortality patterns of chronic diseases and those of all other causes of death, reference to Table XXXVII shows that RADIAT has no association with the urbanization factors (URBW5N and INCM) and has weaker correlations with the population density (DENS50) and weighted population density (WDEN50) variables than does PRELEV. It is more likely that the background radiation level is another component factor in the set of physical environment variables that contribute to the effect of population density measures in state mortality patterns.

VI The Mexican Ethnic Factor

A Cancer Mortality

As inquiry into the possible primary factors underlying the model effects of PRELEV and RADIAT, an ethnic variable representing the proportion of a state's white population born in Mexico, MEXI, was introduced to the variable pool. This is undoubtedly a severely undervalued measure but it is used, as were the other ethnic variables, to reflect each state's relative position in reference to the others in this ethnicity, both native and foreign born. The settlement of the Mexican subpopulation in the states with higher elevation and dry climate suggested a possible explanation of the PRELEV effect by this ethnic factor. The outlier underestimation of New Mexico, the state with the highest Mexican proportion, and the inclusion of Indian ethnicity in the white population through the Mexicans, were further considerations that led to the testing of this ethnic factor.

A subset model for female mortality from cancer of the biliary passages and liver was derived by stepwise regression (BMD) with both MEXI and RADIAT added to the 12-variable pool. Because of the southwestern Indian's high risk of cancer of the gallbladder (40-42), the strong positive RADIAT effect in the model, and the persistence of New Mexico as an underestimated outlier, the emergence of a Mexican factor in the model would indicate ethnicity rather than environment underlying the PRELEV or the RADIAT model effects. Since the model remained unchanged, and the positive RADIAT effect persisted unaltered, the primacy of the radiation factor went unchallenged. Division of this combined category into gallbladder and liver cancer mortality, and division of the radiation factor into its cosmic and terrestrial components produced the same results. The only Mexican effect to emerge was a nonsignificant positive one in the model of male mortality from liver cancer, while the radiation factor remained the same—very significant positive RADTER effects in the gallbladder models, less significant negative RADTER effects in the liver models. It is probable that the failure of the MEXI variable to play a significant role in the gallbladder cancer models is due to the indirectness as well as the inaccuracy of this measure in indicating the mix of the high-risk Indian ethnicity in the white population death records. This variable is more valuable as an index of Mexican ethnicity itself, as is discussed below in the models for certain major categories of disease.

Because of the outlier underestimation of New Mexico in both the male and female mortality models for cancer of the stomach, subset models were derived with the Mexican ethnic variable added to the variable pool. Just as they were unchanged by the addition of RADIAT to the pool, they remained unaltered by the inclusion of MEXI, and New Mexico's male and female death rates from stomach cancer continue as underestimated residual outliers.

B Major Categories of Death

Although the MEXI variable has its second largest correlation with RADIAT (.388) of which .543 is with RADCOS and .110 with RADTER, its closest association is with PRELEV (−.647), and more specifically with the precipitation component (−.661) rather than the elevation component (.562). Given these interrelationships the models for the major categories of death were derived with both RADIAT and MEXI in the variable pool in an attempt to determine whether the Mexican ethnic factor was responsible in part for the role both PRELEV and RADIAT play in separating the mortality patterns of cancer and circulatory system diseases from those of the other causes of death. This division is also related to the urban and the population density factors and additional information on the model effects in this set of major category mortality patterns increases insight into these influential but generalized factors.

The Mexican ethnic variable emerges as a highly significant positive effect in the male and female mortality models for infectious and parasitic diseases[a] and for diseases of the digestive system. In the mortality models for infectious and parasitic diseases a highly significant positive Mexican effect replaces a highly significant negative PRELEV effect, increasing the R^2 in the male mortality model by 9.2% and in the female mortality model by 13.7%. The inclusion of MEXI in the pool brings RADIAT into the models and together they replace the strong negative PRELEV factor, increasing the variation explained by the model and eliminating Texas as an underestimated residual outlier in both models and Wyoming as one in the male mortality model. New Mexico, however, remains in an outlier position of underestimation in the female mortality model for infectious and parasitic diseases.

The Mexican ethnic effect is just as strong in the mortality models for diseases of the digestive system. A highly significant positive MEXI effect and a significant positive RADIAT effect together replace the negative PRELEV effect in both the male and female mortality models for diseases of the digestive system. Combined with other model changes they produce an increase in R^2 of 7.7% in the male mortality model and 12.0% in the female mortality model.

Table XXXVIII summarizes the Mexican ethnic factor in the mortality models for the major categories of death. The inclusion of MEXI as a positive effect in the model for female mortality from diseases of the respiratory system improves the R^2 by 3.3% but it does not replace or change any other model effects. MEXI enters both the male and female mortality models for diseases of the circulatory system and genito-urinary diseases as a negative effect, increasing the R^2 slightly in the female mortality model for circulatory system diseases, but decreasing it in the others. Thus the Mexican ethnicity is primarily a factor in the mortality models for infectious and parasitic diseases and for diseases of the digestive system, presenting with the radiation factor an explanation of the PRELEV effect in those mortality patterns.

Just as additional factors that measure population exposure to background radiation or reflect a state's relative degree of Mexican ethnicity accounted for part or all of the precipitation/elevation effect in some of the mortality patterns, it can be assumed that other factors, ethnic or otherwise, could be found to explain more of this strong and prevalent climatic effect. From the examples in this chapter it would appear that these additional, as yet undetermined, factors would exert their influence in just a few particular mortality patterns, rather

[a] Tuberculosis and influenza were excluded from this category.

TABLE XXXVIII
Mexican Ethnic Factor in Major Categories of Death[a]

	Males		Females	
	Positive	Negative	Positive	Negative
All Malignant Neoplasms (1950-1969)	–	–	–	–
All Malignant Neoplasms (1949-1959)	–	–	–	–
Circulatory System (1949-1959)	–	**	–	*
Respiratory System (1949-1959)	–	–	*	–
Digestive System (1949-1959)	***	–	***	–
Genito-Urinary System (1949-1959)	–	*	–	n.s.
Infectious and Parasitic (1949-1959)	***	–	***	–
Accidental and Violent Causes (1949-1959)	–	–	–	–

[a] Significance of coefficients given by n.s., not significant; *, $.01 < p < .05$; **, $.001 < p < .01$; ***, $p < .001$.

than show the more pervasive influence of the factor variables chosen for the basic variable pools. While it is unlikely that one single factor, not included in the basic variable pools, could be found to enter a large number of the cancer mortality models as a regular member of the team of model effects, it is very probable that there are specialized factors not yet tested which could improve certain individual models, as the RADIAT and MEXI variables have been shown to do. On the other hand the effect of PRELEV could be a true climatic one operating on other factors. For example, air contaminates and nuclear fallout are brought to earth by rainfall (51), so that the positive aspects of this precipitation/elevation variable would indicate higher levels of air pollution and of soil and surface water contamination with long-lived nuclides such as Strontium 90 and Cesium 137. The strength of the positive precipitation/elevation effect throughout the cancer mortality models combined with its relationship to the distribution of radioactive elements in water and milk supplies in the period under study point to the potential of more detailed investigation into the role of radioactive fallout in cancer mortality patterns, particularly in children.

Chapter 9
Summary and Conclusion

I Critique

The arguments against deriving multiple regression models of cancer mortality rates using the factor data available by state are well enumerated by Lave and Seskin (12, 52) and by Speizer *et al.* (53) in the report of the 4th Symposium on Statistics and the Environment in Washington, D. C. (54). Additional caveats have been given throughout the presentation of the mortality models in this study. The arguments for the realization of this study in spite of the problems involved are (1) cancer mortality modeling had not heretofore been carried out by a comprehensive, systematic, and consistent set of procedures; (2) multiple regression is one of the few statistical methodologies that can be applied to the vital statistics gathered regularly in the United States; (3) there are differential state patterns for each type of cancer mortality, which by their consistency and stability imply mass etiological factors in operation; (4) and the successful use of this methodology in other disciplines such as macroeconomics invites its application to the data of macroepidemiology.

The purpose in modeling the cancer mortality patterns was to find one or more subsets of model effects that best explain the variation in the by-state death rates, and then to observe which factors were consistently emphasized for each type of mortality. The regression coefficients are not taken at face value as measures of risk differential due to additional factor units, but rather as a reflection of the relative strength of each model effect as a possible factor in that mortality pattern. Standardization of the factor variables allows this type of comparison. But as Tukey (55) so correctly reminds the practitioner of multiple regression, the definition of a coefficient for a given variable depends on the other variables that have been taken into the regression equation as model effects. In order to limit this problem constant variable pools with controlled additions were used for deriving models uniformly across all mortality patterns, thereby allowing an understanding of the behavior of each variable in the presence of the others and the likelihood of a substitution effect between any two. Thus stress has been laid on the sets of model effects derived from the same variable pool that characterize and differentiate the mortality patterns.

It is true that, as Tukey (55) also points out, the best prediction equations may not imply causation, or that the causation may be directed toward a secondary aspect, such as the recorded death rate rather than the experienced one. This was exemplified in the models of specified primary lung cancer mortality by the positive income effect, relating higher average income level in a state to higher rates of more carefully specified lung cancer deaths. But, again quoting Tukey (55),

> "Difficulties with causal certainty CANNOT be allowed to keep us from making lots of fits, and from seeking lots of alternative explanations of what they might mean.
>
> For most environmental health questions, the best data we will ever get is going to be unplanned, unrandomized, observational data. Perfect, thoroughly experimental data would make our task easier, but only an eternal, monolithic, infinitely cruel tyranny could obtain such data.
>
> We must learn to do the best we can with the sort of data we have. This means that, as statisticians, our job has ONLY BEGUN when we have estimated coefficients and their standard errors.
>
> We cannot live securely in a microcosm where the only things we have to do are clearly specified and where we can sleep well of nights, sure we have done our statistician's duty. We must live in the real world."

II Dynamics of State Mortality Patterns

It is well to make use of these data sets covering the 30-year period in the U. S. from 1940 to 1969, because of their unique and unrepeatable information. Before 1940 the vital statistics on mortality were not uniformly reliable, and after 1969 state differences will continue to diminish. The variance of the state death rates for each type of mortality is in a trend of steady yearly decrease as the states become more alike through the continual interstate movement of their populations and their products. This brief period between inadequate measurement and disappearing differentiation has been used to delineate these state differences and to project them onto a factor surface that, in varying degree, reflects the etiologies of cancer incidence and the causes of cancer death.

The decreasing heterogeneity of state mortality rates is indicated by their decreasing variance. The standard deviations of state age-adjusted death rates for the major causes of death for selected years are shown in Table XXXIX. Since the variance is related to the magnitude of the death rates, the ratio of the standard deviation to the mean, i. e., the coefficient of variation, is used to adjust for overall size. Both measures have steadily decreased from 1940 to 1959 in every major category except diseases of the respiratory system; even

TABLE XXXIX

Standard Deviations[a] and Coefficients of Variation[b] of Age-Adjusted Death Rates for the Major Causes of Death in Selected Years

	Males				Females			
	1940	1946	1949	1959	1940	1946	1949	1959
All Malignant Neoplasms	27.08	24.10	21.33	20.05	18.21	15.63	14.63	11.27
	(21.2)	(18.6)	(15.5)	(13.2)	(13.5)	(12.1)	(11.5)	(9.7)
Respiratory Cancer	4.64	5.21	6.64	7.99	1.05	.93	1.34	1.12
	(44.9)	(32.8)	(32.8)	(23.2)	(29.2)	(21.4)	(27.7)	(20.6)
Intestinal Cancer		5.12	4.25	3.78		4.23	4.06	3.44
		(36.6)	(31.1)	(27.7)		(26.6)	(26.1)	(23.6)
Diseases of the Circulatory System	69.19	58.51	52.49	47.82	52.23	48.19	42.58	39.55
	(17.6)	(15.3)	(12.3)	(10.9)	(19.5)	(19.9)	(16.5)	(15.5)
Diseases of the Respiratory System	18.04	10.18	9.94	10.94	14.10	7.70	8.84	5.19
except Influenza and Asthma	(22.7)	(19.6)	(24.0)	(21.8)	(23.0)	(19.9)	(33.8)	(19.9)
Diseases of the Digestive System	16.53	10.42	8.91	7.66	15.14	8.52	8.46	4.60
	(21.8)	(20.7)	(20.0)	(19.2)	(28.2)	(24.6)	(26.8)	(18.2)
Diseases of the Genito-Urinary System	28.44	16.37	11.15	6.00	20.76	12.62	9.55	4.90
	(24.2)	(20.9)	(19.3)	(18.9)	(24.0)	(23.1)	(24.2)	(24.3)
Infectious and Parasitic Diseases	10.07	5.37	3.96	1.39	9.44	3.53	3.53	.91
except Tuberculosis and Influenza	(30.2)	(24.6)	(26.7)	(22.3)	(47.3)	(29.9)	(39.8)	(21.5)
Accidental and Violent Causes	36.79	27.81	25.04	23.84	12.95	7.01	6.48	6.12
	(25.6)	(21.8)	(21.8)	(23.3)	(22.6)	(14.0)	(14.6)	(16.3)
Total Deaths	158.64	95.32	83.64	68.07	103.38	70.25	64.99	52.80
	(12.1)	(8.5)	(7.6)	(6.6)	(10.4)	(8.7)	(8.6)	(7.9)

[a] Per 100,000. [b] Parenthesis indicates 100 s. d./mean.

in those categories where the death rates were increasing–male mortality from cancer and circulatory system diseases–the variance decreased. The male and female mortality from respiratory system disease decreases in the 1940s and then increases, and the degree of variation in these rates shows no consistent trend. Similarly the respiratory cancer mortality rates do not follow the general trend toward homogeneity; their variation increases with their increasing magnitude, though not as much since the coefficient of variation decreases. In those causes of death whose rates are increasing, the trend of decreasing differentiation among the states may be slowed sufficiently to permit continuing analysis of state patterns, but in most types of mortality state death rates are approaching a similarity that would not sustain the macroepidemiological type of analysis.

The aggregation of mortality rates over the 20-year time period used by Mason and McKay decreases state differentiation because the process of averaging in itself reduces variance. A reduction in state variation and a smoothing of the death rates underestimates the strength of the relationships which are sought in regression modeling (56). In avoiding the chance variation of annual data by averaging over several years, some significant variation may be lost.

The state variation of some factor variables, such as temperature, precipitation, elevation, and background radiation, by their nature changes very little over time. Although the levels of factors associated with urbanization and population density, such as consumption and pollution, increase considerably accompanied by increasing variance, their coefficients of variation show steady decreases, indicating an overall trend to relative homogeneity. The extremely high correlations between individual years of the state indices of these factor variables confirm the stability of their state distributional patterns.

The proportion of white foreign born in the U. S. is decreasing and so is its state variation. Decreasing immigration accompanied by increasing interethnic marriage and decreasing adherence to "old country" customs all contribute to reducing the strength and specificity of ethnic variables used to represent the presence of foreign stock in each state.

Thus the death rates and factor values by state for the time period of this study constitute a unique collection of data for the modeling of state mortality patterns. Even though the models derived from these data are not suitable for the precise forecasting of future state death rates, the information they give concerning the relative importance of a state's factor values to its ranking in each type of mortality can be considered valid into ensuing time periods.

It is possible that state consumption indices for other products such as beef, sugar, and wheat, which might have made valuable contributions to the mortality models if they had been available for the period under study, do not follow the trend of increasing state homogeneity. But including these factors in further modeling of state mortality patterns would be less effective than an analysis of the consumption patterns of those ethnic subpopulations that have been indicated by the models as contributing to the higher state risk of a specific cancer mortality.

Taking the 1949-1959 log linear trend in each state's death rate, i. e., the average percentage change over that period, as the dependent variable, best subset models were derived from variables representing coincident changes in each state's factor values. For most cancer mortality trends, the models accounted for only a small proportion of the state variation in trends, partly due to insufficient time lag between the period of the factor changes and that of the mortality trends. Under the assumption that high levels of a factor variable reflect large increases in previous years and low levels small increases, subset models were then derived using the factor values themselves, rather than the changes in them. Although these models also accounted for very little variation in the state trends of most of the cancer mortalities, the model of the trends in primary lung cancer mortality explained more variation than did the model of the primary lung cancer death rates themselves (males, 44.56 vs. 37.65%; females, 49.96 vs. 28.53%). For both males and females cigarette consumption emerged as a highly significant positive effect in the state mortality increases, while pollution level was another very significant factor in the male model. Thus, states with higher levels of cigarette consumption and pollution experienced larger increases in death rates from primary lung cancer. In the subset models derived for the generally decreasing state trends in stomach cancer mortality, POLLUT and WINE were significantly positive effects for both males and females, indicating that the decreases in stomach cancer death rates were smaller in states with higher levels of pollution and wine consumption. A very highly significant negative income effect in the male model implied that the smaller mortality decreases were also associated with lower income level. It is probable that the subset models of the trends in these two cancer mortalities were more successful because of the consistency of their direction—steadily increasing death rates in specified primary lung cancer and steadily decreasing in stomach cancer.

In comparing the models of the state mortality rates averaged from 1949 through 1959 with the models (derived from the same variable pool) of the state mortality trends over that period, it is of interest to note that cigarette consumption emerges as a very strong factor in the state patterns of increases in primary lung cancer mortality while it represents only a weak effect in the state patterns of the death rates themselves. This characterizes the smoking effect as relatively recent and additional to previous factors. Similarly, pollution emerges as a stronger factor in the trends than in the actual rates of male mortality from primary lung cancer, pointing to an increasing role for this factor also.

III Epidemiological Investigation Suggested by Consumption and Ethnic Effects in the Cancer Mortality Models

Examination of the relationship between the consumption and the ethnic effects in each type of cancer mortality suggests potentially productive epidemiological investigations. In order to focus on the "aliasing" of consumption for ethnic effects and vice versa, best subset models were derived from three variable pools: one pool comprising the environmental and income variables plus the set of consumption variables (CIGS, MALT, WINE, DISP); a second pool replacing the consumption variables with the larger set of ethnic variables (FRAN, BRIT, SCAN, GERM, ITAL, SLAV); a third pool combining the first two. The consumption and ethnic effects which emerged in the models are shown in Table XL, accompanied by the percentage variation in state death rates accounted for by each model. The environmental and income effects are not shown here because they varied little among the models from the three pools, but their influence has been adjusted for. This table shows clearly for each cancer mortality pattern which consumption effects and which ethnic effects are strong before adjustment for each other and which remain strong as net effects after the joint adjustment.

Information as to whether the basis of an ethnic effect is genetic, cultural (e. g., a consumption habit), or environmental can also be gained by comparing its direction and strength with the mortality ranking of the associated country (ies) of origin. A match between U. S. model effect and foreign rank would indicate that either a genetic factor or a cultural pattern, probably of consumption, maintained after migration underlay the ethnic factor. Table XLI presents the relative ranking of the countries of interest given in Segi (26), with the Russian rates taken from the official Soviet statistical journal Vyestnik Statistiki (57) and age-adjusted to Segi's standard population. The common rank for a group of nations, given in parentheses, was calculated as an average of the individual national ranks weighted by the size of each country's contribution to the group's foreign born in the U. S.

Certain background knowledge, useful in planning epidemiological investigations, can be gained from Tables XL and XLI. For example, in cancer of the buccal cavity and pharynx, French males are at very high risk in France and constitute a high risk factor in the U. S. , indicating either genetic or cultural factors in the etiology. All three consumption effects that emerge in the models–CIGS, WINE, and DISP–are most closely associated with the French ethnic variable, but only the last factor, the consumption of distilled spirits, continues to show an important effect after adjustment for the FRAN effect. The same observations are true for male and female mortality from cancer of the larynx: high mortality risk in both France and the U. S.; cigarette and wine consumption effects nullified by the French effect; consumption of distilled spirits the only pre-

TABLE XL Consumption and Ethnic Effects in U. S. Cancer Mortality Models[a]

Cancer site	Effects in male mortality models derived from a variable pool which includes				Effects in female mortality models derived from a variable pool which includes			
	Consumption factors	Ethnic factors	Both consumption and ethnic factors		Consumption factors	Ethnic factors	Both consumption and ethnic factors	
Buc Cav & Ph.	CIGS WINE DISP	FRAN*** –GERM* SLAV	DISP*	FRAN*** –GERM	CIGS* –MALT*** WINE	FRAN* –BRIT –GERM***	–MALT**	FRAN*** –BRIT –GERM**
$100R^2$	81.01%	83.10%	84.25%		58.96%	58.57%	65.43%	
Larynx	CIGS** WINE***	FRAN*** –SCAN –GERM SLAV**	DISP**	FRAN*** –SCAN** SLAV*	CIGS* –MALT WINE**	FRAN*** –GERM**	DISP	FRAN** –GERM*
$100R^2$	81.88%	85.92%	88.23%		54.01%	60.48%	63.58%	
Trachea, Bronchus, and Lung	CIGS*** WINE*** –DISP	FRAN*** –SCAN –GERM SLAV*	CIGS WINE	FRAN*** –SCAN*	CIGS** WINE***	FRAN*** –BRIT –SCAN*** SLAV**	WINE*	FRAN** –BRIT –SCAN*** SLAV**
$100R^2$	80.35%	84.37%	84.35%		62.84%	65.85%	69.26%	
Esophagus	CIGS MALT WINE**	FRAN** SLAV**	DISP***	ITAL* SLAV***	CIGS*** –MALT** WINE*** –DISP	FRAN** –GERM*** SLAV*	CIGS*** –MALT** WINE*** –DISP	
$100R^2$	80.02%	80.44%	83.78%		71.32%	54.32%	71.32%	
Stomach	MALT** WINE** –DISP**	GERM ITAL** SLAV	MALT WINE* –DISP*	ITAL SLAV**	–CIGS MALT* WINE* –DISP*	GERM ITAL* SLAV	–CIGS MALT WINE* –DISP	SLAV**
$100R^2$	74.64%	77.06%	80.51%		63.96%	64.61%	70.14%	
Large Intestine	CIGS* MALT***	BRIT ITAL SLAV**	CIGS MALT** –WINE*	BRIT*** SLAV**	CIGS** MALT** –DISP*	–SCAN* ITAL*** SLAV**	CIGS** MALT –WINE**	ITAL** SLAV*
$100R^2$	81.79%	86.98%	89.37%		80.73%	80.27%	86.33%	

TABLE XL (continued)

Cancer site	Effects in male mortality models derived from a variable pool which includes				Effects in female mortality models derived from a variable pool which includes			
	Consumption factors	Ethnic factors	Both consumption and ethnic factors		Consumption factors	Ethnic factors	Both consumption and ethnic factors	
Rectum	CIGS* MALT**	BRIT* ITAL SLAV**	CIGS* MALT	BRIT* GERM ITAL SLAV	CIGS* MALT** WINE	FRAN* BRIT* –SCAN SLAV**	CIGS**	BRIT ITAL* SLAV*
$100R^2$	80.45%	87.89%	90.88%		76.02%	81.96%	83.86%	
Biliary Passages and Liver	MALT*	–SCAN*** SLAV***	–CIGS** MALT***	FRAN** –BRIT* –SCAN*** SLAV***	MALT*** –DISP**	–FRAN** –SCAN*** GERM*** ITAL*	MALT*** –DISP**	–FRAN* –SCAN*** GERM* SLAV
$100R^2$	42.69%	51.38%	72.67%		59.56%	62.13%	73.06%	
Pancreas	WINE***	FRAN** –BRIT SLAV	WINE***	SCAN	WINE***	FRAN** –BRIT* SCAN* –GERM** SLAV***	WINE***	–BRIT SCAN* –GERM** SLAV***
$100R^2$	38.51%	37.64%	43.01%		43.39%	58.30%	61.41%	
Kidney	MALT*** DISP**	SCAN SLAV**	MALT* DISP**	SCAN –ITAL SLAV**	–CIGS* MALT** –WINE* DISP	–BRIT* –ITAL* SLAV***	MALT**	–BRIT –ITAL** SLAV***
$100R^2$	75.45%	78.05%	84.03%		58.46%	75.41%	79.92%	
Bladder	CIGS MALT*** WINE**	FRAN*** ITAL SLAV*	MALT DISP**	BRIT ITAL* SLAV	CIGS** MALT WINE DISP	FRAN*** –SCAN***	MALT DISP***	–SCAN*** ITAL**
$100R^2$	81.57%	86.70%	89.00%		77.73%	70.06%	81.21%	

Brain	−CIGS**	−FRAN*** SCAN*** −GERM	−CIGS −MALT*	SCAN*** −ITAL	−CIGS**	−FRAN*** SCAN*** −SLAV	−MALT**	−FRAN* SCAN***
$100R^2$	28.01%	46.72%	50.16%		26.23%	40.92%	45.69%	
Lymphosarcoma	MALT*	SCAN** SLAV**	−DISP*	SCAN** −GERM SLAV**		−FRAN* SCAN*** SLAV**		−FRAN* SCAN*** SLAV**
$100R^2$	47.67%	63.11%	64.23%		51.83%	70.14%	70.14%	
Hodgkin's Dis.	CIGS* −DISP	BRIT**	CIGS** −DISP	SCAN** ITAL	MALT*	SCAN** −GERM* SLAV*	CIGS	SCAN*** −GERM SLAV
$100R^2$	35.37%	39.32%	53.49%		45.96%	62.00%	64.03%	
Leukemia	−CIGS*	−BRIT*** SCAN***		−BRIT*** SCAN***	−CIGS**	−FRAN** GERM		−FRAN* −BRIT* SCAN** ITAL
$100R^2$	12.19%	47.29%	47.29%		20.27%	29.91%	38.22%	
Prostate	−WINE DISP*	BRIT* −ITAL**	−WINE* DISP**	SCAN				
$100R^2$	51.00%	51.33%	54.67%					
Female mortality models								
Ovary/Breast		GERM* SLAV**	CIGS**	−FRAN* SCAN GERM* SLAV*	MALT WINE	FRAN BRIT SLAV***		FRAN BRIT SLAV***
$100R^2$	78.11%	85.89%	88.89%		84.21%	89.00%	89.00%	
Cervix/Corpus Ut.	CIGS***	BRIT −SCAN***	−WINE DISP**	−SCAN*** −GERM ITAL	CIGS −DISP*	−FRAN* BRIT*** −SCAN*** GERM*	MALT −WINE*	−FRAN BRIT** −SCAN*** SLAV
$100R^2$	46.30%	66.29%	72.23%		43.75%	60.28%	65.31%	

[a] No asterisk, not significant; *, $.01 < p < .05$; **, $.001 < p < .01$; ***, $p < .001$.

TABLE XLI

Relative Ranking[a] in Cancer Mortality of the Countries of Origin Represented by the Ethnic Variables[b]

Cancer site						
Country (%)[c]	France	Eng. & Wales (49.5) Scotland (18.4) N. Ireland (1.0) Ireland (31.1)	Sweden (44.9) Norway (37.0) Denmark (18.1)	Italy	Germany (66.1) Austria (21.8) Belgium Netherlands (12.1)	Russia (47.4) Poland (39.3) Czechoslovakia (13.3)
	FRAN	BRIT	SCAN	ITAL	GERM	SLAV
Buccal Cavity & Pharynx						
Males	H	M H H H (H)	M M L (M)	H	L M M L (L)	M M M (M)
Females	M	H H H H (H)	H H M (H)	M	L M L L (L)	L M M (M)
Larynx						
Males	H	L M M M (M)	L L L (L)	H	M H H L (M)	H M M (H)
Females	H	M H H H (H)	L L L (L)	M	L L M L (L)	M M L (M)
Trachea, Bronchus, & Lung						
Males	M	H H H M (H)	L L M (L)	M	H H H H (H)	H M H (M)
Females	L	H H H H (H)	L L H (L)	M	M M M L (M)	M M H (M)
Esophagus						
Males	H	H H M H (H)	L L M (L)	H	M M M M (M)	H H M (H)
Females	M	H H H H (H)	M L H (M)	L	M M M M (M)	H M L (H)
Stomach						
Males	L	M M M M (M)	M M L (M)	H	H H M M (H)	H H H (H)
Females	L	L M M M (M)	L M M (M)	M	H H M M (H)	H H H (H)
Intestine except Rectum						
Males	H	H H H H (H)	M M H (M)	M	M M H H (M)	L L M (L)
Females	H	H H H H (H)	H M H (H)	M	M M H H (M)	L L M (L)
Rectum						
Males	H	H H H H (H)	M M H (M)	M	H H H M (H)	L L H (L)
Females	M	H H H M (H)	M M H (M)	M	H H H H (H)	M L H (M)
Leukemia						
Males	M	M M M M (M)	H H H (H)	M	M M M H (M)	– L H
Females	M	M M L M (M)	H H H (H)	H	M M M H (M)	– M M
Prostate						
Males	H	M M M M (M)	H H H (H)	M	M H H H (H)	L L M (L)
Breast						
Females	M	H H H H (H)	M M H (M)	M	M M H H (M)	L L M (L)
Total Uterus						
Females	M	M M L L (M)	L L H (L)	H	H H M L (H)	M H H (H)

[a] H, ranks in the highest third; M, ranks in the middle third; L, ranks in the lowest third; –, data not available.

[b] 1964-1965 except Russia, 1966-1967 and 1968-1969.

[c] Foreign-born from each country as a percentage of group total.

vailing consumption factor after adjustment for the ethnic effects. It should also be noted that the low Germanic risk indicated by the negative GERM effects in male and female mortality from cancer of the buccal cavity and pharynx and in female mortality from laryngeal cancer is paralleled by low ranking in these countries, while the mixed ranking of the Germanic countries in male laryngeal cancer mortality is matched by a null effect in the final model. This precise reflection of the foreign risk in the U. S. models further indicates a genetic or cultural basis to the Germanic factor, possibly the preference of malt over distilled spirits. The other ethnic effects in male mortality from cancer of the larynx also are matched by their associated foreign ranking—negative SCAN by the low ranking of all the Scandinavian countries, and positive SLAV by the high ranking of Russia.

Inspection of the results for the other cancer sites yields similar clues to the probable primacy of the consumption and ethnic factors that emerge in the models of their mortality patterns, thereby suggesting lines of investigation specific to the cancer type and etiological factor. A few examples are offered here.

(1) The risk of mortality from leukemia, lymphosarcoma, Hodgkin's disease and brain cancer is very high in Scandinavian men and women both in the U. S. and abroad. The negative consumption effects in the models (except for smoking in Hodgkin's disease) are weak and appear to be standing in for unknown factors. Thus the consistent Scandinavian ethnic effect is based either on consumption habits other than smoking and alcohol consumption, or on a genetic factor.

(2) The risk of mortality from cancer of the large intestine and of the rectum for males and females is very high in the British countries, and, concomitantly, the British ethnic effect is very significant in the male mortality models for these two related cancers, and to a lesser degree in the female. This would indicate that the British factor, carried over after migration, is less likely to be genetic, but instead, is based on a consumption habit that is continued by the males after migration and to a lesser extent by the females. The consistent effects of cigarette and malt consumption in these models suggest either, or both, as the consumption habit.

(3) The Germanic and the Slavic countries rank very high in stomach cancer mortality, and the associated ethnic factors are significantly positive in the U. S. models. Italy also ranks high in male stomach cancer mortality and is matched by a positive ITAL effect in the male model. However, in the final model the two consumption factors, MALT and WINE, are shown to be stronger than their associated ethnic variables, GERM and ITAL, with the likelihood that each of the ethnic effects was based on its related consumption effect. On the other hand the continued strength of the Slavic factor after adjustment for these two consumption effects indicates that a different factor underlies the high risk of the Slavs before and after migration.

IV Summary of Statistical Procedures

In preliminary analysis, multiple regression, principal components, and discriminant analysis techniques were used to reduce a very large number of factor variables to the smallest set that contained those essential to modeling all different patterns of cancer mortality. From the 12 variables chosen, four graduated sets were constructed for determining the incremental effects of dividing alcohol consumption into its components and including ethnic factors. Using these four variable pools, best subset models were derived for each cancer mortality pattern by the Efroymsen stepwise regression procedure and by the Mallows C_p-statistic search. Using the largest (12-variable) pool, the ridge trace was plotted for the full model to determine the stability of each net effect. A best subset model was nominated for every cancer mortality pattern by considering the models chosen for each pattern from all four variable pools, giving explicit regard to the R^2 value, i. e. , the amount of variation in state death rates explained by the model. Two classes of outlier in the best subset models were inspected, those arising in the influence space and those in the distribution of residuals. The first group concerned those states whose factor values in combination with the coefficient weights of the model indicated exceptional influence or control of the global statistics of the model. The extent of the influence of such a data point was determined by model changes when that state was excluded. The second group involved those states whose death rates were so over- or underestimated by the model that the residual, or difference between the estimated and the observed rate, lay in either 2½% probability tail of the distribution of residuals. These residual outliers were examined to determine which factor values led to their poor conformity to the general model.

Mortality models for the major categories of death, including that of all deaths due to malignant neoplasms, were analyzed in procedures similar to those applied to the individual types of cancer mortality. The same variable pools were used in order that these generalized categories of mortality could provide a type of control or contrast to the specific cancer mortalities with respect to the subsets of model effects chosen to represent their respective patterns.

Because of the potential for its importance, a measure of background radiation was tested as an additional factor in all of the mortality patterns and its contrasting effects presented. Additionally, the role of a Mexican ethnic factor was investigated in a few applicable mortality patterns.

Other statistical analysis not described in the text was used to gain fuller knowledge of the interrelationships in the data, especially among the factor variables themselves. Procedures such as regressing the principal components of the set of factor variables on each mortality pattern, or deriving weights for linear combinations of factor variables that best discriminated between different levels of mortality and observing the misclassified states, all contributed to the researchers' familiarity with the data, but yielded derivative results secondary to those of the multiple regression techniques. Weighting by the size of the white population in each state produced very little change in the regression models for which it was tried and was rejected as contrary to the purpose of explaining state variation in death rates. If, however, the emphasis were on explaining the mortality variation in the U. S. white population as manifested by differences in state death rates, such weighting would have been appropriate.

Interaction terms were added to the variable pools, specifically those between the pollution measure and the level of cigarette consumption, between the pollution measure and the climate factors, and between the levels of cigarette consumption and alcohol consumption. Although these combination variables were standardized as products to reduce correlation with their component variables, their inclusion nevertheless added so much to the collinearity extant in the pools as to confuse the resulting models. The interaction terms appeared to be stronger than the individual factor variables from which they were formed, tending to replace them in the models. These results were not surprising, given the accepted synergism in mortality factors, and further analysis is warranted in this area.

V Summary of Results

By means of multiple regression methodology the patterns of state mortality rates have been transformed into patterns of model effects and their coefficient-weights. This translation of mortality variation into the terminology of factor variables has revealed the interrelationships between mortality level and factor sets and has characterized the interrelationships among the mortality patterns themselves. In spite of the shortcomings of the data, particularly the limitations of the factor measurements that were available, reasonable models, though incomplete, were derived for most of the cancer mortalities.

The sets of model effects that best accounted for the variation in individual mortality patterns also explain the roles of the two umbrella factors, urbanization and population density, at least one of which has usually been included in the derivation of mortality models. In a much earlier study (1) the authors discovered the close association of the urban pattern with many of the cancer mortality patterns, as well as with the mortality pattern for diseases of the circulatory system, while the rural (negative urban) pattern was found to be more closely correlated with the mortality patterns of the other major categories of death, including accidental and violent causes. From the question as to why this urban/rural division existed in the major mortality patterns evolved the concept for this study. Lave and Seskin (52) justify the inclusion of an urban factor by stating that "there is a host of reasons why the mortality rate is higher in large cities (e. g. , tension, stress, and unhealthy personal habits)." Their reference is to mortality in general, without distinction between different causes. Moreover, urbanization and population density are discussed interchangeably and taken to be the same factor, whereas, in fact, their patterns of intercorrelation show them to be only moderately related (Table XXXVII), at most having less than 30% of their variation in common. The goal of this study has been to determine which primary factors are responsible for the urban effect and which for the density effect in the mortality patterns of chronic diseases. It was shown that sociological factors such as income level, alcohol and cigarette consumption levels, and ethnicity are more closely related to, and thus probable components of, the urban effect, while environmental factors such as temperature, precipitation, elevation, pollution, and background radiation are more closely related to, and thus probable components of, the density effect. Although the assumption underlying multiple regression procedures is that all possible factors influencing the dependent variable (death rate) are contained in the variable pool, inclusion of an umbrella factor that represents a combination of basic factors can mask the effect of one or more of these factors by taking their place in the model. Counting on an urban or a density variable to cover a multitude of unknown factors is, in a sense, begging the question. It is not like the traditional inclusion of income level in econometric or sociological models because the reasons for the income effect are well documented or understood. This cannot be said for an urban or density effect in mortality patterns. The most frequently quoted words characterizing the unknowns in this type of effect are tension and stress, but there is no reason to believe that a city dweller who lives there by choice suffers any more stress or tension than a country dweller who lives in the area of his choice. Moreover, if such urban tension were a factor in higher death rates, why are the rates for nonmalignant diseases of the respiratory system, the digestive system, and the genito-urinary system, for infectious and parasitic diseases, and even for accidental and violent deaths lower in the urban areas? Either the time-honored procedure for age-adjustment does not adequately correct for age differences between urban and rural population, or there are some lower mortality risks in urban life.

Of the urban factors, income level proved to be primarily a correctional or adjustment factor, while alcohol consumption factors displayed considerable influence in many of the digestive cancer mortality patterns. The net effect of cigarette consumption was weakened by the inclusion of the ethnic variables, with which all the consumption variables were closely related. The surprising consistency of the ethnic effects was revealed by the relationship between the U. S. cancer mortality risks associated with the model ethnic effects and those risks in their population counterparts abroad.

Of the environmental factors the climate variable combining precipitation and elevation levels emerged as the strongest of all factors. It was shown that in some models this variable was forced to represent a missing factor, such as background radiation or Mexican ethnicity, and it may be presumed that there are other such factors not yet identified. The variable combining the weighted population exposures to each of six air pollutants showed strength but undoubtedly not as much as a more accurate measure might have. The temperature effect though not strong proved to be an interesting discriminator between respiratory cancer and the other major types of cancer mortality patterns.

Individual states were pinpointed which exhibit very high or very low recorded mortality levels that are not sufficiently explained by the factors which do so for the majority of states. Also, individual states with exceptional influence in deriving a model were noted and the degree and type of their influence inspected.

Although the variable pools were tailored to the cancer mortality patterns, mortality models derived from these pools for the other major categories of death were used to cast new light on the major division between the patterns of chronic disease and those of other causes of mortality, and on the urban/rural nature of this dichotomy.

REFERENCES

Cited References

1. Macdonald, E. J., Wellington, D. G., and Wolf, P. F. Regional patterns in mortality from cancer in the United States. *Cancer 20*(5): 617-622, 1967.
2. Mason, T. J., and McKay, F. W. "U. S. Cancer Mortality by County: 1950-1969." DHEW Publ. No. (NIH)74-615, USGPO, Washington, D. C., 1973.
3. Mason, T. J., McKay, F. W., Hoover, R., Blot, W. J., and Fraumeni, J. F., Jr. "Atlas of Cancer Mortality for U. S. Counties: 1950-1969." DHEW Publ. No. (NIH)75-780, USGPO, Washington, D. C., 1975.
4. Erhardt, C. L. The underutilization of vital statistics. *Am. J. Publ. Health 67*(4):325-326, 1977.
5. McDonald, G. C., and Schwing, R. C. Instabilities of regression estimates relating air pollution to mortality. *Technometrics 15*(3): 463-481, 1973.
6. Breslow, N. E., and Enstrom, J. E. Geographic correlations between cancer mortality rates and alcohol-tobacco consumption in the United States. *J. Nat. Cancer Inst. 53*(3): 631-639, 1974.
7. Carnow, B. W., and Meier, P. Air pollution and pulmonary cancer. *Arch. Environ. Health 27*: 207-218, 1973.
8. Mason, T. J., and Miller, R. W. Cosmic radiation at high altitudes and U. S. cancer mortality, 1950-1969. *Radiation Res. 60*: 302-306, 1974.
9. Hoover, R., and Fraumeni, J. F., Jr. Cancer mortality in U. S. counties with chemical industries. *Environ. Res. 9*: 196-207, 1975.
10. Blot, W., Brinton, L. A., Fraumeni, J. F., Jr., and Stone, B. J. Cancer mortality in U. S. counties with petroleum industries. *Science 198*: 51-53, 1977.
11. Blot, W., and Fraumeni, J. F., Jr. Geographic patterns of lung cancer: Industrial correlations. *Am. J. Epidemiol. 103*(6): 539-550, 1976.
12. Lave, L. B., and Seskin, E. P. Does air pollution cause mortality? *In* "Statistics and the Environment," *Proc. 4th Symp., March 3-6, 1976,* pp. 25-34. American Statistical Association, Washington, D. C., 1976.
13. Burbank, F. Patterns in cancer mortality in the United States: 1950-1967. *Nat. Cancer Inst. Monogr. 33*: 199-216, 1971.
14. Marquardt, D. W., and Snee, R. D. Ridge regression in practice. *Am. Statist. 29*(1): 3-20, 1974.
15. Dixon, W. J., ed. "Biomedical Computer Programs." Univ. of California Press, Los Angeles, 1975. Programs developed at the Health Sciences Computing Facility, UCLA, sponsored by NIH Special Research Resources Grant RR-3, Program revised 10/7/74.

16. SHARE Library, Number 360D-13.6.008 (revised 3/72). Triangle Universities Computation Center, P. O. Box 12175, Research Triangle Park, North Carolina 27709.
17. Daniel, C., and Wood, F. S. "Fitting Equations to Data." Wiley (Interscience), New York, 1971.
18. Mallows, C. L. Some comments on C_p. *Technometrics 15*(4): 661-675, 1973.
19. Wood, F. S. The use of individual effects and residuals in fitting equations to data. *Technometrics 15*(4): 677-695, 1973.
20. Larsen, W. A., and McCleary, S. J. The use of partial residual plots in regression analysis. *Technometrics 14*(3): 781-790, 1972.
21. Hoerl, A. E., and Kennard, R. W. Ridge regression: Applications to nonorthogonal problems. *Technometrics 12*(1): 55-67, 1970.
22. Hoerl, A. E., and Kennard, R. W. Ridge regression: Biased estimation for nonorthogonal problems. *Technometrics 12*(1): 69-82, 1970.
23. Pybus, F. C. Cancer and atmospheric pollution. *Newcastle Med. J. 28*: 31-66, 1963.
24. Oakley, D. T. "Natural Radiation Exposure in the United States." U. S. Environmental Protection Agency Publ. No. ORP/SID 72-1, Washington, D. C., June, 1972, reprinted October, 1974.
25. Kuzma, R. J., Kuzma, C. M., and Buncher, C. R. Ohio drinking water source and cancer rates. *Am. J. Publ. Health 67*(8): 725-729, 1977.
26. Segi, M. "Cancer Mortality for Selected Sites in 24 Countries, No. 5 (1964-1965)." Department of Public Health, Tohoku Univ. School of Medicine, Sendai, Japan, 1969.
27. Doll, R., Muir, C., and Waterhouse, J., eds. "Cancer Incidence in Five Continents," Volume II. Springer-Verlag, Berlin, 1970.
28. Haenszel, W. Cancer mortality among the foreign-born in the United States. *J. Nat. Cancer Inst. 26*: 37-132, 1961.
29. Macdonald, E. J. Report to the Committee on Gastric Cancer Research of the National Advisory Cancer Council. San Francisco, California, 1948.
30. Macdonald, E. J. Epidemiology of gastric cancer. *In* "Cancer of the Gastrointestinal Tract," a Collection of Papers Presented at the Tenth Annual Clinical Conference on Cancer, 1965, at The University of Texas, M. D. Anderson Hospital and Tumor Institute, pp. 233-268. Year Book Medical Publishers, Chicago, 1967.
31. Wellington, D. G. Epidemiological association among diseases of the liver and gallbladder. Unpublished paper, 1971.
32. Macdonald, E. J. Unpublished M. D. Anderson Study.
33. Macdonald, E. J. The epidemiology of skin cancer. *J. Investigative Dermatol. 32*(2): 379-382, 1959.
34. Macdonald, E. J. Epidemiology of skin cancer, 1975. *In* "Neoplasms of the Skin and Malignant Melanoma," pp. 27-42. Year Book Medical Publishers, Chicago, 1976.
35. Macdonald, E. J. Incidence and epidemiology of melanoma in Texas. *In* "Neoplasms of the Skin and Malignant Melanoma," pp. 279-292. Year Book Medical Publishers, Chicago, 1976.
36. Anscombe, F. J. Rejection of outliers. *Technometrics 2*(2): 123-147, 1960.
37. Cook, R. D. Detection of influential observation in linear regression. *Technometrics 19*(1): 15-18, 1977.
38. Steiner, P. E. "Cancer/Race and Geography." Williams & Wilkins, Baltimore, Maryland, 1954.
39. Hauch, E. W., and Lichstein, J. The clinical problem of primary carcinoma of the liver. *Gastroenterology 27*(3):292-299, 1954.

40. Lam, R. C. Gallbladder disease among the American Indians. *Lancet 74*: 305-309, 1954.
41. Hesse, F. G. Incidence of cholecystitis and other diseases among the Pima Indians of Southern Arizona. *J. Am. Med. Assoc. 170*: 1789-1790, 1959.
42. Sievers, M. L., and Marquis, J. R. The Southwestern American Indian's burden: Biliary disease. *J. Am. Med. Assoc. 182*: 570-572, 1962.
43. Beeson, P. B., and McDermott, W., eds. "Cecil-Loeb Textbook of Medicine." W. B. Saunders, Philadelphia, 1967.
44. Hartley, H. O. In discussion of the session on residuals. 1977 American Statistical Association and Biometric Society Annual Meeting, Chicago, Illinois, August 15-18, 1977.
45. Segi, M. "Mortality for Selected Causes in 30 Countries." Department of Public Health, Tohoku Univ. School of Medicine, Sendai, Japan, 1966.
46. "The Effects on Populations of Exposure to Low Levels of Ionizing Radiations." Report of the Advisory Committee on the Biological Effects of Ionizing Radiations. National Academy of Sciences. National Research Council, Division of Medical Sciences, Washington, D. C., November 1972.
47. Frigerio, N. A., Eckerman, K. F., and Stowe, R. S. "The Argonne Radiological Impact Program," Part 1. Carcinogenic Hazard from Low-Level, Low-Rate Radiation. Argonne National Laboratory, Argonne, Illinois, 1973.
48. Jacobson, A. P., Plato, P. A., and Frigerio, N. A. The role of natural radiation in human leukemogenesis. *Am. J. Publ. Health 66*(1): 31-37, 1976.
49. Mason, T. J., Fraumeni, J. F., and McKay, F. W. Uranium mill tailings and cancer mortality in Colorado. *J. Nat. Cancer Inst. 49*: 661-664, 1972.
50. Wagoner, J. K., Archer, V. E., Lundin, F. E., Holaday, D. A., and Lloyd, J. W. Radiation as the cause of lung cancer among uranium miners. *N. Engl. J. Med. 273*: 181-188, 1965.
51. "Report of the United Nations Scientific Committee on the Effects of Atomic Radiation." General Assembly Official Records; Seventeenth Session Supplement No. 16 (A/5216). United Nations, New York, 1962.
52. Lave, L. B., and Seskin, E. P. Air pollution and human health. *Science 169*(3947): 723-733, 1970.
53. Speizer, F. E., Bishop, Y., and Ferris, B. G., Jr. Epidemiologic approach to the study of air pollution. *In* "Statistics and the Environment," *Proc. 4th Symp., March 3-6, 1976*, pp. 56-68. American Statistical Association, Washington, D. C., 1976.
54. "Statistics and the Environment," *Proc. 4th Symp., March 3-6, 1976*. American Statistical Association, Washington, D. C., 1976.
55. Tukey, J. W. Discussion of paper by Lave and Seskin. *In* "Statistics and the Environment," *Proc. 4th Symp., March 3-6, 1976*, pp. 37-41. American Statistical Association, Washington, D. C., 1976.
56. Hopkins, C. E. Personal communication, 1977.
57. Vyestnik Statistiki–Organ Tsentralnovo Statisticheskovo Upravlenia Pree Sovietye Ministrov. SSSR No. 2, 1969, p. 92, and No. 2, 1971, p. 94 (in Russian).

Additional Bibliography

Abt, K. On the identification of the significant independent variables in linear models. *Biometrika 12*:2-15, 81-96, 1967.

Ahern, W. R., Jr. Health effects of automotive air pollution. *In* "Clearing the Air, Federal Policy on Automotive Emissions Control" (Jacoby, H. D., and Steinbruner, J. D., eds.), pp. 139-174. Ballinger Publ. Co., Cambridge, Massachusetts, 1973.

Aitkin, M. A. Simultaneous inference and the choice of variable subsets in multiple regression. *Technometrics 16*(2):221-227, 1974.

Allen, D. M. Mean square error of prediction as a criterion for selecting variables. *Technometrics 13*(3):125-127, 1971.

Altshuller, A. P. Evaluation of oxidant results at CAMP sites in the United States. *J. Air Pollution Control Assoc. 25*:19-24, 1975.

Anderson, D. O. Current progress: The effects of air contamination on health, Part 1. *Can. Med. Assoc. J. 97*:528-536, 1967.

Anderson, R. L., Allen, D. M., and Cady, F. D. Selection of predictor variables in linear multiple regression. *In* "Statistical Papers in Honor of George W. Snedecor" (Bancroft, T. A., ed.), pp. 3-17. Iowa State Univ. Press, Des Moines, 1970.

Andrews, D. F. A robust method for multiple linear regression. *Technometrics 16*(4):523-531, 1974.

Anscombe, F. J. Examination of residuals. *In* "Proc. 4th Berkeley Symp. Math. Statist. Probability" (Neyman, J., ed.), pp. 1-36. Univ. of California Press, Berkeley, California, 1961.

Anscombe, F. J. Topics in the investigation of linear relations fitted by the method of least squares. *J. Roy. Statist. Soc. 29*:1-52, 1967.

Anscombe, F. J., and Tukey, J. W. The examination and analysis of residuals. *Technometrics 5*(2):141-160, 1963.

Aranda, R. G. The Mexican American syndrome. *Am. J. Publ. Health 61*(1):104-109, 1971.

Arvesen, J. N., and McCabe, G. P., Jr. Subset selection problems for variances with applications to regression analysis. *J. Am. Statist. Assoc. 70*(349):166-170, 1975.

Banerjee, K. S., and Carr, R. N. A comment on ridge regression. Biased estimation for nonorthogonal problems. *Technometrics 13*(4):895-898, 1971.

Barrett, J. P. The coefficient of determination—Some limitations. *Am. Statist. 28*(1):19-20, 1974.

Beale, E. M. L. Note on procedures for variable selection in multiple regression. *Technometrics 12*(4):909-914, 1970.

Beale, E. M. L., Kendall, M. G., and Mann, D. W. The discarding of variables in multivariate analysis. *Biometrika 54*(3, 4):357-366, 1967.

Belcher, J. R. The changing pattern of bronchial carcinoma. The London Chest Hospital and Middlesex Hospital, London. *Br. J. Dis. Chest 69*(247):217-258, 1975.

"Biological and Environmental Effects of Low Level Radiation," Vols. I and II. *Proc. Symp. Chicago, 3-7 November 1975.* International Atomic Energy Agency, Vienna, 1975.

Birch, M. W. A note on the maximum likelihood estimation of a linear structural relationship. *J. Am. Statist. Assoc. 59*:1175-1178, 1964.

Blot, W. J., and Fraumeni, J. F., Jr. Arsenical air pollution and lung cancer. *Lancet 2* (7926):142-144, 1975.

Box, G. E. P. Use and abuse of regression. *Technometrics 8*(4):625-629, 1966.

Breaux, H. J. A modification of Efroymsen's technique for stepwise regression analysis. *Comm. Assoc. Comput. Mach. 11*(8):556-557, 1968.

Brenner, M. H. Trends in alcohol consumption and associated illnesses—Some effects of economic changes. *Am. J. Publ. Health 65*(12):1279-1292, 1975.

Brues, A. M. Critique of the linear theory of carcinogenesis. *Science 128*(3326):693-699, 1958.

Buell, P., Dunn, J. E., and Breslow, L. Cancer of the lung and Los Angeles-type air pollution. *Cancer 20*(12):2139-2147, 1967.

Chiacchierini, R. P., Landau, E., and Mills, W. A. On the role of radiation in leukemogenesis (letter to the editor). *Am. J. Publ. Health 66*(9):908-909, 1976.

Cohen, J. Multiple regression as a general data-analytic system. *Psychol. Bull. 70*(6):426-443, 1965.

Comess, L. J., Bennett, P. H., and Burch, T. A. Clinical gallbladder disease in Pima Indians. *N. Engl. J. Med. 277*:894-898, 1967.

"Considerations of Health Benefit-Cost Analysis for Activities Involving Ionizing Radiation Exposure and Alternatives." A Report of Advisory Committee on the Biological Effects of Ionizing Radiations. Assembly of Life Sciences. National Research Council. National Academy of Sciences. Washington, D. C., Environmental Protection Agency, 1977.

The contribution of air pollution to the aetiology of lung cancer. *In* "Air Pollution and Respiratory Disease" (Holland, W. W., ed.), pp. 89-100. Technomic Publ. Co., Westport, Connecticut, 1971.

Crocker, D. C. Some interpretations of the multiple correlation coefficient. *Am. Statist. 27*: 31-33, 1972.

Cutler, S. J., and Devesa, S. S. Trends in cancer incidence and mortality in the USA. *In* "Host Environmental Interactions in the Etiology of Cancer in Man," pp. 15-33. IARC Scientific Publication No. 7, Lyon, France, 1973.

Daling, J. R., and Tamura, H. Use of orthogonal factors for selection of variables in a regression equation–An illustration. *Appl. Statist. 19*:260-268, 1970.

Davidson, J. Alcohol and cholelithiasis: A necropsy survey of cirrhotics. *Am. J. Med. Sci. 244*:703-705, 1962.

Diehr, G., and Hoflin, D. R. Approximating the distribution of the sample R^2 in best subset regressions. *Technometrics 16*(2):317-320, 1974.

Dunham, L. J., and Bailar, J. C. World maps of cancer mortality rates and frequency ratios. *J. Nat. Cancer Inst. 41*:155-203, 1968.

Dunn, J. E., Jr. Geographic considerations of endometrial cancer. *Gynecol. Oncol. 2*:114-121, 1974.

Eckhoff, N. D., Shultis, J. K., Clack, R. W., and Ramer, E. R. Correlation of leukemia mortality rates with altitude in the United States. *Health Phys. 27*:377-380, 1974.

Editorial. Gallstones: A new liver disease? *N. Engl. J. Med. 283*(2): 96-97, 1970.

Effects on populations of exposure to low levels of ionizing radiation. *Bull. Atomic Sci. 29*(3):47-49, 1973.

Enstrom, J. E. Strikingly low cancer mortality among Mormons. *UCLA Cancer Bull. 1*(4): 1, 5-6, 1974.

Enstrom, J. E., and Austin, D. F. Interpreting cancer survival rates. *Science 195*(4281): 847-851, 1977.

"Environmental Factors in Respiratory Disease," *Fogarty Int. Center Proc. 11*(Lee, D. H. K., ed.). Academic Press, New York, 1972.

Epstein, S. S. Environmental determinants of human cancer. *Cancer Res. 34*:2425-2435, 1974.

Forsythe, A. B., Engelman, L., Jennrich, R., and May, P. R. A. A stopping rule for variable selection in multiple regression. *J. Am. Statist. Assoc. 68*(341):75-77, 1973.

Friedman, G. D., Kannel, W. B., and Dawbar, T. R. The epidemiology of gallbladder disease: Observations in the Framingham study. *J. Chronic Dis. 19*:273-292, 1966.

Garside, M. J. The best subset in multiple regression. *Appl. Statist. 14*:196-200, 1965.

Gentlemen, J. F., and Forbes, W. F. Cancer mortality for males and females and its relation to cigarette smoking. *J. Gerontol. 29*(5):518-533, 1974.

Glenn, F. Calculous biliary tract disease an increasing burden on surgical facilities. *Ann. Surg. 17*:163-164, 1970.

Gorman, J. W., and Toman, R. J. Selection of variables for fitting equations to data. *Technometrics 8*(1):27-51, 1966.

Gross, P. Asbestos fibers in drinking water. *J. Am. Med. Assoc. 229*(7):767, 1974.

Guilkey, D. K., and Murphy, J. L. Directed ridge regression techniques in cases of multicollinearity. *J. Am. Statist. Assoc. 70*(352):769-775, 1975.

Gunst, R. F., Webster, J. T., and Mason, R. L. A comparison of least squares and latent root regression estimators. *Technometrics 12*(1):75-83, 1976.

Hanushek, E. A. Efficient estimators for regressing regression coefficients. *Am. Statist. 28* (2):66-67, 1974.

Harris, R. H. "Implications of Cancer Causing Substances in Mississippi River Water." Environmental Defense Fund, Washington, D. C., 1974.

Hart, J., Shani, M., and Modan, B. Epidemiological aspects of gallbladder and biliary tract neoplasm. *Am. J. Publ. Health 62*(1):36-39, 1972.

"Health Hazards of the Human Environment." World Health Organization, Geneva, Switzerland, 1972.

Hickey, R. J., Schoff, E. P., and Clelland, R. C. Relationship between air pollution and certain chronic disease death rates. *Arch. Environ. Health 15*:728, 1967.

Higginson, J., MacLennan, R., and Muir, C. S. Aetiological factors in human cancer. *In* "The Physiopathology of Cancer: Diagnosis, Treatment, Prevention" (Homburger, F., ed.), pp. 281-299. Karger, New York, 1976.

Higginson, J., and Muir, C. S. Geographical variation in cancer distribution. *In* "The Physiopathology of Cancer: Diagnosis, Treatment, Prevention" (Homburger, F., ed.), pp. 300-322. Karger, New York, 1976.

Hocking, R. R. The analysis and selection of variables in linear regression. *Biometrics 32*: 1-49, 1976.

Hocking, R. R., and Leslie, R. N. Selection of the best subset in regression analysis. *Technometrics 9*(4):531-540, 1967.

Honeyman, M. C., and Menser, M. A. Ethnicity is a significant factor in the epidemiology of rubella and Hodgkin's disease. *Nature 251*:441-442, 1974.

Hoover, R., Mason, T. J., McKay, F. W., and Fraumeni, J. F., Jr. Cancer by county: New resource for etiologic clues. *Science 189*(4207):1005-1007, 1975.

Hoover, R., McKay, F. W., and Fraumeni, J. F., Jr. Unpublished data.

Hotelling, H. The selection of variates for use in prediction with some comments on the general problem of nuisance parameters. *Ann. Math. Statist. 11*:271-283, 1940.

How air pollution may affect the respiratory tract. *In* "Pollution Primer," pp. 62-79. National Tuberculosis and Respiratory Disease Association, New York, 1969.

Howell, M. A. Factor analysis of international cancer mortality data and per capita food consumption. *Br. J. Cancer 29*:328-336, 1974.

Jones, H. L. Linear regression functions with neglected variables. *J. Am. Statist. Assoc. 41*: 356-369, 1946.

Kennard, R. W. A note on the C_p statistic. *Technometrics 13*(4):899-900, 1971.

Kennedy, W. J., and Bancroft, T. A. Model building for prediction in regression based upon repeated significance tests. *Ann. Math. Statist. 42*(4):1273-1284, 1971.

Kmet, J. The role of migrant populations in studies of selected cancer sites. A review. *J. Chronic Dis. 23*:305-324, 1970.

Kotin, P. The role of atmospheric pollution in the pathogenesis of pulmonary cancer. A review. *Cancer Res. 16*:375-393, 1956.

Krasnow, S. Geographic patterns of large intestine and rectal malignancy mortality in Virginia. *Virginia Med. Month. 97*:226-227, 1970.

LaMotte, L. R., and Hocking, R. R. Computational efficiency in the selection of regression variables. *Technometrics 12*(1):83-93, 1970.

Landsberg, H. E. The city and the weather. *Sciences 15*(8):11-13, 1975.

Larson, H. J., and Bancroft, T. A. Sequential model building for prediction in regression analysis. *Ann. Math. Statist. 34*(1):462-479, 1963.

"Late Effects of Radiation." *Proc. Colloq. Center for Continuing Education, Univ. of Chicago, Chicago, Illinois.* Von Nostrand Reinhold, New York, 1970.

Levy, B. S., Sigurdson, E., Mandel, J., Laudon, E., and Pearson, J. Investigating possible effects of asbestos in city water: Surveillance of gastrointestinal cancer incidence in Duluth, Minnesota. *Am. J. Epidemiol. 103*(4):362-368, 1976.

Li, C. C., Mazumdar, S., and Rao, B. R. Partial correlation in terms of path coefficients. *Am. Statist. 29*(2):89-90, 1975.

Lieber, M. M. The incidence of gallstones and their correlation with other diseases. *Ann. Surgery 135*(3):394-405, 1952.

Mahboubi, E., Emet, J., Cook, P. J., Day, N. E., Ghadirian, P., and Salmasizadeh, S. Oesophageal cancer studies in the Caspian littoral of Iran: The Caspian Cancer Registry. *Br. J. Cancer 28*: 197-214, 1973.

Malnasi, G., Jakab, S., Incze, A., Apostol, A., Csapo, J. M., Szabo, E., Csapo, J. J., and Jakab, K. An assay for selecting high risk population for gastric cancer by studying environmental factors. *Neoplasms 23*(3):333-341, 1976.

Mancuso, T. F., and Mordell, J. S. Proposed initial studies of the relationship of community air pollution to health. *Environ. Res. 2*(2):102-133, 1969.

Marx, J. L. Drinking water: Another source of carcinogens? *Science 186*(4166):809-811, 1974.

Mason, R. L., and Gunst, R. F. Some additional indices for selection of variables in regression (abstr.). *Biometrics 30*:382, 1974.

Mason, T. J., McKay, F. W., and Miller, R. W. Asbestos-like fibers in Duluth water supply. *J. Am. Med. Assoc. 228*(8):1019-1020, 1974.

Mickey, M. R., Dunn, O. J., and Clark, V. Note on the use of stepwise regression in detecting outliers. *Comput. Biomed. Res. 1*:105-111, 1967.

Modan, B. Role of ethnic background in cancer development. *Israel J. Med. Sci. 10*:1112-1116, 1974.

Morgan, R. W., and Jain, M. G. Bladder cancer: Smoking, beverages and artificial sweeteners. *Can. Med. Assoc. J. 111*:1067-1070, 1967.

"Persons at High Risk of Cancer; An Approach to Cancer Etiology and Control" (Fraumeni, J. F., Jr., ed.). Academic Press, New York, 1975.

Petersen, G. R., and Milham, S., Jr. Brief communication: Hodgkin's disease mortality and occupational exposure to wood. *J. Nat. Cancer Inst. 53*(4):957-958, 1974.

Philippe, P. Correlation and causation in epidemiology (letter to the editor). *Int. J. Epidemiol. 5*(4):391-392, 1976.

Priester, W. A., and Mason, T. J. Human cancer mortality in relation to poultry population, by county, in 10 southeastern states. *J. Nat. Cancer Inst. 53*(1):45-49, 1974.

Radhakrishnan, S. Selection of variables in multiple regression–An analysis of contemporary techniques. Abstract of a Dissertation presented to the Faculty of the College of Business of the University of Houston, Houston, Texas, 1974.

Rossiter, C. E., and Weill, H. Ethnic differences in lung function: Evidence for proportional differences. *Int. J. Epidemiol. 3*(1):55-61, 1974.

Sampliner, R. E., Bennett, P. H., Comess, L. J., Rose, F. A., and Burch, T. A. Gallbladder disease in Pima Indians. *N. Engl. J. Med. 283*:1358-1364, 1970.

Sauer, H. I., and Donnell, H. D., Jr. Age and geographic differences in death rates. Unpublished paper for presentation at 8th International Congress of Gerontology, Biology Section 6, August 1969.

Sawicki, E., Elbert, W. C., Hauser, T. R., Fox, F. T., and Stanley, T. W. Benzo(a)pyrene content of the air of American communities. *Am. Ind. Hyg. J. 21*:443-451, 1960.

Schultz, R. Geographic distribution of carcinogenic sun radiation. *In* "Cancer of the Skin: Biology, Diagnosis, Management" (Andrade, R., Gumport, S. L., Popkin, G. L., and Rees, T. D., eds.), pp. 172-188. Saunders, Philadelphia, Pennsylvania, 1976.

Shapley, D. Nitrosamines: Scientists on the trail of prime suspect in urban cancer. *Science 191*(4224):268-270, 1976.

Sievers, M. L. Cigarette and alcohol usage by southwestern American Indians. *Am. J. Publ. Health 58*(1):71-82, 1968.

Sievers, M. L. Disease patterns among southwestern Indians. *Publ. Health Rep. 81*(12):1075-1083, 1966.

Small, D. M. Prestone gallstone disease–Is therapy safe? *N. Engl. J. Med. 284*(4):214-216, 1971.

Small, D. M., and Rapo, S. Source of abnormal bile in patients with cholesterol gallstones. *N. Engl. J. Med. 283*(2):53-57, 1970.

"The Sources of Air Pollution and Their Control." Public Health Service Publ. No. 1548, USGPO, Washington, D. C., 1968.

Staszewski, J. Cancer of the upper alimentary tract and larynx in Poland and in Polish-born Americans. *Br. J. Cancer 29*:389-399, 1974.

Staszewski, J., Slomska, J., Muir, C. S., and Jain, D. K. Sources of demographic data on migrant groups for epidemiological studies of chronic diseases. *J. Chronic Dis. 23*:351-373, 1970.

Stocks, P. Lung cancer and bronchitis in relation to cigarette smoking and fuel consumption in twenty countries. *Br. J. Prevent. Soc. Med. 21*:181-185, 1967.

Swindel, B. F. Instability of regression coefficients–Illustrated. *Am. Statist. 28*(2): 63-65, 1974.

Tabor, E. C., Hauser, T. E., Lodge, J. P., and Burttschell, R. H. Characteristics of the organic particulate matter in the atmosphere of certain American cities. *Am. Med. Assoc. Arch. Ind. Health 17*:58-63, 1958.

Thistle, J. L., and Schoenfield, L. J. Lithogenic bile among young Indian women. *N. Engl. J. Med. 284*(4): 177-181, 1971.

Thomson, J. G. Primary carcinoma of the liver in the three ethnic groups in Cape Town. *Acta Unio Int. Contra Cancer 17*:632-638, 1961.

Totter, J. R. Research programs of the Atomic Energy Commission's Division of Biology and Medicine Relevant to Problems of Health and Pollution. *In Proc. 6th Berkeley Symp. Math. Statist. Probability 6, Effects of Pollution on Health,* pp. 71-100. Univ. of California Press, Berkeley, California, 1972.

Tuyns, A. J., and Masse, G. Cancer of the oesophagus in Brittany: An incidence study in Ille-et-Vilaine. *Int. J. Epidemiol. 4*:55-59, 1975.

Tuyns, A. J., and Obradovic, M. Brief communication: Unexpected high incidence of primary liver cancer in Geneva, Switzerland. *J. Nat. Cancer Inst. 54*(1):61-64, 1975.

Waugh, F. V. The analysis of regression in subsets of variables. *J. Am. Statist. Assoc. 31*: 729-730, 1963.

Weitzner, S., and Smith, D. E. Cancer of the stomach in New Mexico: A preliminary report. *Am. Surgeon 40*:161-163, 1974.

Williams, R. R., and Horm, J. W. Association of cancer sites with tobacco and alcohol consumption and socioeconomic status of patients: Interview study from the Third National Cancer Survey. *J. Nat. Cancer Inst. 58*(3): 525-547, 1977.

Winkelstein, W., Kantor, S., Davis, E. W., Maneri, C. S., and Mosher, W. E. The relationship of air pollution and economic status to total mortality and selected respiratory system mortality in men: 1. Suspended particulates. *Arch. Environ. Health 14*:162-171, 1967.

Wong, J. K. Notes on the elimination of variables in multiple correlation. *J. Am. Statist. Assoc. 32*:357-360, 1937.

Wright, G. W. An appraisal of epidemiologic data concerning the effect of oxidants, nitrogen dioxide and hydrocarbons upon human populations. *J. Air Pollution Control Assoc. 19*: 679-682, 1969.

Zavon, M. R., Hoegg, U., and Bingham, E. Benzidine exposure as a cause of bladder tumors. *Arch. Environ. Health 27*:1-7, 1973.

SUBJECT INDEX

F

G

H

I

J

K

L

M

N

O

P

R

S